T0226645

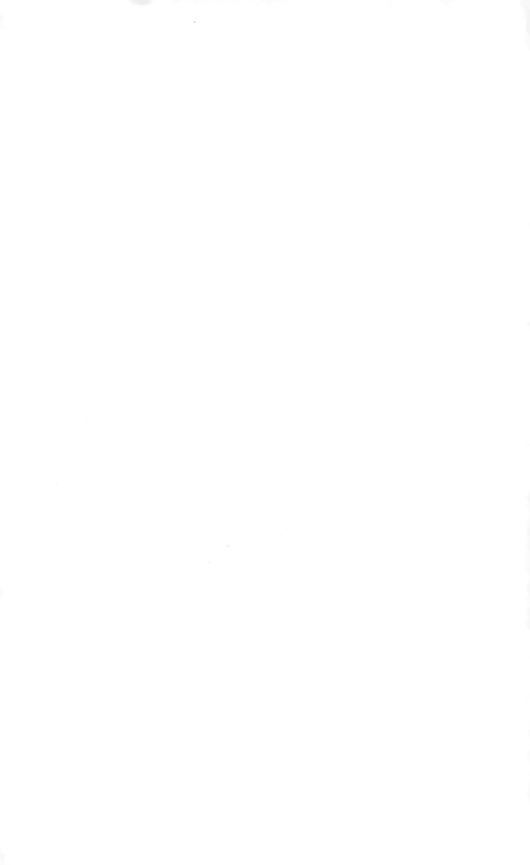

Dysphagia: Diagnosis and Management

Editor

KENNETH W. ALTMAN

OTOLARYNGOLOGIC CLINICS OF NORTH AMERICA

www.oto.theclinics.com

December 2013 • Volume 46 • Number 6

ELSEVIER

1600 John F. Kennedy Boulevard • Suite 1800 • Philadelphia, Pennsylvania, 19103-2899

http://www.oto.theclinics.com

OTOLARYNGOLOGIC CLINICS OF NORTH AMERICA Volume 46, Number 6
December 2013 ISSN 0030-6665, ISBN-13: 978-0-323-26116-6

Editor: Joanne Husovski
Development Editor: Susan Showalter

© **2013 Elsevier Inc. All rights reserved.**

This periodical and the individual contributions contained in it are protected under copyright by Elsevier, and the following terms and conditions apply to their use:

Photocopying
Single photocopies of single articles may be made for personal use as allowed by national copyright laws. Permission of the Publisher and payment of a fee is required for all other photocopying, including multiple or systematic copying, copying for advertising or promotional purposes, resale, and all forms of document delivery. Special rates are available for educational institutions that wish to make photocopies for non-profit educational classroom use. For information on how to seek permission visit www.elsevier.com/permissions or call: (+44) 1865 843830 (UK)/(+1) 215 239 3804 (USA).

Derivative Works
Subscribers may reproduce tables of contents or prepare lists of articles including abstracts for internal circulation within their institutions. Permission of the Publisher is required for resale or distribution outside the institution. Permission of the Publisher is required for all other derivative works, including compilations and translations (please consult www.elsevier.com/permissions).

Electronic Storage or Usage
Permission of the Publisher is required to store or use electronically any material contained in this periodical, including any article or part of an article (please consult www.elsevier.com/permissions). Except as outlined above, no part of this publication may be reproduced, stored in a retrieval system or transmitted in any form or by any means, electronic, mechanical, photocopying, recording or otherwise, without prior written permission of the Publisher.

Notice
No responsibility is assumed by the Publisher for any injury and/or damage to persons or property as a matter of products liability, negligence or otherwise, or from any use or operation of any methods, products, instructions or ideas contained in the material herein. Because of rapid advances in the medical sciences, in particular, independent verification of diagnoses and drug dosages should be made.

Although all advertising material is expected to conform to ethical (medical) standards, inclusion in this publication does not constitute a guarantee or endorsement of the quality or value of such product or of the claims made of it by its manufacturer.

Otolaryngologic Clinics of North America (ISSN 0030-6665) is published bimonthly by Elsevier, Inc., 360 Park Avenue South, New York, NY 10010-1710. Months of issue are February, April, June, August, October, and December. Business and Editorial Offices: 1600 John F. Kennedy Blvd., Suite 1800, Philadelphia, PA 19103-2899. Customer Service Office: 6277 Sea Harbor Drive, Orlando, FL 32887-4800. Periodicals postage paid at New York, NY and additional mailing offices. Subscription prices is $365.00 per year (US individuals), $692.00 per year (US institutions), $175.00 per year (US student/resident), $485.00 per year (Canadian individuals), $876.00 per year (Canadian institutions), $540.00 per year (international individuals), $876.00 per year (international institutions), $270.00 per year (international & Canadian student/resident). Foreign air speed delivery is included in all *Clinics*' subscription prices. All prices are subject to change without notice. **POSTMASTER:** Send address changes to *Otolaryngologic Clinics of North America*, Elsevier Health Sciences Division, Subscription Customer Service, 3251 Riverport Lane, Maryland Heights, MO 63043. **Telephone: 1-800-654-2452 (U.S. and Canada); 314-447-8871 (outside U.S. and Canada). Fax: 314-447-8029. E-mail: journalscustomerservice-usa@elsevier.com (for print support); journalsonlinesupport-usa@elsevier.com (for online support).**

Reprints. For copies of 100 or more of articles in this publication, please contact the Commercial Reprints Department, Elsevier Inc., 360 Park Avenue South, New York, NY 10010-1710. Tel.: 212-633-3874; Fax: 212-633-3820; E-mail: reprints@elsevier.com.

Otolaryngologic Clinics of North America is also published in Spanish by McGraw-Hill Interamericana Editores S.A., P.O. Box 5-237, 06500 Mexico D.F., Mexico.

Otolaryngologic Clinics of North America is covered in *MEDLINE/PubMed (Index Medicus), Current Contents/Clinical Medicine, Excerpta Medica, BIOSIS, Science Citation Index,* and *ISI/BIOMED.*

Printed and bound by CPI Group (UK) Ltd, Croydon, CR0 4YY

Transferred to digital print 2012

Contributors

EDITOR

KENNETH W. ALTMAN, MD, PhD
Professor of Otolaryngology, Department of Otolaryngology Head and Neck Surgery, Icahn School of Medicine at Mount Sinai, Director, Eugen Grabscheid MD Voice Center, New York, New York

AUTHORS

LATIFAT ALLI-AKINTADE, MD
Clinical Fellow, Division of Gastroenterology, University of California, Davis Medical Center, Sacramento, California

KENNETH W. ALTMAN, MD, PhD
Professor of Otolaryngology, Department of Otolaryngology Head and Neck Surgery, Icahn School of Medicine at Mount Sinai, Director, Eugen Grabscheid MD Voice Center, New York, New York

LONI C. ARRESE, MS
Clinical Instructor, Department of Otolaryngology, Manager of Speech Pathology, JamesCare Head and Neck Clinic, JamesCare Voice and Swallowing Disorders Clinic, The Ohio State University Comprehensive Cancer Center, Arthur G. James Cancer Hospital, Richard J. Solove Research Institute, The Ohio State University, Columbus, Ohio

PETER C. BELAFSKY, MD, MPH, PhD
Professor, Department of Otolaryngology/Head and Neck Surgery, Center for Voice and Swallowing, University of California, Davis, Sacramento, California

DONALD C. BOLSER, PhD
Professor, Department of Physiological Sciences, College of Veterinary Medicine, University of Florida, Gainesville, Florida

SUSAN BRADY, MS, CCC-SLP, BRS-S
Board Recognized Swallowing and Swallowing Disorders Specialist, Research Coordinator, Departments of Speech-Language Pathology and Clinical Education, Swallowing Center, Marianjoy Rehabilitation Hospital, Wheaton, Illinois

SITA CHOKHAVATIA, MD
Professor of Medicine, Division of Gastroenterology, Rutgers-Robert Wood Johnson School of Medicine, New Jersey

PAUL W. DAVENPORT, PhD
Professor, Department of Physiological Sciences, College of Veterinary Medicine, University of Florida, Gainesville, Florida

JOSEPH DONZELLI, MD
Department of Otolaryngology, Midwest ENT, Springbrook Medical Center, Naperville, Illinois

STEVEN FRUCHT, MD
Department of Neurology, Icahn School of Medicine at Mount Sinai, New York, New York

ERIC M. GENDEN, MD, FACS
Professor and Chairman, Otolaryngology–Head and Neck Surgery, Professor of Neurosurgery and Immunology, Department of Otolaryngology, Director, The Head Neck, and Thyroid Center, The Mount Sinai Medical Center, Icahn School of Medicine at Mount Sinai, New York, New York

CHRISTIAN GESTREAU, PhD
Associate Professor, Center of Research in Neurobiology and Neurophysiology of Marseille, Aix Marseille Universite, CRN2M-UMR7286, Marseille, France

LAUREANO A. GIRALDEZ-RODRIGUEZ, MD
Fellow, Department of Otolaryngology–Head and Neck Surgery, Emory Voice Center, Atlanta, Georgia

LEANNE GOLDBERG, MS, CCC-SLP
Department of Otolaryngology Head and Neck Surgery, Icahn School of Medicine at Mount Sinai, New York, New York

NOAM HARPAZ, MD, PhD
Professor, Department of Pathology, Icahn School of Medicine at Mount Sinai, New York, New York

KAREN W. HEGLAND, PhD, CCC-SLP
Assistant Professor, Department of Speech, Language and Hearing Sciences, College of Public Health and Health Professions, University of Florida, Gainesville, Florida

MICHAEL JOHNS, III, MD
Director, Department of Otolaryngology–Head and Neck Surgery, Emory Voice Center, Atlanta, Georgia

MAGGIE A. KUHN, MD
Assistant Professor, Department of Otolaryngology/Head and Neck Surgery, Center for Voice and Swallowing, University of California, Davis, Sacramento, California

JEFFREY T. LAITMAN, PhD, DMedSc. (Hon), FAAAS, FAAA, FALA
Distinguished Professor, Professor and Director, Center for Anatomy and Functional Morphology, Professor of Otolaryngology, Professor of Medical Education, Icahn School of Medicine at Mount Sinai, New York, New York

CATHY L. LAZARUS, PhD
Associate Professor, Department of Otorhinolaryngology Head and Neck Surgery, Albert Einstein College of Medicine of Yeshiva University; Research Director, Thyroid Head and Neck Research Center, Thyroid Head and Neck Cancer (THANC) Foundation, Beth Israel Medical Center, New York, New York

ROSEMARY MARTINO, MA, MSc, PhD, CCC-SLP, Reg CASLPO
Associate Professor and Associate Chair, Department of Speech-Language Pathology, University of Toronto; Associate Professor, Department of Otolaryngology–Head and Neck Surgery, University of Toronto; Director of the Swallowing Disorders Laboratory, University Health Network, University of Toronto, Toronto, Ontario, Canada

DANIEL J. MCCABE, DMA, CCC-SLP
Department of Otolaryngology Head and Neck Surgery, Icahn School of Medicine
at Mount Sinai, New York, New York

JEFFREY I. MECHANICK, MD, FACP, FACE, FACN
Clinical Professor of Medicine, Director, Metabolic Support, Division of Endocrinology,
Diabetes and Bone Disease, Icahn School of Medicine at Mount Sinai, New York,
New York

KENDALL F. MORRIS, PhD
Professor, Department of Molecular Pharmacology and Physiology, Morsani College
of Medicine, University of South Florida, Tampa, Florida

THOMAS MURRY, PhD
Professor of Speech Pathology in Otolaryngology, Department of Otolaryngology–Head
and Neck Surgery, Weill Cornell Medical College, New York, New York

DHYANESH PATEL, MD
Department of Internal Medicine, Vanderbilt University Medical Center, Nashville,
Tennessee

TERESA E. PITTS, PhD
Assistant Professor, Department of Physiological Sciences, College of Veterinary
Medicine, University of Florida, Gainesville, Florida

EITAN PRISMAN, MD, FRCSC
Clinical Assistant Professor, Division of Otolaryngology Head and Neck Surgery, Gordon
and Leslie Diamond Health Care Centre, Vancouver General Hospital, University of British
Columbia, Vancouver, British Columbia, Canada

JOY S. REIDENBERG, PhD
Professor, Center for Anatomy and Functional Morphology, Professor of Medical
Education, Icahn School of Medicine at Mount Sinai, New York, New York

AMANDA RICHARDS, MBBS, FRACS
Department of Otolaryngology Head and Neck Surgery, Icahn School of Medicine
at Mount Sinai, New York, New York

DYLAN F. RODEN, MD, MPH
Department of Otolaryngology–Head and Neck Surgery, Mount Sinai School of Medicine,
New York, New York

STEPHANIE M. SHAW, MS, CCC-SLP
PhD Candidate, Department of Speech-Language Pathology, University of Toronto,
Toronto, Ontario, Canada

RENÉE SPEYER, PhD
Associate Professor and Head, Discipline of Speech Pathology, School of Public Health,
Tropical Medicine and Rehabilitation Sciences, James Cook University, Townsville,
Queensland, Australia; Department of Otorhinolaryngology and Head and Neck Surgery,
Leiden University Medical Center, Leiden, The Netherlands

RICHARD STERN, MD
Assistant Professor, Department of Radiology, Icahn School of Medicine at Mount Sinai,
New York, New York

MICHAEL F. VAEZI, MD, PhD, MSc (Epi), FACG
Director, Division of Gastroenterology, Hepatology and Nutrition, Center for Swallowing and Esophageal Disorders, Professor of Medicine, Clinical Director, Vanderbilt University Medical Center, Nashville, Tennessee

MICHAEL A. VIA, MD
Assistant Professor of Medicine, Division of Endocrinology and Metabolism, Albert Einstein College of Medicine, Beth Israel Medical Center, New York, New York

Contents

The mammalian larynx gained importance in new activities such as controlling intra-abdominal pressure during the evolutionary transition from egg-laying to birthing, and intrathoracic stabilization allowing rib stabilization for upper limb movements during climbing. Proper laryngeal development and positioning is crucial to its later normal function. Permanent intersection of the respiratory and digestive pathways creates a de novo aerodigestive tract; a first of its kind in mammals. The lowered position of the adult human larynx provides a greatly expanded supralaryngeal portion of the pharynx, enabling speech abilities. The intersection of respiratory and digestive tracts increases risk for choking in adults.

Swallowing is a complex physiologic function that involves precisely coordinated movements within the oral cavity, pharynx, larynx, and esophagus. This article reviews the anatomy, muscular control, and neurophysiological control of normal, healthy swallowing.

The purpose of this article is to update the otolaryngologic community on recent developments in the basic understanding of how cough, swallow, and breathing are controlled. These behaviors are coordinated to occur at specific times relative to one another to minimize the risk of aspiration. The control system that generates and coordinates these behaviors is complex, and advanced computational modeling methods are useful tools to elucidate its function.

Dysphagia is a common problem that has the potential to result in severe complications such as malnutrition and aspiration pneumonia. Based on the complexity of swallowing, there may be many different causes. This

with food propulsion, and it may be caused by oropharyngeal or esophageal disorders. Radiological modalities, endoscopy, and manometry play an important role in both the diagnosis and management of esophageal disorders.

OTOLARYNGOLOGIC CLINICS OF NORTH AMERICA

FORTHCOMING ISSUES

Asthma
Karen Calhoun, MD, *Editor*

Headache
Howard Levine, MD, and
Michael Setzen, MD, *Editors*

TransOral Robotic Surgery (TORS)
Neil Gross, MD, and
F. Christopher Holsinger, MD, *Editors*

Thyroid Cancer: Diagnosis, Treatment, Prognostication
Robert L. Witt, MD, *Editor*

RECENT ISSUES

Surgical Management of Facial Trauma
Kofi Derek O. Boahene, MD,
Anthony E. Brissett, MD, FACS, *Editors*
October 2013

Oral Cavity and Oropharyngeal Cancer
Jeffrey N. Myers, MD, PhD, and
Erich M. Sturgis, MD, MPH, *Editors*
August 2013

Complementary and Integrative Therapies for ENT Disorders
John Maddalozzo, MD,
Edmund A. Pribitkin, MD, and
Michael D. Seidman, MD, FACS, *Editors*
June 2013

Endoscopic Ear Surgery
Muaaz Tarabichi, MD, João Flávio
Nogueira, MD, Daniele Marchioni, MD,
Livio Presutti, MD, and
David D. Pothier, MD, *Editors*
April 2013

RELATED INTEREST

Dysphagia as a Cause of Chest Pain: An Otolaryngologist's View
Julia Vent, Simon F. Preuss, Guy D. Eslick
in Medical Clinics of North America, Volume 94, Issue 2, March 2010
Guy D. Eslick and Michael Yelland, Editors

DOWNLOAD
Free App!

Review Articles
THE CLINICS

NOW AVAILABLE FOR YOUR iPhone and iPad

Preface

Understanding Dysphagia: A Rapidly Emerging Problem

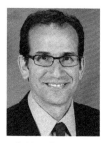

Kenneth W. Altman MD, PhD
Editor

Swallowing and deglutition are among the most primitive of animal life functions. These are driven by hard-wired innate connections in the brainstem, as well as a strong drive for nutrition and satiety originating in the deep recesses of the brain. As animals have evolved, the functions of swallowing have become increasingly complex. Dating back more than 300 million years with the evolution of the larynx in the African lungfish, tight pharyngeal constrictor muscles and sensory reflexes arose to protect against aspiration of food contents when swallowing. These mechanisms still hold true today, although they have become increasingly complex across the species, in addition to different developmental stages in mammals.

Humans advanced from hunter-gatherers following the retreat of the pleistocene ice age 10,000 BC, but it wasn't until the Neolithic revolution 5000–8000 BC where the development of tools allowed for planned agriculture. This led to crop cultivation and increased the diversity of food materials available, ultimately leading to the concept of recipes to include bread, beer, and soup by about 4000 BC. We have since come to use food to define our cultures, and the act of sitting at a meal with family, friends, and business relationships helps determine our pleasures and success in life. Thus, the impact of impaired swallowing (dysphagia) has profound quality-of-life as well as the expected nutritional consequences.

There are new challenges as we enter an era beyond the agricultural and industrial revolutions. Technological advances are facilitating increased life expectancy, where there is a growing aging population with increased medical problems. Oropharyngeal dysphagia is present in as many as 35% of the population older than 75,[1] as associated with muscle atrophy, cognitive decline, and increased aspiration risk. While the world population is expected to have 1 billion people older than 65 years by 2020, this number is forecasted to grow to 2 billion by 2050.[2] People are also living to older ages, so the prevalence and impact of dysphagia are also expected to increase.

Otolaryngol Clin N Am 46 (2013) xiii–xvi
http://dx.doi.org/10.1016/j.otc.2013.09.012
0030-6665/13/$ – see front matter © 2013 Elsevier Inc. All rights reserved.

Our fast-paced lifestyles have shifted commitments from standard meal times, and there's an associated increased likelihood of gastroesophageal reflux (GERD), which can contribute to dysphagia. In one 12-year period from 1990 to 2001, there was a documented four-fold increase in visits to physicians in the United States for GERD,[3] emphasizing its significant epidemiologic impact. Food supplies and sources are increasingly diverse, not only the types of products available through modern transportation that overcomes the historic seasonal limitations but also the increasing array of natural and synthetic ingredients. These issues offer a mixed blessing, diminishing a holistic natural existence, yet offering an amazing set of opportunities to address nutrition.

The consequences of dysphagia are also staggering. Long disqualified as an unfortunate complication of aging, stoke, and other degenerative illnesses, dysphagia affects both nutrition and quality of life. The idea of a family member dependent on enteral feeding when others are eating is depressing to them and counters their natural drives to eat. Social isolation is another severe consequence. And costs to the health care system are significant. In a study using the National Hospital Discharge Survey from 2005 to 2006, the presence of dysphagia was shown to be associated with a 40% increased length of stay (4 days compared to 2.4 days hospitalization in patients without dysphagia), with greater than $500 million of direct costs annually.[4] Mortality was 13 times higher in rehabilitation patients with dysphagia compared to those with no dysphagia, and 1.8 to 2.6 times higher during hospitalizations associated with cardiac dysrhythmias and atherosclerosis, respectively. Also, the rate of dysphagia was double (0.73% of all hospitalizations) in the age group 75 years and older compared to 45 to 64 years old.

Our traditional understanding of the swallowing mechanism is changing.[5] In the following list, there is renewed appreciation for central neurologic control, and the role of the larynx:

1. **Oral preparatory phase**: mastication and tongue manipulation of food, soft palate seal against the posterior tongue
2. **Oral transport phase**: tongue thrust and propulsion of the bolus to the oropharynx
3. **Pharyngeal phase**: pharyngeal constrictor contraction with peristalsis, laryngeal and pharyngeal elevation, false vocal fold closure, cricopharyngeus muscle relaxation
4. **Esophageal phase**: cricopharyngeus muscle contraction following passage of the bolus, esophageal peristalsis, secondary peristalsis. This phase should also address lower esophageal relaxation and competence (to be able to relax, or conversely, to prevent regurgitation)
5. **Central neurologic control**: brainstem deglutition reflexes, coordination with cessation of respiration, nutritional drive, urge for satiety, cognitive awareness of food bolus, social influence
6. **Laryngeal roles**: sensation of the bolus aids aspiration protection, and the cricopharyngeus is a shared muscle with the pharynx and larynx. Also, when there is penetration or microaspiration, glottal closure is essential for a competent cough reflex that produces accelerative flow for expulsion from the lungs rather than linear flow.

Dysphagia can be classified by the location, generally oral/pharyngeal versus esophageal phases. Also, the basic etiology of the dysphagia may be considered to be neuromuscular or obstructive. Some specific medical disorders of these divisions are listed in **Table 1**. The most common etiologies of dysphagia in different age groups also help the clinician diagnose the underlying causes of dysphagia. In this

Table 1
Classifications of dysphagia, with some examples of medical disorders

	Neuromuscular	Obstructive
Oropharyngeal	CVA, PD, ALS, MS, MG, MD, polio, syphilis	Tonsillitis, tumor
Esophageal	Achalasia, cricopharyngeus/ esophageal spasm, motility disorders (dermatomyositis, scleroderma)	Esophagitis (XRT, GERD, Candida), Zenker diverticulum, webs, Schiatzki ring, extrinsic compression

Abbreviations: ALS, amyotrophic lateral sclerosis; CVA, stroke; MD, muscular dystrophy; MG, myasthenia gravis; MS, multiple sclerosis; PD, Parkinson disease; XRT, radiation therapy.

classification, infancy is associated with neurodevelopmental delay; childhood and adolescence is associated with pharyngitis; young adult to middle age is associated predominantly with GERD; and older adults are at significantly higher risk because of medical comorbidities and neurodegenerative disease.

A systematic or protocolized approach is needed to screen high-risk groups, identify those needing further evaluation, include nutrition assessment, and intervene using an interdisciplinary approach. Specifically, these measures partly include

- Dysphagia screening and assessment instruments/questionnaires to address the presence of dysphagia as well as quality of life
- Bedside screening options, including nursing-administered water swallow test, and speech therapy–administered bedside or office-based swallow tests
- The Modified Barium Swallow and Functional Endoscopic Evaluation of swallowing (possibly with sensory testing) to quantify oropharyngeal dysphagia
- Understanding the presence of esophageal pathology through barium esophagogram, transnasal esophagoscopy, esophagogastroduodenoscopy
- Addressing esophageal function and reflux through manometry and pH/impedance testing
- Assessment for malnutrition and dehydration and determination of the role for ancillary feeding options depending on aspiration risk versus quality of life
- Swallowing rehabilitation with principles of care to assess aspiration risk, add muscular reconditioning strategies, reintroduce oral care and sensory stimulation, and suggest compensatory safe-swallow techniques
- Management of cricopharyngeal dysfunction with the use of botulinum toxin in the office and operating room, dilation, and consideration of endoscopic and open cricopharyngeal myotomy
- Surgical intervention for Zenker's diverticulum, with both endoscopic and open approaches
- Recognizing vocal paresis and paralysis in patients with aspiration risk, and being able to offer injection or medialization laryngoplasty. There is also a role for pharyngoplasty and cricopharyngeal myotomy in patients with impaired laryngeal sensation

High-risk groups are particularly interesting and more complicated as dysphagia patients. As with the aging and stroke populations, muscular atrophy predisposes to presbypharynges and subsequent oropharyngeal dysphagia. Decreased pharyngeal and laryngeal sensation, as well as impaired cognition, and increased aspiration risk. There is also reduced aspiration protection in the way of weaker glottal closure for a less expulsive cough, and reduced pulmonary reserve is associated with advancing age. There is an interesting paradox with these patients, where the aging process and muscular atrophy requires a relatively higher nutritional intake. Yet, the presence of dysphagia limits the patient's ability to meet their nutritional goals, and pushing these limits increases the likelihood of aspiration.

Other special populations are complicated and interesting as well. Advances in surgical and chemo-radiation treatments for head and neck cancer have resulted in a group of patients with altered anatomy. Chemo-radiation therapy also causes dysphagia in the short term through mucositis and edema. We are now beginning to recognize long-term consequences to include fibrosis that results in a dysfunctional laryngopharynx. Neurodegenerative diseases and dementia are likewise challenging conditions to treat when they are associated with dysphagia. In these situations, it is imperative to monitor decline with the overall disease, offer targeted consistencies and techniques that reduce aspiration risks, and consider patient goals with quality of life when deciding on a role for adjunctive nutrition.

Dysphagia is an important and interesting part of otolaryngology practice, and it needs to be structured in the right context. Although speech pathologists play a crucial role in assessment and behavioral modifications, the interdisciplinary partnership helps create the best outcomes in complicated patients. Furthermore, diagnostic and therapeutic procedures offered by the otolaryngologist can be pivotal in patient care.

This edition is expected to provide a useful and concise reference for care of dysphagia patients, with the goal of helping to translate the wealth of basic science literature to clinical relevance. Increasing the otolaryngologist's appreciation for dysphagia should heighten their role in patient care and serve as a conduit for further interest and research. The set of recommendations presented here should help standardize the approach to these complicated patients and inspire the use of clinical care pathways for dysphagia.

Kenneth W. Altman, MD, PhD
Professor of Otolaryngology
Department of Otolaryngology Head and Neck Surgery
The Icahn School of Medicine at Mount Sinai
Director, Eugen Grabscheid MD Voice Center
One Gustave L. Levy Place, Box 1189
New York, NY 10029, USA

E-mail address:
Kenneth.altman@mountsinai.org

REFERENCES

1. Barczi SR, Sullivan PA, Robbins J. How should dysphagia care of older adults differ? Establishing optimal practice patterns. Semin Speech Lang 2000;21:347–61.
2. Ageing and Life Course. WHO 2013. World Health Organization. Accessed on 3 January 2013. Available at: http://www.who.int/ageing/en/.
3. Altman KW, Stephens RM, Lyttle CS, et al. Changing impact of gastroesophageal reflux in medical and otolaryngology practice. Laryngoscope 2005;115:1145–53.
4. Altman KW. Dysphagia evaluation and care in the hospital setting: the need for protocolization. Otolaryngol Head Neck Surg 2011;145:895–8.
5. Altman KW, Yu GP, Schaeffer SD. Consequence of dysphagia in the hospitalized patient: impact on prognosis and hospital resources. Arch Otolaryngol Head Neck Surg 2010;136:784–9.

Fundamentals of Swallowing

The Evolution and Development of Human Swallowing
The Most Important Function We Least Appreciate

Jeffrey T. Laitman, PhD, DMedSc (Hon)*, Joy S. Reidenberg, PhD

KEYWORDS

- Aerodigestive tract • Swallowing • Deglutition • Larynx • Evolution

KEY POINTS

- As mammals morphed from their amphibian and reptilian ancestors, their larynx accrued added importance in new activities such as effectuating intra-abdominal pressure control during the transition from egg-laying to birthing and control of intrathoracic stabilization as movement of the upper limb required rib stabilization during climbing.
- The proper development of the larynx during the embryonic period is crucial to its later normal function, with miscues during this phase of development resulting in a range of serious congenital, often life-incompatible, anomalies.
- The permanent intersection of the respiratory and digestive pathways has created a de novo "aerodigestive" tract, a first of its kind in mammals.
- The lowered position of the human larynx has provided one major positive aspect: a greatly expanded supralaryngeal portion of the pharynx that enables speech production.
- The panoply of swallowing problems seen today was starting to come to the fore as the unique human ADT evolved.

Of all human activities, the function we probably least appreciate is swallowing. We must breathe and are always acutely aware of our breathing patterns. The slightest disruption or sniffle causes immediate reactions. Bathroom needs and activities are also high on our list (particularly as we age; can you say "prostate"). And we protect and monitor our senses - from smell to sight to hearing and balance - scrupulously. We infrequently, however, think about the many manifestations of swallowing, or of a swallow, unless, of course, one cannot do it.

The ability to swallow is arguably the "Rodney Dangerfield" of human aerodigestive functions: it receives little respect. The movement of a bolus from initial contact with our external lips through the various oral and pharyngeal portals, sphincters,

Center for Anatomy and Functional Morphology, Icahn School of Medicine at Mount Sinai, One Gustave Levy Place, New York, NY 10029-6574, USA
* Corresponding author.
E-mail address: Jeffrey.laitman@mssm.edu

Otolaryngol Clin N Am 46 (2013) 923–935
http://dx.doi.org/10.1016/j.otc.2013.09.005
0030-6665/13/$ – see front matter © 2013 Elsevier Inc. All rights reserved.

and way-stations en route to our gastro-esophageal processing chambers is given nary a thought. Whether we swallow saliva or transport a heavy density bolus of meat, whether we are young or old, male or female, from New York or New Delhi, the expectation is that our swallowing mechanism will function, and function constantly and well.

We humans arguably sit at the pinnacle of the mammalian world. Linnaeus unabashedly anointed our biological order, Primates, the "firsts." Our feline or cetacean brethren may take some umbrage, but since they can't speak we will never know. We are the masters of our planet and our evolution has endowed us with incomparable cognitive and communicative abilities that have allowed us the pre-eminence of culture and mastery of our world.

As our kind meandered through the corridors of evolution our basic body plan morphed and changed through genetics and environmental necessity to arrive at the masterful visage reflected in the mirror each morning. We evolved our distinctive habitually bipedal mode of locomotion, derived dentognathic arrangements commensurate with our dietary palate and unrivaled intricacies of our brain in the entangled evolutionary dance. Tied with all this, was an equally remarkable re-arrangement and functional redesign of the region of our interests, the aerodigestive tract, the unwieldy handle most have come to use for this mixed-use realm.

Indeed, we humans are arguably the only mammal – assuredly, only living primate (prosimians, monkeys, apes and us) – that has a constantly communal respiratory, digestive, vocal, aeration, olfactory and pressure control "tract." The very fact that we have no scientifically precise name for this noisy confluence of functions – it is neither purely respiratory, purely digestive, nor purely vocal – speaks to how the region has morphed and changed in starts and stops during eons of our evolution. All these changes have produced the unique substrate that allows for our distinctive modes of swallowing.

THE AERODIGESTIVE TRACT AMONG MAMMALS

One cannot understand the function of the human "aerodigestive" tract (ADT), let alone its evolution or unique ontogenetic development, without first viewing it in a comparative mammalian context. To gain some handle on the ADT it is necessary to have a focal point for that discussion, and that touchstone is the larynx – arguably one of the key structures in mammalian anatomy and function. As air-breathing mammals, the need to protect the lungs from incursions became paramount.[1] Although we have ascended the evolutionary ladder, the primary function of our larynx remains true to its heritage: it is still essentially a valve, regulating and guarding the airway. As mammals morphed from their amphibian and reptilian ancestors their larynx also accrued added importance in new activities such as effectuating intra-abdominal pressure control during the transition from egg-laying to birthing, and control of intrathoracic stabilization as movement of the upper limb required rib stabilization during climbing. Although the larynx of diverse mammalian species share many homologous components, the specifics of structure for larynges of species that inhabit often vastly differing environments have been modified extensively during the course of evolution.[2–4]

While mammals exhibit great variation in body plan, the general template for their throat region is remarkably similar (**Fig. 1**).[5,6] A hallmark of most mammals is that the epiglottis can make contact, or overlap the soft palate, during both normal respiration and deglutition. This is effectuated in most species due to a larynx positioned, at all stages of postnatal development, relatively "high" in the neck when related to the

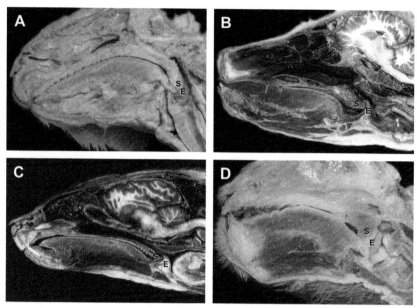

Fig. 1. Midsagittal sections of the head and neck regions of: (*A*) adult rabbit Oryctolagus cuniculus, (*B*) juvenile cattle Bos primigenius Taurus, (*C*) adult sea lion Zalophus californianus, (*D*) adult patas monkey Erythrocebus patas. E = epiglottis, S = soft palate. Note the high position of the larynx and the apposition or overlap of the epiglottis and soft palate.

basicranium and/or cervical vertebrae. Its position, measured from the cranial aspect of the epiglottis to the caudal border of the cricoid cartilage, corresponds to the level of the basiocciput or first cervical vertebra (C1) to the third or fourth cervical vertebrae (C3 or C4) in most terrestrial mammals. The hyoid bone and associated suprahyoid and infrahyoid muscles (i.e., muscles largely responsible for raising or lowering the larynx) are also relatively high. The tongue at rest lies almost entirely within the oral cavity, with no portion of it forming part of the anterior pharyngeal wall. Because of this high position of the larynx, the supralaryngeal region of the pharynx is noticeably small; the pharynx has little or no oral portion and significantly reduced nasal and laryngeal segments. Inferiorly, the striated muscle fibers of the pharynx blend with the longitudinal striated fibers of the esophagus to form a continuous functional unit.

As noted, the high position of the larynx enables the epiglottis to pass upward behind the soft palate and lock the larynx directly into the nasopharynx. This configuration provides a direct air channel from the external nares through the nasal cavities, nasopharynx, larynx, and trachea to the lungs. Liquids, and in some species even chewed or solid material, can pass on either side of the interlocked larynx and nasopharynx by way of the isthmus faucium, through the piriform sinuses to the esophagus, following the so-called "lateral food channels." This anatomic configuration allows streams of liquid or semisolid food to be transmitted around each side of the larynx during swallowing, while also maintaining patency of the laryngeal airway. Two largely separate pathways are created: a digestive tract from the oral cavity to the esophagus and a respiratory tract from the nose to the lungs. This arrangement confers on mammals the ability to use these two pathways simultaneously, including enabling simultaneous breathing while: (1) young are suckling, (2) ruminants are regurgitating cud, (3) carnivores have their mouth clamped tightly closed around the neck of their prey, and (4) a variety of animals use the mouth as a tool (e.g., beavers gnawing trees, felines or rodents grasping and carrying young). In addition, as many mammals are macrosmatic (i.e., largely dependent on olfaction for communication with their environment), the two-tube system is particularly valuable as this arrangement allows, for example, grazing or drinking herbivores to simultaneously detect the scent of a predator.

Although the larynx is consistently high in most mammals, its exact position and the extent of its placement in the nasopharynx can vary considerably among species. For example, studies of cetaceans (i.e., whales, dolphins, porpoises) have shown that the larynx is positioned so high (rostral) that it is no longer solely in the neck but rather lies largely within the head.[7] The epiglottis lies under the presphenoidal synchondrosis, while the caudal border of the cricoid is positioned approximately opposite the occipital condyles or perhaps C1. The compressed cervical vertebrae characteristic of these mammals makes it difficult to determine a corresponding cervical position, as there is very little neck region for the larynx to occupy. The anterior portion of the larynx is elongated into a tube that is encircled by a strong palatopharyngeal sphincter muscle (homologous to the soft palate and palatopharyngeal arch in humans). This sphincter grips the laryngeal tube and keeps its aditus intranarial, thus effectively sealing the respiratory tract from the digestive route. Although they exhibit the baseline mammalian pattern of a high larynx, odontocetes appear to have exaggerated it by placing the larynx even higher (or more rostral) than their terrestrial relatives. This extra high position ensures these mammals of a larynx fitted snugly into the nasopharynx, and indeed may make it permanently intranarial—that is, it is not normally retracted from its position behind the soft palate. This arrangement may allow them to swallow whole fish while keeping the airway patent for generating sounds for communication or navigation (echolocation).

Although cetaceans demonstrate an example of larynges that have both migrated cranially and elongated their rostral cartilages, some terrestrial species have larynges that have expanded their caudal components (e.g., thyroid cartilage) so that they appear to extend considerably into the neck. For example, some male artiodactyls (red and fallow deer, Mongolian gazelle) exhibit particularly large larynges that seem to be located more caudally in the neck compared with other related species.[8] However, although the larynges of these animals are elongated, they still retain roughly the same position opposite the cervical vertebrae as most other terrestrial mammals (extending from the basiocciput to C2-C3). Maintenance of this typical mammalian position is due to concomitant elongation of the cervical vertebrae. These animals also exhibit an elongated and elastic velum (red and fallow deer) and an elongated epiglottis (Mongolian gazelle) that appear to assist in epiglottic/palatal contact and, therefore, the maintenance of the two-pathway system. Thus, while larynges differ considerably in position, the ancestral "two-tube" configuration is essentially maintained. These animals have modified a basic plan; they have not changed it.[1]

Postmortem dissections and a range of imaging studies, including cineradiography, CT, and MR, of our closest relatives the nonhuman primates show that their upper respiratory anatomy is also similar to the general mammalian pattern.[1,9–11] As in other mammals, nonhuman primates exhibit a larynx positioned high in the neck, usually corresponding to the first to third cervical vertebrae (**Fig. 1**). This position allows for epiglottic-soft palate apposition and the possibility of an intranarial larynx, thus providing a continuous airway from the nose to the lungs, while the alimentary tract passes around the larynx en route to the esophagus. Cineradiographic studies have confirmed that nonhuman primates exhibit mostly separate respiratory and digestive routes and the ability to breathe and swallow almost simultaneously.[10,12] Because of this configuration, nonhuman primates, like other mammals, appear strongly, if not totally, dependent on nasal breathing. As occurs in many mammals, the connection between the epiglottis and the soft palate can be broken, as the larynx exhibits extensive mobility and can be transiently lowered. This can occur for a number of reasons, including some vocalizations, swallowing certain foods (e.g., a large bolus of meat), or due to disease.

Although this anatomic arrangement may enable almost simultaneous breathing and swallowing, it severely limits the array of sounds an animal can produce. The high position of the larynx means that only a small supralaryngeal portion of the pharynx exists. In turn, only a very reduced area is available to modify the initial sounds generated at the vocal folds. Due to this limitation, most mammals therefore depend primarily on altering the shape of the oral cavity and lips to modify laryngeal sounds. Although some animals can approximate some human speech sounds, they are anatomically incapable of producing the range of sounds necessary for human speech.[13,14]

UNIQUE DEVELOPMENT OF THE HUMAN AERODIGESTIVE TRACT

The human ADT, particularly the larynx and its positional relationships to contiguous structures, undergoes dramatic changes during development. Indeed, the highly derived characteristics of the adult human ADT reflect both a distinctive developmental path as well as an evolutionary one.

Embryonic Period

The major morphologic events in embryonic development (0–8 weeks) of the human larynx have been well documented and new data from homeobox genes are shedding further light on the mechanisms of early spatial establishment in the head and neck.[15,16] The proper development of the larynx during the embryonic period is obviously crucial to its later normal function, with miscues during this phase of development resulting in a range of serious congenital, often life-incompatible, anomalies.

Fetal Period

Although aspects of laryngeal development during the embryonic period have been well studied, changes during the fetal period (8 weeks to birth) have not been as extensively explored. To elucidate the latter, studies by our laboratory and others have investigated fetal laryngeal development both through postmortem study employing precise means of age determination and ultrasonography of living fetuses.[17–19] These studies have shown that the fetal period is a time of extensive laryngeal growth and of significant changes in the positional relationships of the larynx. The second trimester (13–26 weeks), in particular, is an active period for laryngeal development:

- By week 15, earlier than was previously reported, the epiglottis is already present, indicating that the epiglottic primordium may appear earlier in development than classically believed. Throughout this period, the larynx is found high in the neck, generally corresponding, from the epiglottic tip to the inferior border of the cricoid, to the level of the basioccipital bone to the third cervical vertebra.
- By week 21, the epiglottis is found to be almost in apposition to the uvula of the soft palate.
- Between weeks 23 and 25, the epiglottis and soft palate overlap for the first time, providing the anatomical "interlocking" of the larynx into the nasopharynx characteristic of mammals described previously.

Larynx-Nasopharynx Interlocking

The attainment of larynx-nasopharynx interlocking is a significant maturational horizon in the development of the ADT. Establishment of this anatomic relationship allows the creation of essentially separate respiratory and digestive routes that will function as such in the newborn infant. Our ultrasound investigations have shown upper respiratory activity patterns that strongly suggest an operational "two-tube" system is beginning to function prenatally, in which the larynx remains highly positioned and intranarial during fetal swallowing movements. A critical time in the development of the entire upper respiratory region may take place during the period between weeks 23 and 25. Not only does the larynx attain an intranarial position, but also contiguous portions of the skull base—the de facto roof of the upper respiratory tract—appear to be undergoing remodeling at this time. As portions of the cranial base are intimately related to the larynx and its contiguous musculature[17] shape development and ADT positions may also be linked, although the precise extent and relationships are still unclear. What may be beginning during this period is a remodeling and refinement of the positional anatomy of the entire ADT—soft tissue and cartilaginous structures, such as the larynx, and bony skeletal parameters, such as the skull base—to provide the anatomical framework for the newborn's independent respiratory and digestive functions.

Lower Respiratory Tract Concomitant Development

It should be noted that while laryngeal and basicranial modifications are occurring in the *upper* respiratory region, concomitant changes are also occurring in the *lower* respiratory tract. For example, the period from weeks 23 to 25 corresponds to the maturation of the alveolar cells in the pulmonary epithelium.[1] This alveolar epithelium is responsible for the production of fetal lung surfactant, a substance that is essential for independent respiratory function. The contemporaneous development of the fetal larynx to permit soft palate–epiglottic overlap with increasing levels of lung surfactant suggests that the time frame for the maturation of the upper and lower respiratory tracts are synchronized. Normal fetal maturation of the larynx may be an essential factor in determining the onset of respiratory function and overall fetal viability.

High Laryngeal Position

The morphologic pattern of high laryngeal position established during fetal life continues past the perinatal period and into infancy (**Fig. 2**A). Indeed, the newborn/young infant period may more accurately be seen as an extension of the pattern established

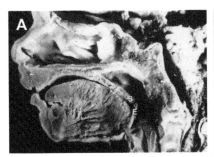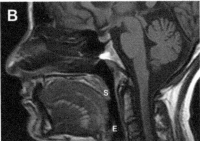

Fig. 2. (*A*) Midsagittal section of the head and neck of a newborn human infant, (*B*) Midsagittal MR image of the head and neck of an adult human. E = epiglottis, S = soft palate. Note the apposition of the epiglottis in *A*, and the descent of the larynx and posterior tongue in *B*.

during the late second and early third fetal trimesters rather than as a distinct entity. Postmortem dissections and imaging studies have shown that the positional relationships in the aerodigestive region of human newborns and young infants closely resemble the baseline primate and mammalian pattern. In newborns and infants until approximately $1\frac{1}{2}$ to 2 years of age, the larynx remains high in the neck.[1,6,20–24] Its position corresponds opposite the level of basiocciput/C1 through the superior border of C4 in newborns, and descends slightly to the level between C2 and C5 by approximately 2 years of age. The tongue can be found entirely within the oral cavity at rest, with no portion of it forming the upper anterior wall of the pharynx.

Largely separate respiratory and digestive pathways, similar to those described in most other terrestrial mammals, are effectuated by the high laryngeal position in newborns and young infants. This arrangement prevents the mixing of ingested food and inhaled air, thereby enabling the baby to swallow liquids and breathe almost simultaneously in a manner similar to that of monkeys. Thus the baby can breathe through the nose with only minimal, if any, cessations as liquid flows from the oral cavity around the larynx into the esophagus (**Fig. 3**A). Because of this high laryngeal position, newborns are essentially, if not obligatorily, nose breathers. As with nonhuman primates, the connection between the epiglottis and the soft palate is usually constant, but may be interrupted during the swallowing of a particularly large or dense bolus of food or liquid, during vocalization or crying, or because of disease as noted above.

Although the high position of the larynx in a human newborn or young infant effectuates the dual-pathway ADT, it severely limits the array of sounds babies produce. Many studies have shown that the high position of the larynx greatly restricts the supralaryngeal portion of the pharynx/tongue available to modify the initial, or

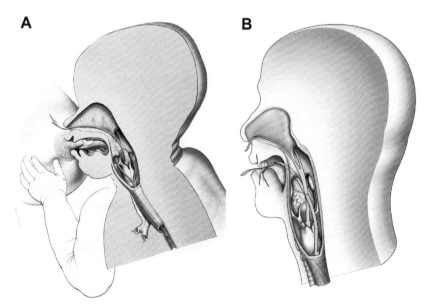

Fig. 3. Drawings depicting: (A) the aerodigestive tract of a newborn human during suckling, and (B) the aerodigestive region in an adult human. Respiratory route = arrows from nose to larynx, digestive route = arrows from mouth to esophagus. Note the high laryngeal position in the infant effectuates largely distinct pathways, whereas the lowered position of the larynx and tongue in the adult mandates crossing of the pathways.

fundamental, sounds produced at the vocal folds.[14] Thus, an individual with a larynx situated high in the neck, as is found in a newborn human or monkey, would have a more restricted range of vocalizations available than would individuals with larynges and tongues placed lower in the neck. Indeed, linguistic analyses have[14] identified the quantal vowels [i], [u], and [a] as sounds that human infants and nonhuman primates cannot produce. As these vowels are the limiting articulations of a vowel triangle that is language universal, their absence considerably restricts speech capabilities.

Although the larynx remains high in the neck until around the second year, functional changes, such as the first occasional instances of oral respiration, have been noted to occur considerably earlier, indeed within the first 6 months of life.[21] The period between 4 and 6 months, in particular, may represent a crucial stage in upper respiratory activity. At this time, neural control of laryngeal and pharyngeal musculature is beginning to change even before true structural "descent" of the larynx has occurred. This changeover period may also indicate a time of potential respiratory instability because of the transition from one respiratory pattern to another.

The time and manifestation of both prenatal and postnatal maturation within the central nervous system relates directly to normal and abnormal upper respiratory and swallowing functions. For example, studies from our laboratory have suggested that there are crucial prenatal periods for the development of mammalian upper respiratory motor nuclei in the brainstem, and that insults *in utero* could affect postnatal functions.[25,26] The combination of subsequent, postnatal CNS maturation and developmental changes in respiratory patterns may predispose the infant to several developmentally related problems. The sudden infant death syndrome (SIDS), for example, may be related to the fragility of these first postnatal upper respiratory changes, reflecting prenatal insults to the brainstem nuclei involved in aerodigestive neuromuscular control.[25,27] The precise time of the shifts that occur in breathing patterns, their relationship to laryngeal changes, and the neurophysiologic mechanisms that accompany them are obviously crucial questions that are still poorly understood and require more specific and detailed study.

Descent of the Larynx

The larynx of human infants may remain high in the neck until approximately $1\frac{1}{2}$ to 2 years of age. Our studies and others have confirmed that around the second year, children begin to show positional rearrangements of the ADT that differ sharply from the condition in newborns and early infants. Around this period the larynx begins its permanent, structural descent into the neck. Minor topographic changes in laryngeal position continue until puberty and beyond, however, the major qualitative change probably occurs between the second to third years of life. The exact timing of laryngeal descent has yet to be fully determined, but imaging and postmortem observations indicate that the position of the larynx has been significantly lowered by the third year.

Although the internal nature of the larynx changes relatively little after the third year (except for normal maturational changes at puberty), positional changes relative to contiguous upper respiratory structures are considerable. The tongue no longer lies entirely within the oral cavity at rest, as in the newborn infant or nonhuman primate. The posterior portion of the tongue, from the foramen cecum caudally, has descended into the neck. It bends at a right angle relative to the oral portion, and lies in a vertical plane where it now forms the upper anterior wall of the pharynx. The larynx is now situated considerably lower in the neck. For example, in a 7-year-old child, the larynx is positioned between the upper border of C3 and the lower border of C5. In the adult, the larynx has further descended, lying between the lower border of C3/upper part of C4 to the upper border of C7. Concomitantly, the hyoid bone and its associated suprahyoid and infrahyoid muscles are relatively lower in the neck (**Fig. 2**B).

Due to the descent of the larynx, tongue, and hyoid apparatus in children after the second to third year, the epiglottis can no longer approximate the soft palate, even during maximal laryngeal elevation. As the larynx cannot lock into the nasopharynx, there no longer exists the possibility of a continuous, tubelike airway from the external nares to the lungs. The lower position of the larynx alters dramatically the way humans, after the early years of life, breathe and swallow. The loss of the ability of the epiglottis to make contact with the soft palate means that the possibility of having two separate pathways, one for air and one for liquid - the baseline ancient terrestrial template - no longer exists. Unlike this general mammalian pattern, the respiratory and digestive tracts now cross each other in the area of the pharynx (**Fig. 3**B). This low position of the larynx also results in a large supralaryngeal portion of the pharynx. A permanently enlarged oropharynx is now present even during maximal laryngeal elevation. These changes have pronounced effects upon our respiratory behavior. For example, we are habitual nose breathers but, unlike newborn infants, adults have a greater ability for oral respiration and do so more frequently. Loss of the two-pathway system has now made it imperative that the respiratory tract be sealed off during swallowing.

EVOLUTION OF THE AERODIGESTIVE TRACT IN THE COURSE OF HUMAN EVOLUTION: CHOKING TO DEATH ALONG THE WAY

The permanent intersection of the respiratory and digestive pathways has created a *de novo* "aerodigestive" tract, a first of its kind in mammals. This has created many problems, which, if not unique, are certainly accentuated in us. A major problem is that a bolus of food can easily become lodged in the laryngeal aditus leading to the common occurrence of food "going down the wrong pipe." However, if the bolus is large or not expelled rapidly enough one may choke to death. This event is often referred to as a "cafe coronary," because it frequently occurs in restaurants and may be mistaken for a heart attack. Similarly, another disadvantage of the crossed pathways is the relative ease with which vomitus can be aspirated into the larynx and trachea and passed into the lungs.

Not only has a permanently lowered larynx proven to be a danger in the ingestion of material, but this anatomy underlies why stomach contents enter the pharyngeal or oral cavities during bouts of gastroesophageal reflux.[28,29] The human aerodigestive tract has clearly not been selected evolutionarily for the purpose of efficiently dealing with constant, retrograde incursions into the supraesophagus. Indeed, our ADT appears to be particularly poorly designed to handle any esophageal or gastroesophageal reflux. This is most clearly demonstrated by two features: (1) our uniquely low laryngeal position, and (2) our relatively unprotected posterior larynx. Low laryngeal position, by creating a permanent oropharynx, has by definition created a greatly expanded supraesophageal region. It should also be noted that as the larynx has migrated caudally, so too has the location of the cricopharyngeal sphincter (i.e., the upper esophageal sphincter) at the caudal-most extent of the pharynx. Thus, adult humans have a relatively shorter esophagus and relatively longer supraesophagus than most other mammals. At the very least, then, the highly acidic contents of human gastroesophageal reflux have gained access to a proportionally greater surface area of pharyngeal mucosa with which it interacts negatively.

Clearly, laryngeal descent in humans has altered considerably the way we breathe and swallow. From an evolutionary perspective, we have lost the basic mammalian ability to breathe and swallow simultaneously or almost simultaneously. We have also accrued a number of most unwanted guests, including the relative ease of lodging material in the airway or refluxing contents to the supraesophagus and other portals. A litany of other diseases and/or incoordination clinicopathologies, ranging from otitis media and frequent rhinosinusitis[30] to SIDS and aspects of obstructive sleep-apnea (OSA),[31] may also be a price we pay for peripheral and central neuromuscular rearrangements that accompany ADT modifications.

The lowered position of our larynx has, however, provided one major positive aspect: a greatly expanded supralaryngeal portion of the pharynx. This enlarged supralaryngeal pharynx has "liberated" the tongue from oral cavity confinement. Its posterior portion now forms the movable anterior wall of this enlarged pharyngeal chamber. This configuration allows for enhanced oral tidal respiration, which may have occurred in temperate environments for our early ancestors. In addition, pharyngeal/lingual modification of sounds produced at the vocal folds is considerably greater than that possible for newborns, early infants, or any nonhuman mammal. In essence, it is the unique marked descent of the larynx, and the resultant expansion of the pharynx and liberation of the posterior tongue, that gives us the anatomic ability to produce fully articulate speech.

When, how and why our uniquely derived ADT came about during the course of our species' evolution is a source of much discussion. While fossilized throats do not remain, some researchers, our lab included, have developed methods to reconstruct the anatomy of the region through the use of remnant portions of the cranial base, the de facto "roof" of the ADT, as a guide.[32–35]

Reconstruction of the ADT of fossil human ancestors (known in anthropologic parlance as "hominids")—ranging in age from our earliest direct relatives known as australopiths (who came on the scene arguably over four million years ago), to early members of our own genus *Homo* (appearing over a million and a half years ago), to our own species *Homo sapiens* (arriving perhaps 200,000 to 300,000 years before the present)—have enabled us to trace the changes in the region through our evolutionary history. For example, our reconstructions have suggested that the earliest hominids likely exhibited an ADT largely similar to those of the extant apes, with the larynx positioned high in the throat and the epiglottis able to contact the soft palate during normal tidal respiration. These early ancestors likely breathed and swallowed essentially as do our living monkey and ape relatives, being nasal breathers with a modified two-tube system. The high position of their larynx would by necessity limit the supralaryngeal area of the pharynx and the freedom of the tongue to modify sounds as extensively as modern adult humans can. This suggests that they were restricted in the types of sounds that they could make, probably being incapable of producing a number of the universal vowel sounds found in human speech patterns.[33,34]

If our earliest relatives were still "ape-like" in their ADT, when did things change en route to us? This is a key question in our evolution and while definitive answers in evolution are rare, we have unearthed some good clues. Our fossil data – and by extension reconstructions – suggest that the region was starting to change with the first members of our own genus, *Homo*, some million-plus years before the present on the plains of Africa. It was at this time that the ancient, two-tube system in place for millennia was morphing into something different. The basicranium was changing, indicating that the larynx was also changing in position, likely becoming disengaged from the nasopharynx. Such a shift would have radically altered the way our ancestors breathed (e.g., increasing oral respiration possibilities) and, most important for our purposes here, dramatically altered deglutition. No longer, for example, would such ancestors have had the ability to breathe and swallow almost simultaneously. A new paradigm would have come in place. Such a shift would have required not only obvious anatomical uncoupling and rearrangements, but also a "rewiring" of central and peripheral neural control. As with developmental shifts noted previously, change has its costs, and many of our early ancestors likely paid the ultimate price. Scenarios such as increased choking and other upper respiratory and upper digestive maladies probably evolved along with our laryngeal shifts. Indeed, the predecessor of a "café coronary" – perhaps a "savanna coronary" - was coming on the scene.[5]

While changes may have begun with early members of our genus, it was not until the appearance of early members our own species Homo sapiens, some 200–300,000 years before the present, that an ADT similar to ours appeared.[34] These early H. sapiens probably functioned much as we do today as regards their breathing, swallowing, and vocal patterns, and accordingly, likely accrued the unpleasant baggage of many swallowing disorders. Fortunately, or more likely unfortunately as per your perspective, since early members of our species did not live anywhere near the life-span we exhibit today, many of the age-related aspects of swallowing problems likely did not visit them. None-the-less, the panoply of swallowing problems exhibited today was undeniably starting to come to the fore as our uniquely odd ADT evolved. Our species has paid many an expensive ticket to reach our level of uniqueness, perhaps none more so than those related to swallowing.

REFERENCES

1. Laitman JT, Reidenberg JS. Evolution of the human larynx: Nature's great experiment. In: Fried M, Ferlito A, editors. The larynx. 3rd edition. San Diego (CA): Plural; 2009. p. 19–38.
2. Harrison DF. The anatomy and physiology of the mammalian larynx. Cambridge (United Kingdom): Cambridge University Press; 1995.
3. Reidenberg JS, Laitman JT. Morphophysiology of the larynx. In: Van De Water T, Staecker H, editors. Basic science review for otolaryngology. New York: Thieme; 2005. p. 505–15.
4. Kirchner JA. The vertebrate larynx: adaptations and aberrations. Laryngoscope 1993;103:1197–201.
5. Laitman JT, Reidenberg JS. Specializations of the human upper respiratory and upper digestive systems as seen through comparative and developmental anatomy. Dysphagia 1993;8:318–25.
6. Laitman JT, Reidenberg JS. Comparative and developmental anatomy of human laryngeal position. In: Bailey B, editor. Head and Neck Surgery – Otolaryngology, vol. 1, 2nd edition. Philadelphia: Lippincott Company; 1998. p. 45–52.
7. Reidenberg JS, Laitman JT. The position of the larynx in Odontoceti (toothed whales). Anat Rec 1987;218:98–106.
8. Frey R, Gebler A. The highly specialized vocal tract of the male Mongolian gazelle (Procapra gutturosa Pallas, 1777- Mammalia, Bovidae). J Anat 2003;203(5): 451–71.
9. Laitman JT, Crelin ES, Conlogue GJ. The function of the epiglottis in monkey and man. Yale J Biol Med 1977;50:43–9.
10. Laitman JT, Crelin ES. Tantalum markers as an aid in identifying the upper respiratory structures of experimental animals. Lab Anim Sci 1980;30(2):245–8.
11. Flugel C, Rohen JW. The craniofacial proportions and laryngeal position in monkeys and man of different ages. (A morphometric study based on CT scans and radiographs.). Mech Ageing Dev 1991;61:65–83.
12. German RZ, Crompton AW. Integration of swallowing and respiration in infant macaques (Macaca fascicularis). Am J Phys Anthropol 1993;(Suppl 16):94.

13. Laitman JT. The evolution of the hominid upper respiratory system and implications for the origins of speech. In: de Grolier E, editor. Glossogenetics: The Origin and Evolution of Language. Paris: Harwood Academic Press; 1983. p. 63–90.
14. Lieberman P, Laitman JT, Reidenberg JS, et al. The anatomy, physiology, acoustics and perception of speech: essential elements in analysis of the evolution of human speech. J Hum Evol 1992;23:447–67.
15. Som PM, Smoker WR, Reidenberg JS, et al. Embryology and anatomy of the neck. In: Som PM, Curtin HD, editors. Head and neck imaging. 5th edition. New York: Mosby; 2011. p. 2117–64.
16. Laitman JT, Noden DM, Van De Water TR. Formation of the larynx: from homeobox genes to critical periods. In: Rubin JS, Sataloff RT, Korovin GS, et al, editors. Diagnosis and treatment of voice disorders. 4th edition. San Diego (CA): Plural Publishing; 2013.
17. Magriples U, Laitman JT. Developmental change in the position of the fetal human larynx. Am J Phys Anthropol 1987;72:463–72.
18. Wolfson VP, Laitman JT. Ultrasound investigation of fetal human upper respiratory anatomy. Anat Rec 1990;227:363–72.
19. Isaacson G, Birnholz JC. Human fetal upper respiratory tract function as revealed by ultrasonography. Ann Otol Rhinol Laryngol 1991;100:743–7.
20. Laitman JT, Crelin ES. Developmental change in the upper respiratory system of human infants. Perinatology/Neonatology 1980;4:15–22.
21. Sasaki CT, Levine PA, Laitman JT, et al. Postnatal descent of the epiglottis in man: a preliminary report. Arch Otolaryngol 1977;103:169–71.
22. Westhorpe RN. The position of the larynx in children and its relationship to the ease of intubation. Anaesth Intensive Care 1987;15:384–8.
23. Schwartz D, Keller M. Maturational descent of the epiglottis. Arch Otolaryngol Head Neck Surg 1997;123:627–8.
24. Vorperian HK, Kent RD, Linstrom MJ, et al. Development of vocal tract length during early childhood: a magnetic resonance imaging study. J Acoust Soc Am 2005;117:338–50.
25. Friedland DR, Eden AR, Laitman JT. Naturally occurring motoneuron cell death in rat upper respiratory tract motor nuclei: a histological, Fast-DiI and immunocytochemical study in the nucleus ambiguus. J Neurobiol 1995;26:563–78.
26. Friedland DR, Eden AR, Laitman JT. Naturally occurring motoneuron cell death in rat upper respiratory tract motor nuclei: a histological, Fast-DiI and immunocytochemical study in the hypoglossal nucleus. J Neurobiol 1995;27:520–34.
27. Tonkin SL, Gunn TR, Bennet L, et al. A review of the anatomy of the upper airway in early infancy and its possible relevance to SIDS. Early Hum Dev 2002;66:107–21.
28. Laitman JT, Reidenberg JS. The human aerodigestive tract and gastroesophageal reflux: an evolutionary perspective. Am J Med 1998;103:3–11.
29. Lipan M, Reidenberg JS, Laitman JT. The anatomy of reflux: a growing healthproblem affecting structures of the head and neck. Anat Rec B New Anat 2006;289: 261–70.
30. Bluestone CD, Pagano AS, Swarts JD, et al. Consequences of evolution: Is rhinosinusitis, like otitis media, a unique disease of humans? Otolaryngol Head Neck Surg 2012;147:986–91, 62.
31. Davidson T. The Great Leap Forward: the anatomic basis for the acquisition of speech and obstructive sleep apnea. Sleep Med 2003;4:185–94.
32. Laitman JT, Heimbuch RC, Crelin ES. Developmental change in a basicranial line and its relationship to the upper respiratory system in living primates. Am J Anat 1978;152:467–83.

33. Laitman JT, Heimbuch RH, Crelin ES. The basicranium of fossil hominids as an indicator of their upper respiratory systems. Am J Phys Anthropol 1979;51:15–34.
34. Laitman JT, Heimbuch RC. The basicranium of Plio-Pleistocene hominids as an indicator of their upper respiratory systems. Am J Phys Anthropol 1982;59: 323–44.
35. Reidenberg JS, Laitman JT. Effect of basicranial flexion on larynx and hyoid position in rats: an experimental study of skull and soft tissue interactions. Anat Rec 1991;220:557–69.

The Normal Swallow
Muscular and Neurophysiological Control

Stephanie M. Shaw, MS, CCC-SLP[a],
Rosemary Martino, MA, MSc, PhD, CCC-SLP, SLP Reg CASLPO[a,b,c,*]

KEYWORDS

- Dysphagia • Deglutition • Swallowing • Anatomy • Physiology • Neurophysiology

KEY POINTS

- Swallowing is a rapid yet complex sequence of movements with 4 primary phases: oral preparatory, oral transport, pharyngeal, and esophageal.
- These phases are primarily coordinated by 5 cranial nerves and 3 peripheral nerves, which are mediated centrally via the medulla oblongata of the brain stem.
- In addition to the brain stem, the cortical and subcortical regions of the brain play an integral part in mediating the swallow, especially the oral preparatory and oral transport phases.
- Impaired sensory or motor ability at any level impairs the efficiency of swallow physiology; impairment that affects the mechanisms responsible for airway protection also affects swallow safety.

INTRODUCTION

Swallowing is a normal physiologic function that is often taken for granted. As humans, we swallow an average of 500 times per day.[1] A normal swallow requires the precise coordination of more than 30 muscles located within the oral cavity, pharynx, larynx, and esophagus (**Table 1**). Muscle movements are controlled by several cranial (CN V, VII, and IX-XII) and peripheral (C1-C3)[2] nerves and are coordinated within the brain stem (mainly medulla oblongata, where a network of sensory nuclei, motor nuclei, and interneurons form what is known as the "swallowing center"[3]). Often, individuals with neurologic and/or structural abnormalities of the head and neck due to causes

Funding Sources: Ms Shaw, Connaught Scholarship; Dr Martino, CRC, CIHR, CCSRI, NCIC.
Conflict of Interest: None.
[a] Department of Speech-Language Pathology, University of Toronto, 160-500 University Avenue, Toronto, Ontario M5G 1V7, Canada; [b] Department of Otolaryngology–Head & Neck Surgery, University of Toronto, 190 Elizabeth Street, Rm 3S-438, R. Fraser Elliott Building, Toronto, Ontario M5G 2N2, Canada; [c] Swallowing Disorders Laboratory, University Health Network, University of Toronto, 399 Bathurst Street, Main Pavilion 11-327, Toronto, Ontario M5T 2S8, Canada
* Corresponding author. Department of Speech-Language Pathology, University of Toronto, 160-500 University Avenue, Toronto, Ontario M5G 1V7, Canada.
E-mail address: rosemary.martino@utoronto.ca

0030-6665/13/$ – see front matter Crown Copyright © 2013 Published by Elsevier Inc. All rights reserved.

Abbreviations	
CN	Cranial nerve
DSG	Dorsal swallowing group
FEESST	Fiberoptic endoscopic evaluation of swallowing with sensory testing
ISLN	Internal branch of the superior laryngeal nerve
LAR	Laryngeal adductor response
LCA	Lateral cricoarytenoid
LCR	Laryngeal cough reflex
LES	Lower esophageal sphincter
SLN	Superior laryngeal nerve
UES	Upper esophageal sphincter
VSG	Ventral swallowing group

such as stroke, Parkinson's disease, or cancer, experience problems with swallowing, or dysphagia. Dysphagia can lead to several negative outcomes, including pneumonia,[4] malnutrition,[5] dehydration,[6] and reduced quality of life.[7] As a result, rehabilitation is often required to prevent negative outcomes and ensure, where possible, safe and adequate oral intake. To understand the processes involved in rehabilitating a disordered swallow, it is imperative to first understand the anatomy, muscular control, and neurophysiological control of a normal, healthy swallow.

ANATOMY AND CONTRIBUTING LANDMARKS

Many structures within the oral cavity, pharynx, and esophagus are involved in swallowing, including several bones, cartilages, teeth, spaces, salivary glands, and muscles. Familiarity with these structures is a necessary first step to differentiate between normal and disordered swallowing (**Fig. 1**).

Bones and Cartilages

Bones such as the mandible, maxilla, hard palate, hyoid bone, cervical vertebrae (C1-C7), and skull (specifically the styloid and mastoid processes of the temporal bone) are critical during swallowing in that they support and stabilize the involved muscles and aid in mastication. Similarly, cartilages such as the thyroid cartilage, cricoid cartilage, arytenoids, and epiglottis are important during swallowing. Cartilages, like bones, provide support for several of the muscles that are involved in mastication as well as lingual and pharyngeal bolus transport. They anchor the muscles that protect the airway as the liquid or food bolus traverses the pharynx. In particular, the epiglottis deflects downward, thereby directing the oncoming bolus away from the airway and into the esophagus.[8]

Teeth

A healthy adult has 32 permanent teeth,[9] all of which are critical to bolus preparation. The incisors are used for cutting and biting, and the molars are used for grinding solid food. Any disruption to an individual's dentition can affect his/her ability to consume a typical adult diet.

Spaces

As a point of reference when describing the swallow, the upper aerodigestive tract is divided into 4 main areas or spaces: the oral cavity, nasopharynx, oropharynx, and hypopharynx (**Fig. 2**). Within each of these main spaces, there are several smaller spaces

Table 1
Swallowing-related musculature

Category	Muscle Name	Innervation	Attachments	Function
Muscles of the face	Orbicularis oris	CN VII	Maxilla; mandible; mucous membrane of lips	Closes and protrudes lips
	Buccinator	CN VII	Maxilla and mandible (alveolar process); pterygomandibular raphe; orbicularis oris	Flattens and compresses cheek
Muscles of mastication	Temporalis	CN V	Temporal fossa of the parietal bone; mandible (coronoid process)	Elevates mandible
	Masseter	CN V	Zygomatic bone; zygomatic arch; lateral surface of ramus of mandible	Elevates mandible
	Medial pterygoid	CN V	Medial surface of lateral plate (pterygoid process); palatine bone (pyramidal process); maxilla (tuberosity and pyramidal process)	Elevates mandible
	Lateral pterygoid	CN V	Greater wing of sphenoid bone; lateral surface of lateral plate (pterygoid process); mandible (condolyoid process)	Moves mandible laterally (rotary chew); depresses and protrudes mandible
Intrinsic muscles of the tongue	Superior longitudinal	CN XII	Median septum of tongue; submucosal connective tissue of tongue; mucous membrane of tongue	Shortens tongue; raises tip and lateral margins of tongue
	Inferior longitudinal	CN XII	Root of tongue; hyoid bone; apex of tongue	Shortens tongue; pulls tongue tip down
	Transverse	CN XII	Median septum of tongue; submucosal connective tissue on lateral margins of tongue	Narrows and elongates tongue
	Verticalis	CN XII	Submucosal connective tissue on dorsal surface and ventral regions of tongue	Flattens and widens tongue
Extrinsic muscles of the tongue	Genioglossus	CN XII	Mandible (superior mental spine); hyoid bone; dorsum of tongue	Depresses center of tongue (groove); protrudes tongue
	Hyoglossus	CN XII	Hyoid bone; lateral aspect of tongue	Depresses and retrudes tongue
	Styloglossus	CN XII	Styloid process; styloid ligament; lateral surface of tongue	Elevates and retracts tongue
	Palatoglossus	CN X	Palatine aponeurosis; lateral margin of tongue	Depresses soft palate; moves palatoglossal fold toward midline; elevates back of tongue

(continued on next page)

Table 1
(continued)

Category	Muscle Name	Innervation	Attachments	Function
Muscles of the soft palate	Levator veli palatini	CN X	Temporal bone; palatine aponeurosis	Elevates soft palate
	Musculus uvulae	CN X	Posterior nasal spine; palatine aponeurosis; mucosa of uvula	Elevates and retracts uvula
	Tensor veli palatini	CN V	Medial pterygoid plate (sphenoid bone); palatine aponeurosis	Tenses soft palate; opens pharyngotympanic tube
Pharyngeal musculature	Superior pharyngeal constrictor	CN X	Pharyngeal raphe; medial pterygoid plate (pterygoid hamulus); pterygomandibular raphe; mandible	Constricts pharynx
	Middle pharyngeal constrictor	CN X	Pharyngeal raphe; hyoid bone; stylohyoid ligament	Constricts pharynx
	Inferior pharyngeal constrictor	CN X	Pharyngeal raphe; cricoid cartilage; thyroid cartilage; crosses cricothyroid muscle	Constricts pharynx
	Stylopharyngeus	CN IX	Styloid process (temporal bone); pharyngeal wall	Elevates pharynx
	Salpingopharyngeus	CN X	Pharyngotympanic tube; pharyngeal wall	Elevates pharynx
	Palatopharyngeus	CN X	Palatine aponeurosis; lateral pharyngeal wall	Elevates pharynx; moves posterior pharyngeal wall toward midline
Suprahyoid muscles	Mylohyoid	CN V	Medial body of mandible; hyoid bone	Elevates hyoid, floor of mouth
	Geniohyoid	CN XII; C1-2	Anterior body of mandible; hyoid bone	Fixed mandible, pulls hyoid forward; fixed hyoid, depresses and retracts mandible
	Digastric (anterior)	CN V	Anterior body of mandible; intermediate tendon; hyoid bone	Fixed mandible, elevates hyoid; fixed hyoid, depresses mandible
	Digastric (posterior)	CN VII	Temporal bone (mastoid process); intermediate tendon; hyoid bone	Elevates and retracts hyoid bone
	Stylohyoid	CN VII	Temporal bone (styloid process); hyoid bone	Elevates hyoid

Muscles of the larynx	Lateral cricoarytenoid	CN X	Arch of cricoid cartilage; vocal process of arytenoid cartilage	Adducts vocal folds and closes off/protects airway
	Transverse arytenoid	CN X	Arytenoid cartilage on one side; contralateral arytenoid cartilage	Adducts vocal folds and closes off/protects airway (especially at posterior commissure)
	Thyroarytenoid	CN X	Inner surface of thyroid cartilage (anterior); arytenoid cartilage (anterior surface)	Helps to close off airway by narrowing laryngeal inlet
Infrahyoid muscles	Sternothyroid	Ansa cervicalis (C1-C3)	Manubrium of sternum; thyroid cartilage	Depresses larynx (and hyoid)
	Sternohyoid	Ansa cervicalis (C1-C3)	Manubrium of sternum; hyoid bone	Depresses hyoid
	Thyrohyoid	CN XII; C1	Thyroid cartilage; hyoid bone	Depresses hyoid; elevates larynx
	Omohyoid (superior and inferior bellies)	Ansa cervicalis (C1-C3)	Scapula; hyoid bone	Depresses and retracts hyoid
Muscles of the upper esophagus	Inferior fibers of the inferior pharyngeal constrictor	CN X	Cricoid cartilage; pharyngeal raphe	—
	Cricopharyngeus	CN IX, X	Lateral aspects of cricoid cartilage	Contracted at rest to prevent reflux; relaxes during swallow to allow bolus to pass from pharynx into esophagus
	Upper fibers of the esophagus	CN X	Lower borders of cricoid cartilage	—

Data from Moore KL, Dalley AF, Agur AM. Clinically oriented anatomy. 5th edition. Lippincott Williams & Wilkins; 2006; and Drake RL, Vogl AW, Mitchell AW. Gray's anatomy for students. 2nd edition. Churchill Livingstone; 2010.

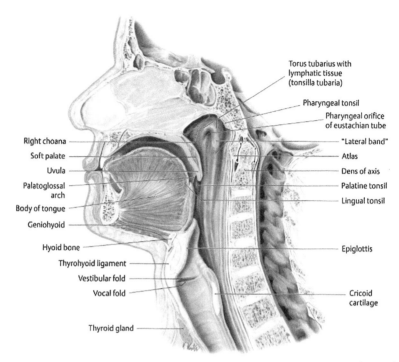

Fig. 1. Midsagittal view of head and neck. (*From* Schuenke M, Schulte E, Schumacher U. Thieme atlas of anatomy: neck and internal organs. New York (NY): Georg Thieme Verlag; 2010. p. 36; with permission.)

through which fluids and foods pass during a normal swallow, namely, the valleculae and pyriform sinuses. There are other spaces that are effectively sealed during the swallow and hence make no contact with the ingested bolus. These include the lateral and anterior sulci, laryngeal vestibule, and laryngeal ventricle. After the completion of the swallow, residue of the liquid or solid bolus in any of these spaces indicates dysphagia.

Salivary Glands

Three pairs of major salivary glands are housed within the oral cavity and produce 95% of the saliva: parotid, sublingual, and submandibular.[10] Additional saliva is produced by minor salivary glands located within the lining of the oral mucosa. Saliva is critical during mastication as it assists with bolus formation and transport, especially with dry and particulate solid foods. Although the composition of saliva is mostly water, it also contains proteins, enzymes, and electrolytes. These substances serve 2 main purposes: to promote oral and dental health and to start the digestive process.[11]

MUSCULAR CONTROL

As previously mentioned, there are more than 30 pairs of muscles that are active during swallowing. These muscles are listed in **Table 1** and are organized according to their primary function. All the muscles involved in swallowing are striated, with the exception of the medial and distal esophagus, which have segments that are partially and completely smooth muscle.[12,13] Somatic afferent and efferent feedback is provided

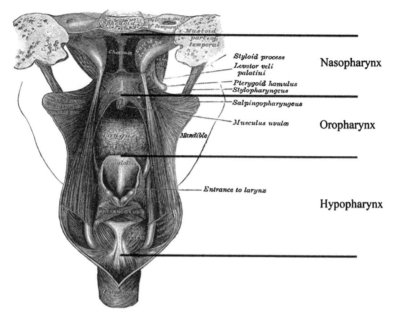

Styloid process
Levator veli palatini
Pterygoid hamulus
Stylopharyngeus
Salpingopharyngeus
Musculus uvulæ
Mandible
Entrance to larynx

Nasopharynx

Oropharynx

Hypopharynx

Fig. 2. Major cavities and spaces within the head and neck. (*From* Belafsky PC, Lintzenich CR. Development, anatomy, and physiology of the pharynx. In: Shaker R, Belafsky PC, Postma GN, et al, editors. Principles of deglutition: a multidisciplinary text for swallowing and its disorders. Springer; 2013. p. 167; with permission.)

primarily via cranial and peripheral nerves (for striated musculature) and an autonomic enteric system (for smooth muscle within the medial and distal esophagus).

Despite the fact that swallowing is a continuous and well-coordinated event, swallow physiology is traditionally described in 4 discrete yet sequential phases: (1) the oral preparatory phase, (2) the oral transport phase, (3) the pharyngeal phase, and (4) the esophageal phase.[2,14,15] The first 2 phases are modulated primarily by voluntary control, whereas the latter 2 phases are under involuntary control. Within each phase, the timing and extent of movements can vary slightly, depending on the type and amount of input (ie, liquid vs solid, large vs small bolus), as well as the age and gender of the individual.[16] For example, the elderly often have a longer oral preparatory phase and take longer to trigger the pharyngeal phase[17] than their younger counterparts. In the following section, unique features of the muscular control for each phase are reviewed.

Oral Preparatory Phase

The oral preparatory phase is the first phase of swallowing, during which food is broken down (via mastication) and a cohesive bolus is formed.[14,15,18–20] Many muscles are active during this phase and help to contain liquid and/or food within the oral cavity. In particular, the muscles of the face (orbicularis oris and buccinators) seal the lips and close off the lateral and anterior sulci.[21] Likewise, the soft palate is depressed toward the base of the tongue (via contraction of the palatoglossus muscle), sealing off the oral cavity posteriorly. This posterior seal prevents premature spillage of liquid or food into the oropharynx, and is therefore critical for airway protection.[22] When consuming solid food, the muscles of mastication (masseter, temporalis, and medial and lateral pterygoid muscles) are also engaged and serve to stabilize and actively move the jaw during mastication (**Fig. 3**).[18,23] Lateral and vertical movements of the tongue help to position the food between the teeth, thereby facilitating mastication. During mastication, food particles are reduced and softened with saliva until a cohesive ball, or bolus, is formed. Once mastication is complete, the bolus is contained between the dorsal surface of the tongue and the hard palate.[18] The intrinsic muscles of the tongue and genioglossus muscle transform its shape into one with a central trough or groove so as to better contain the newly formed liquid or food bolus.[24]

Oral Transport Phase

On successful formation of a cohesive bolus, the oral transport phase commences. During this phase, the bolus is propelled posteriorly through the oral cavity and into the oropharynx.[14] The muscles of the face (orbicularis oris and buccinators) remain contracted to contain the bolus within the oral cavity. The soft palate is elevated (via contraction of the levator veli palatini and musculus uvulae) and seals off the nasal cavity from the oropharynx (**Fig. 4**). These oral and nasopharyngeal seals are important in that they create a closed pressure loop within the oral cavity, pharynx, and esophagus. During the oral transport and pharyngeal phases of swallowing, sequential points of high pressure, generated by lingual and pharyngeal movements within this closed loop system, travel in a rostral-caudal direction, thereby facilitating bolus transport.

   At the outset of the oral transport phase, the bolus is contained between the lingual dorsum and hard palate by contraction of the superior longitudinal muscle (**Fig. 5**), which raises the anterior tip and lateral edges of the tongue toward the alveolar ridge. With the lateral edges and anterior tip of the tongue in contact with the alveolar ridge, the tongue is prepared to initiate posterior transport of the bolus. It does so by pressing the tongue blade upward against the hard palate and moving in an anterior-to-posterior wavelike motion. This wavelike motion occurs as a result of activity within the intrinsic and extrinsic muscles of the tongue (ie, genioglossus, hyoglossus, styloglossus, palatoglossus, superior longitudinal) and is both centripetal and centrifugal in nature,[25] meaning that it first directs the bolus toward the midline of the central groove and then posteriorly toward the oropharynx.

   Entry of the bolus into the oropharynx is further facilitated by depression of the posterior tongue (via contraction of the hyoglossus muscle) and elevation of the soft palate, or velum (via contraction of levator veli palatini and musculus uvulae). The muscles

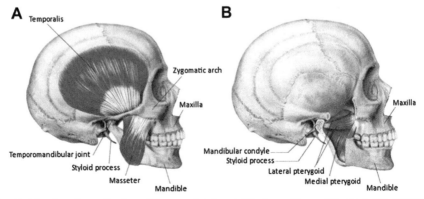

Fig. 3. Muscles of mastication, (*A*) superficial and (*B*) deep. (*From* Albertine KH. Barron's anatomy flash cards. 2nd edition. Hauppauge (NY): Barron's Educational Series; 2008; with permission.)

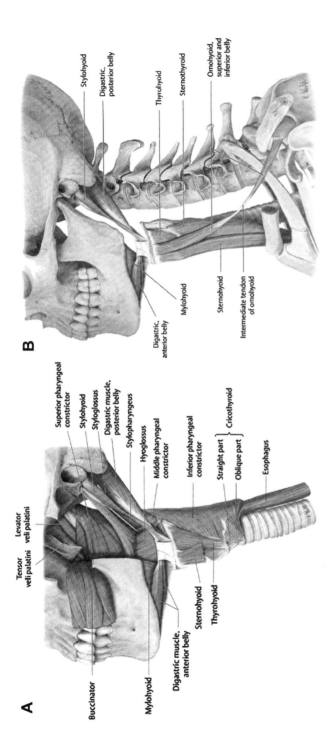

Fig. 4. Lateral view of the head and neck showing (*A*) facial, soft palate, pharyngeal, suprahyoid, extrinsic tongue, and esophageal muscles and (*B*) suprahyoid and infrahyoid muscles. (*From* Schuenke M, Schulte E, Schumacher U. Thieme atlas of anatomy: neck and internal organs. New York (NY): Georg Thieme Verlag; 2010. p. 7, 32; with permission.)

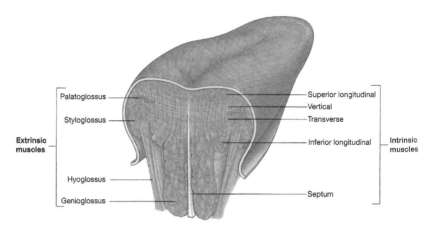

Fig. 5. Intrinsic and extrinsic muscles of the tongue. (*From* Drake RL, Vogl AW, Mitchell AW. Gray's anatomy for students. 2nd edition. Philadelphia (PA): Churchill Livingstone; 2010. p. 1038; with permission.)

of mastication (temporalis, masseter, and medial and lateral pterygoids), as well as the submental or suprahyoid muscles (mylohyoid, geniohyoid, anterior digastric, posterior digastric, and stylohyoid), are active during the oral transport phase and serve to stabilize the jaw and tongue.[15,19,26]

PHARYNGEAL PHASE

The third phase of swallowing is the pharyngeal phase. Once triggered, this phase lasts for approximately 1 second.[15,27] Despite its brief duration, the pharyngeal phase of swallowing is the most complex of all the phases and requires the precise and rapid coordination of nearly all the muscles listed in **Table 1**.

As the oral transport phase ends, the bolus passes into the oropharynx and crosses over the area of the anterior faucial pillars. This contact initiates the involuntary "trigger" of the pharyngeal phase. Unlike a true reflex, the pharyngeal swallow response can be modulated in part by how the bolus is transported in the preceding phase, also known as the leading complex[2] (**Fig. 6**). Food properties such as texture, taste, and volume can also alter the timing of the trigger. For example, more viscous liquids[28] may delay the pharyngeal trigger, whereas sour foods[29] may initiate an earlier trigger. In addition, larger boluses during sequential liquid drinking may pass the faucial pillars and reach the valleculae before the trigger is initiated.[30]

Once triggered, the pharyngeal phase of the swallow proceeds as follows. First, respiration ceases in favor of airway protection; this is achieved by adduction of the true vocal folds, via contraction of the laryngeal musculature (lateral cricoarytenoid, transverse arytenoid, and thyroarytenoid).[31] Next, the pharyngeal muscles (palatopharyngeus, stylopharyngeus, and salpingopharyngeus) contract, raising the pharynx superiorly (**Fig. 7**). At the same time, the tongue base is retracted toward the posterior pharyngeal wall (via contraction of hyoglossus and styloglossus), and the pharyngeal constrictors (superior, middle, and inferior) are activated in a rostral-caudal direction.[20,32] As a result, pharyngeal constrictor contraction occurs in a wavelike motion that descends inferiorly from the level of the nasopharynx to the level of the upper esophageal sphincter (UES) at a rate of between 9 and 25 cm/s.[33] This wave is termed pharyngeal peristalsis, or the pharyngeal stripping wave, because it strips along the

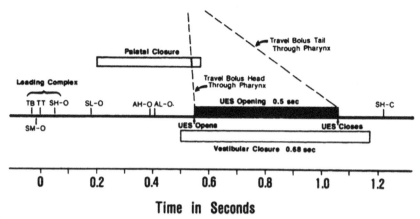

Fig. 6. Diagram illustrating the timing of events for the oral transport and pharyngeal phases of swallowing. AH-O, onset of anterior hyoid movement; AL-O, onset of anterior laryngeal movement; SH-C, completion of superior hyoid movement; SH-O, onset of superior hyoid movement; SL-O, onset of superior laryngeal movement; SM-O, onset of submental electric activity; TB, tongue base movement; TT, onset of propulsive tongue tip. (*From* Dodds WJ, Stewart ET, Logemann JA. Physiology and radiology of the normal oral and pharyngeal phases of swallowing. AJR Am J Roentgenol 1990;154(5):962; with permission.)

tail of the bolus, squeezing the bolus through the pharynx and into the upper esophagus. The pharyngeal stripping wave generates an average pressure of 22 mmHg[33] and an average force of 1.2 mmHg*s.[32]

As the pharynx elevates, the suprahyoid muscles (mylohyoid, stylohyoid, geniohyoid, and anterior and posterior bellies of digastric) contract, directing the hyoid bone superiorly and anteriorly.[34] Simultaneously, the thyrohyoid muscle contracts, moving the larynx superiorly toward the hyoid bone.[2] Anterior and superior movements of the larynx and the hyoid bone are important for several reasons. First, these movements provide airway protection by directing the larynx under the tongue base and by inverting the epiglottis, thereby directing the bolus away from the laryngeal inlet. Second, laryngeal elevation, coupled with simultaneous elevation of the hypopharynx, creates a negative pressure source below the level of the bolus,[32] which helps to "suck" the bolus inferiorly toward the esophagus. Third, as the larynx and pharynx elevate, they create a biomechanical force that pulls the cricoid cartilage up and away from the posterior pharyngeal wall, thereby pulling open the cricopharyngeal muscle and the UES. Assuming that the labial and nasopharyngeal seals have remained intact, the opening of the UES creates an additional source of negative pressure, or "suction force," in the upper esophagus.[32] This suction force, combined with the driving force of the tongue and pharyngeal stripping wave, greatly enhances the efficiency of pharyngeal bolus transit.

As with the oral preparatory and oral transport phases of swallowing, the muscles of mastication remain active throughout the pharyngeal phase and ensure that the tongue and jaw remain stabilized.[15]

ESOPHAGEAL PHASE

Once the bolus passes through the UES, the esophageal phase of swallowing begins. In addition to the biomechanical forces involved in opening the UES, relaxation of the cricopharyngeal muscle further facilitates UES opening.[35] Relaxation lasts for

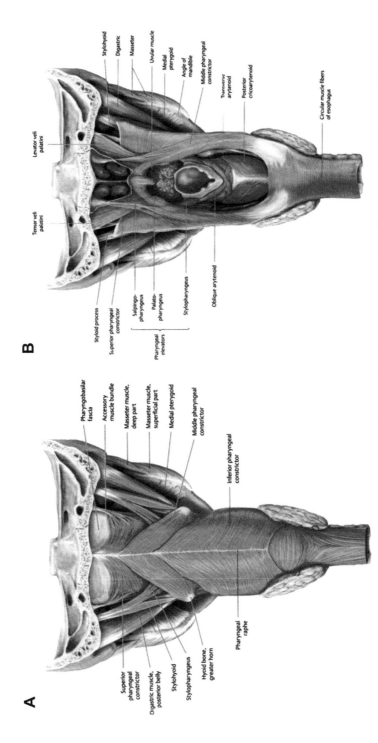

Fig. 7. Posterior view of the head and neck, illustrating (A) superficial muscles of the pharynx, suprahyoid region, and esophagus and (B) deep muscles of the soft palate, pharynx, suprahyoid region, and esophagus. (*From* Schuenke M, Schulte E, Schumacher U. Thieme atlas of anatomy: neck and internal organs. New York (NY): Georg Thieme Verlag; 2010. p. 33; with permission.)

approximately 0.5 to 1.2 seconds,[36] just enough time for food to pass through the UES and into the esophagus.

Once the bolus has successfully entered the esophagus, the cricopharyngeal muscle returns to its contracted state, thereby sealing off the esophagus and preventing any retrograde bolus entry into the hypopharynx. At that point, esophageal peristalsis is activated, and the bolus is propelled toward the lower esophageal sphincter (LES) and stomach.[37] This esophageal peristaltic wave travels inferiorly at a rate of approximately 3 to 4 cm/s[38] and serves to squeeze the bolus through the esophagus. Approximately 0.5 to 1.4 seconds after hypopharyngeal pressure peaks,[39] the LES is triggered to relax, at which point the peristaltic waves squeeze the bolus into the stomach. Several secondary peristaltic waves also occur up to an hour after the swallow and help to clear any remaining esophageal residue.[40] Transit times during this phase vary with age, bolus size, and bolus texture. However, in healthy adults, esophageal transit times should be between 8 and 13 seconds.[41]

IMPORTANCE OF AIRWAY PROTECTION

Airway protection is a vital part of a normal, healthy swallow. When food is misdirected toward the airway (rather than toward the esophagus), aspiration occurs. Aspiration of food or liquid places an individual at risk for developing aspiration pneumonia,[4] which can be a life-threatening condition.

The first step to ensuring adequate airway protection is proper coordination and timing of the swallow. Because respiration and swallowing use similar anatomic pathways, respiration and deglutition must, of necessity, be well coordinated to prevent aspiration. To this end, the pharyngeal phase of swallowing typically occurs as an individual is starting to exhale.[42,43] Once swallowing begins, respiration ceases for a time, resulting in a brief period of apnea. Once the bolus has successfully cleared the hypopharynx and entered the esophagus, the halted exhalation resumes.[42,43]

There are also several physical movements that occur, which help to protect the airway, including true and false vocal fold closure and epiglottic deflection. First, vocal fold closure is achieved when the true and/or false vocal folds are adducted just before the initiation of the pharyngeal phase of swallowing. Closure of the vocal folds serves 2 main purposes: it ceases respiration, and it seals off the airway, preventing any misdirected food or liquid from entering the lungs.[44,45] Epiglottic deflection is also vital to airway protection. During epiglottic deflection, the inferior surface of the epiglottis makes contact with the arytenoid cartilages and directs the food and liquid past the airway and into the esophagus. In effect, the epiglottis and true and false vocal folds act as shields for the airway, protecting it against penetration and aspiration of food or liquid.

A third aspect of airway protection involves sensory innervation of the vocal folds. Sensation is provided primarily by the internal branch of the superior laryngeal nerve (ISLN) of CN X.[46] The ISLN serves 2 main purposes: to ensure that the airway is completely closed during swallowing[44,47] and to trigger the reflexes that help eject or clear any penetrated or aspirated bolus material from the airway.

One of these clearing reflexes, mediated by the ISLN, is the laryngeal adductor response (LAR). When the LAR is triggered (via tactile stimulation of the laryngeal mucosa), the vocal folds involuntarily respond via rapid adduction.[48,49] This healthy response can be tested using fiberoptic endoscopic evaluation of swallowing with sensory testing.[50] During this examination, puffs of air are administered to the aryepiglottic folds at gradually increasing thresholds until the LAR is triggered. There is evidence that normal thresholds approximate less than 4.0 mmHg.[51] This test yields important clinical insights because, as the threshold of the LAR increases above normal or expected levels, the risk of silent aspiration during meal intake also increases.[51–53]

A second reflex that is mediated by the ISLN is the laryngeal cough reflex (LCR). This reflex is triggered by tactile or chemical stimulation (via capsaicin[54] or citric acid[55]) of the larynx and/or trachea. A typical LCR results in an involuntary cough response that lasts for several seconds and is accompanied by significant alterations in an individual's breathing pattern (ie, slower breathing or rapid and shallow breathing).[56,57] If the LCR is below expected levels (ie, <5 coughs within 60 seconds of citric acid inhalation[55]) or is completely absent,[58] the individual is considered to be at risk for silent aspiration during oral intake and for developing aspiration pneumonia.

Although the gag reflex has historically been associated with airway protection, research has consistently shown that a reduced or absent gag response is not in fact correlated with an increased risk for aspiration.[59] Nevertheless, any deficit that affects this motor response may provide useful insights into general sensory and/or motor cranial nerve function.[51,52]

NEUROPHYSIOLOGICAL CONTROL

Initially, the process of swallowing was thought to be purely reflexive in nature; however, recent research has shown that it is actually a dynamic, multilayered process involving a complex neuronal network with both volitional and reflexive components (**Fig. 8**).[12,60]

This network includes portions of the supratentorium (cortical and subcortical), infratentorium (brain stem), and peripheral nervous system (motor and sensory). The next section reviews the contribution of the central nervous system to swallowing

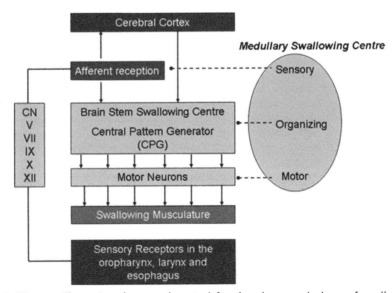

Fig. 8. Diagram illustrating the neural control for the pharyngeal phase of swallowing. (*From* Diamant NE. Firing up the swallowing mechanism. Nat Med 1996;2(11):1191; with permission.)

physiology and highlights how this central system serves to mediate the process of swallowing throughout each phase.

Supratentorium

As stated earlier, swallowing physiology is influenced and controlled by several cortical and subcortical structures. Cortical regions (such as the primary and secondary sensorimotor cortices) are especially active during the oral preparatory and oral transport phases of swallowing.[61–63] These 2 phases consist mainly of voluntary feeding behaviors (ie, bolus preparation and mastication), as well as a series of movements that constitute the leading complex (eg, pressing of the tongue tip against the hard palate and posterior movement on the tongue base during the oral transport phase).[2]

In addition, several cortical and subcortical sites are involved in the pharyngeal phase of swallowing, including the primary and secondary sensorimotor cortices, insula, anterior and posterior cingulate cortices, basal ganglia, amygdala, hypothalamus, and substantia nigra.[63–65] Each of these neuronal influences is either excitatory or inhibitory in nature. For example, the amygdala and lateral hypothalamus are thought to facilitate swallowing by means of dopaminergic mechanisms, whereas structures such as the periaqueductal gray and ventrolateral pontine reticular formation are thought to inhibit swallowing.[66] Swallowing inhibition is important, particularly during the oral preparatory and oral transport phases of swallowing, in that it prevents premature trigger of the pharyngeal swallow during bolus preparation.

Studies in healthy individuals have shown that cortical representation of swallowing is bilateral and asymmetrical, particularly in the motor and premotor cortices.[67] This asymmetric bilaterality is not related to handedness; therefore, it has been attributed to the presence of a dominant swallowing hemisphere.[67] The concept of bilaterality, as it relates to the cortical representation of swallowing, has important therapeutic implications and is influencing the development of new dysphagia interventions, especially for patients with hemispheric stroke. For example, Hamdy and colleagues[68] are currently investigating whether dysphagia due to unilateral stroke can be rehabilitated via cortical stimulation to the unaffected cerebral hemisphere.

Infratentorium

The second level of neurophysiological control for swallowing involves the infratentorium (mainly the medulla oblongata within the brain stem). The infratentorium is active during swallowing, especially during the involuntary pharyngeal and esophageal phases. A central pattern generator (CPG), housed within the medulla oblongata, helps to regulate and coordinate these 2 phases. CPGs are neuronal pools that contain sensory, motor, and interneurons that work together to control sequential, rhythmic, and somatic events within the body. Examples of events that are regulated by CPGs include locomotion, respiration, and deglutition.[69]

The swallowing CPG can be viewed as a linearlike chain of neurons that fire sequentially and according to the rostral-caudal nature of swallowing physiology. In addition, the CPG involves bilateral representation within the medulla oblongata. Previous studies, involving midline splitting of the medulla, have shown that unilateral stimulation of the superior laryngeal nerve (SLN) triggers a swallow on the ipsilateral oropharyngeal side only. This finding suggests that both CPG halves are tightly synchronized and that the CPG also organizes and coordinates contraction from a bilateral perspective.[69,70]

Motor neurons that are involved in the swallowing CPG are localized within the brain stem. They include the trigeminal (V), facial (VII), and hypoglossal (XII) motor nuclei; the nucleus ambiguus (NA) (IX, X) and the dorsal motor nucleus of the vagus nerve (X); and 2 cervical spinal neurons (C1 and C3).[69–72] Not all of these motor neurons participate to an equal extent during the swallow. For example, motor nuclei V and VII (which innervate some of the suprahyoid muscles, muscles of mastication, facial muscles, and muscles of the soft palate) deal mainly with orofacial activity, such as mastication, licking, and sucking.[69,70,72,73] Although these motor nuclei (V and VII) are important, the main motor nuclei involved in swallowing are the hypoglossal motor nucleus (XII) and the NA. These nuclei are critical for swallowing in that they provide innervation for the intrinsic and extrinsic muscles of the tongue (ie, genioglossus, geniohyoid, styloglossus, and hyoglossus), as well as for the pharynx, larynx, and upper esophagus (specifically its striated musculature).[12,70,71] Motor output for the lower esophagus (smooth muscle) is provided by the dorsal motor nucleus.[12]

Sensory neurons that regulate the pharyngeal and esophageal phases of swallowing are also housed within the brain stem. They include the nucleus of the solitary tract and the neighboring reticular formation. General sensory information from the oral, pharyngeal, and esophageal mucosa is sent to these sensory neurons via CN X (specifically via the SLN).[3,44,46,64,74–76] For the tongue, general sensory information is provided by 2 cranial nerves: the lingual nerve (CN V) for the anterior two-thirds and the glossopharyngeal nerve (CN IX) for the posterior one-third.[77] Special sensory information (taste) has also been shown to alter swallowing physiology in both oral and pharyngeal phases.[24,78] Taste is provided by CN VII for the anterior two-thirds of the tongue and by CN IX for the posterior one-third.[77]

As mentioned previously, both motor and sensory neurons are represented bilaterally within the medulla oblongata and form what is known as the swallowing center (ie, swallowing CPG). Dorsal sensory and ventral motor signals[69] are integrated within this swallowing center via 2 groups of interneurons: the dorsal swallowing group (DSG), and the ventral swallowing group (VSG). First, sensory signals from the oropharyngeal area (via CN IX and X) are sent to the nucleus of the solitary tract and the neighboring reticular formation. These sensory signals trigger interneurons housed within the DSG. The DSG responds by sending motor signals to the neighboring VSG. The VSG takes these motor signals from the DSG and ensures that they are properly sequenced and coordinated. The VSG then passes these signals on to the hypoglossal motor nucleus (XII) and the nucleus ambiguous (X), which then trigger the muscles involved in swallowing. The result is a rapid and well-coordinated sequence of muscle movements. Swallowing neurons are located in the same medullary sites as neurons that control respiration and cardiovascular processes.[79] This location enables swallowing to be efficiently coordinated with these other autonomic functions.

The trigger of the pharyngeal swallow described earlier is semireflexive in that the sequence of muscle activity is fixed and once triggered cannot be reversed[69]; for this reason, the oropharyngeal motor response that occurs during the pharyngeal phase of swallowing has been classically described as a dedicated fixed circuit.[69] This traditional viewpoint, however, is now being challenged. As evidence mounts in support of functional plasticity within the cortical hemispheres, emerging evidence has also suggested that there is neuronal redundancy and hence the potential for such neuronal flexibility, within the swallowing CPG.[80] Additional research has shown that, even during normal swallowing, the duration and intensity of muscular contractions can be modulated by incoming sensory information[81] pertaining to bolus temperature, size, texture, and flavor.[46]

Many aspects of the neuropharyngeal control of swallowing are yet unknown. Research in this area is ongoing and will likely lead to increased understanding and improved intervention for individuals with dysphagia.

SUMMARY

Swallowing is a complex process that involves well-coordinated movements within the oral cavity, pharynx, larynx, and esophagus. Any impairment within this system (structural or neural) can lead to problems with swallowing, or dysphagia. Understanding normal anatomy and physiology is critical to treating dysphagia and improving intervention techniques.

REFERENCES

1. Lear C, Flanagan J, Moorrees C. The frequency of deglutition in man. Arch Oral Biol 1965;10(1):83–99.
2. Dodds WJ, Stewart ET, Logemann JA. Physiology and radiology of the normal oral and pharyngeal phases of swallowing. AJR Am J Roentgenol 1990; 154(5):953–63.
3. Miller A. Neurophysiological basis of swallowing. Dysphagia 1986;1(2):91–100.
4. Martino R, Foley N, Bhogal S, et al. Dysphagia after stroke: incidence, diagnosis, and pulmonary complications. Stroke 2005;36(12):2756–63.
5. Foley NC, Martin RE, Salter KL, et al. A review of the relationship between dysphagia and malnutrition following stroke. J Rehabil Med 2009;41(9): 707–13.
6. Leibovitz A, Baumoehl Y, Lubart E, et al. Dehydration among long-term care elderly patients with oropharyngeal dysphagia. Gerontology 2007;53(4): 179–83.
7. Funk GF, Karnell LH, Christensen AJ. Long-term health-related quality of life in survivors of head and neck cancer. Arch Otolaryngol Head Neck Surg 2012; 138(2):123.
8. Ekberg O, Sigurjónsson SV. Movement of the epiglottis during deglutition. Gastrointest Radiol 1982;7(1):101–7.
9. Moore KL, Dalley AF, editors. Clinically oriented anatomy. 5th edition. Philadelphia: Lippincott Williams & Wilkin; 2006.
10. Edgar W. Saliva: its secretion, composition and functions. Br Dent J 1992; 172(8):305–12.
11. Humphrey SP, Williamson RT. A review of saliva: normal composition, flow, and function. J Prosthet Dent 2001;85(2):162–9.
12. Diamant N. Physiology of esophageal motor function. Gastroenterol Clin North Am 1989;18(2):179.
13. Meyer GW, Austin RM, Brady CE, et al. Muscle anatomy of the human esophagus. J Clin Gastroenterol 1986;8(2):131–4.
14. Logemann JA. Evaluation and treatment of swallowing disorders. San Diego (CA): College-Hill Press; 1983.
15. Palmer JB, Rudin NJ, Lara G, et al. Coordination of mastication and swallowing. Dysphagia 1992;7(4):187–200.
16. Ryan C. Gustation, olfaction, and deglutition. In: Shaker R, Belafsky PC, Postma GN, et al, editors. Principles of deglutition: a multidisciplinary text for swallowing and its disorders. New York: Springer; 2013. p. 19–24.
17. Robbins J, Hamilton JW, Lof GL, et al. Oropharyngeal swallowing in normal adults of different ages. Gastroenterology 1992;103(3):823–9.
18. Abd-El-Malek S. The part played by the tongue in mastication and deglutition. J Anat 1955;89(Pt 2):250–4.
19. Gay T, Rendell JK, Spiro J. Oral and laryngeal muscle coordination during swallowing. Laryngoscope 1994;104(3):341–9.

20. McKeown MJ, Torpey DC, Gehm WC. Non-invasive monitoring of functionally distinct muscle activations during swallowing. Clin Neurophysiol 2002;113(3): 354–66.
21. Dutra EH, Caria P, Rafferty KL, et al. The buccinator during mastication: a functional and anatomical evaluation in minipigs. Arch Oral Biol 2010;55(9):627–38.
22. Dodds W. The physiology of swallowing. Dysphagia 1989;3(4):171–8.
23. Mittal S, Koshal N, Kumar M, et al. Masticatory performance and chewing cycle kinematics: an overview. Int J Physiol 2013;1(1):62–4.
24. Lund J. Mastication and its control by the brain stem. Crit Rev Oral Biol Med 1991;2(1):33–64.
25. Ergun GA, Kahrilas PJ, Lin S, et al. Pattern and modulation of tongue surface movement during deglutition. Paper presented at the Dysphagia Research Society (DRS) Annual Meeting. Milwaukee, WI, November 6–8, 1992.
26. Cook I, Dodds W, Dantas R, et al. Timing of videofluoroscopic, manometric events, and bolus transit during the oral and pharyngeal phases of swallowing. Dysphagia 1989;4(1):8–15.
27. Sonies BC, Parent LJ, Morrish K, et al. Durational aspects of the oral-pharyngeal phase of swallow in normal adults. Dysphagia 1988;3(1):1–10.
28. Robbins J, Gensler G, Hind J, et al. Can thickened liquids or chin-down posture prevent aspiration? Ann Intern Med 2008;148(7):I39.
29. Logemann JA, Pauloski BR, Colangelo L, et al. Effects of a sour bolus on oropharyngeal swallowing measures in patients with neurogenic dysphagia. J Speech Hear Res 1995;38(3):556–63.
30. Martin-Harris B, Brodsky MB, Michel Y, et al. Delayed initiation of the pharyngeal swallow: normal variability in adult swallows. J Speech Lang Hear Res 2007; 50(3):585–94.
31. Shaker R, Dodds WJ, Dantas RO, et al. Coordination of deglutitive glottic closure with oropharyngeal swallowing. Gastroenterology 1990;98(6):1478–84.
32. McConnel FM. Analysis of pressure generation and bolus transit during pharyngeal swallowing. Laryngoscope 1988;98(1):71–8.
33. Dodds WJ, Hogan WJ, Lydon SB, et al. Quantitation of pharyngeal motor function in normal human subjects. J Appl Physiol 1975;39(4):692–6.
34. Pearson WG Jr, Langmore SE, Yu LB, et al. Structural analysis of muscles elevating the hyolaryngeal complex. Dysphagia 2012;27:1–7.
35. Ertekin C, Aydogdu I. Electromyography of human cricopharyngeal muscle of the upper esophageal sphincter. Muscle Nerve 2002;26(6):729–39.
36. Ingelfinger FJ. Esophageal motility. Physiol Rev 1958;38(4):533–84.
37. Miller A. Swallowing: neurophysiologic control of the esophageal phase. Dysphagia 1987;2(2):72–82.
38. Humphries TJ, Castell DO. Pressure profile of esophageal peristalsis in normal humans as measured by direct intraesophageal transducers. Am J Dig Dis 1977;22(7):641–5.
39. Holloway RH, Penagini R, Ireland AC. Criteria for objective definition of transient lower esophageal sphincter relaxation. Am J Physiol Gastrointest Liver Physiol 1995;268(1):G128–33.
40. Goyal RK, Cobb BW. Chapter 11: Motility of the pharynx, esophagus, and esophageal sphincters. In: Johnson LR, editor. Physiology of the gastrointestinal tract. New York: Raven Press; 1981. p. 359–91.
41. De Vincentis N, Lenti R, Pona C, et al. Scintigraphic evaluation of the esophageal transit time for the noninvasive assessment of esophageal motor disorders. J Nucl Med Allied Sci 1984;28:137–42.

42. Martin BJ, Logemann JA, Shaker R, et al. Coordination between respiration and swallowing: respiratory phase relationships and temporal integration. J Appl Physiol 1994;76(2):714–23.

43. Klahn MS, Perlman AL. Temporal and durational patterns associating respiration and swallowing. Dysphagia 1999;14(3):131–8.

44. Jafari S, Prince RA, Kim DY, et al. Sensory regulation of swallowing and airway protection: a role for the internal superior laryngeal nerve in humans. J Physiol 2003;550(1):287–304.

45. Ardran GM, Kemp FH. The protection of the laryngeal airway during swallowing. Br J Radiol 1952;25(296):406–16.

46. Steele CM, Miller AJ. Sensory input pathways and mechanisms in swallowing: a review. Dysphagia 2010;25(4):323–33.

47. Sulica L, Hembree A, Blitzer A. Swallowing and sensation: evaluation of deglutition in the anesthetized larynx. Ann Otol Rhinol Laryngol 2002;111(4):291–4.

48. Ambalavanar R, Tanaka Y, Selbie WS, et al. Neuronal activation in the medulla oblongata during selective elicitation of the laryngeal adductor response. J Neurophysiol 2004;92(5):2920–32.

49. Ludlow C, Van Pelt F, Koda J. Characteristics of late responses to superior laryngeal nerve stimulation in humans. Ann Otol Rhinol Laryngol 1992;101(2 Pt 1): 127.

50. Aviv JE, Martin JH, Kim T, et al. Laryngopharyngeal sensory discrimination testing and the laryngeal adductor reflex. Ann Otol Rhinol Laryngol 1999; 108(8):725–30.

51. Aviv JE, Spitzer J, Cohen M, et al. Laryngeal adductor reflex and pharyngeal squeeze as predictors of laryngeal penetration and aspiration. Laryngoscope 2002;112(2):338–41.

52. Setzen M, Cohen MA, Mattucci KF, et al. Laryngopharyngeal sensory deficits as a predictor of aspiration. Otolaryngol Head Neck Surg 2001;124(6):622–4.

53. Setzen M, Cohen MA, Perlman PW, et al. The association between laryngopharyngeal sensory deficits, pharyngeal motor function, and the prevalence of aspiration with thin liquids. Otolaryngol Head Neck Surg 2003;128(1):99–102.

54. Niimi A, Matsumoto H, Ueda T, et al. Impaired cough reflex in patients with recurrent pneumonia. Thorax 2003;58(2):152–3.

55. Sato M, Tohara H, Iida T, et al. Simplified cough test for screening silent aspiration. Arch Phys Med Rehabil 2012;93(11):1982–6.

56. Nishino T, Tagaito Y, Isono S. Cough and other reflexes on irritation of airway mucosa in man. Pulm Pharmacol 1996;9:285–92.

57. Yoshida Y, Tanaka Y, Hirano M, et al. Sensory innervation of the pharynx and larynx. Am J Med 2000;108(4 Suppl 1):51–61.

58. Sekizawa K, Ujiie Y, Itabashi S, et al. Lack of cough reflex in aspiration pneumonia. Lancet 1990;335(8699):1228–9.

59. Bleach NR. The gag reflex and aspiration: a retrospective analysis of 120 patients assessed by videofluoroscopy. Clin Otolaryngol 1993;18(4):303–7.

60. Diamant NE. Firing up the swallowing mechanism. Nat Med 1996;2(11):1190–1.

61. Hamdy S, Mikulis DJ, Crawley A, et al. Cortical activation during human volitional swallowing: an event-related fMRI study. Am J Physiol Gastrointest Liver Physiol 1999;277(1):G219–25.

62. Martin RE, Goodyear BG, Gati JS, et al. Cerebral cortical representation of automatic and volitional swallowing in humans. J Neurophysiol 2001;85(2):938–50.

63. Humbert I, Robbins J. Normal swallowing and functional magnetic resonance imaging: a systematic review. Dysphagia 2007;22(3):266–75.

64. Dziewas R, Sörös P, Ishii R, et al. Cortical processing of esophageal sensation is related to the representation of swallowing. Neuroreport 2005;16(5): 439–43.

65. Sörös P, Inamoto Y, Martin RE. Functional brain imaging of swallowing: an activation likelihood estimation meta-analysis. Hum Brain Mapp 2009;30(8): 2426–39.

66. Kessler J, Jean A. Identification of the medullary swallowing regions in the rat. Exp Brain Res 1985;57(2):256–63.

67. Hamdy S, Aziz Q, Thompson D, et al. Physiology and pathophysiology of the swallowing area of human motor cortex. Neural Plast 2001;8(1–2):91–7.

68. Hamdy S. Chapter 20: The organisation and re-organisation of human swallowing motor cortex. In: Paulus W, Tergau F, Nitsche MA, et al, editors. Supplements to clinical neurophysiology. Amsterdam: Elsevier; 2003. p. 204–10.

69. Jean A. Brain stem control of swallowing: localization and organization of the central pattern generator for swallowing. In: Taylor A, editor. Neurophysiology of the jaws and teeth. London: Macmillan; 1990. p. 294–321.

70. Doty R. Neural organization of deglutition. In: Charles FC, Werner H, editors. Handbook of physiology: alimentary canal. Washington, DC: American Physiological Society; 1968. p. 1861–902.

71. Miller AJ. Deglutition. Physiol Rev 1982;62(1):129–84.

72. Dubner R, Sessle BJ, Storey A. The neural basis of oral and facial function. New York: Plenum Press; 1978.

73. Cunningham E Jr, Donner M, Jones B, et al. Anatomical and physiological overview. In: Jones B, Donner MW, editors. Normal and abnormal swallowing. New York: Springer; 1991. p. 7–32.

74. Miller A. The neuroscientific principles of swallowing and dysphagia. San Diego (CA): Singular Pub Group; 1999.

75. Lang IM. Brain stem control of the phases of swallowing. Dysphagia 2009;24(3): 333–48.

76. Miller AJ, Bowman JP. Precentral cortical modulation of mastication and swallowing. J Dent Res 1977;56(10):1154.

77. Catalanotto FA, Bartoshuk LM, Östrom KM, et al. Effects of anesthesia of the facial nerve on taste. Chem Senses 1993;18(5):461–70.

78. Leow L, Huckabee ML, Sharma S, et al. The influence of taste on swallowing apnea, oral preparation time, and duration and amplitude of submental muscle contraction. Chem Senses 2007;32(2):119–28.

79. Bianchi AL, Denavit-Saubié M, Champagnat J. Central control of breathing in mammals: neuronal circuitry, membrane properties, and neurotransmitters. Physiol Rev 1995;75(1):1–45.

80. Jean A, Dallaporta M. Brain stem control of deglutition: swallowing pattern generator. In: Shaker R, Belafsky PC, Postma GN, et al, editors. Principles of deglutition: a multidisciplinary text for swallowing and its disorders. New York: Springer; 2013. p. 89–113.

81. Teismann I, Steinstraeter O, Stoeckigt K, et al. Functional oropharyngeal sensory disruption interferes with the cortical control of swallowing. BMC Neurosci 2007; 8(1):62.

Central Neural Circuits for Coordination of Swallowing, Breathing, and Coughing
Predictions from Computational Modeling and Simulation

Donald C. Bolser, PhD[a],*, Christian Gestreau, PhD[b],
Kendall F. Morris, PhD[c], Paul W. Davenport, PhD[a],
Teresa E. Pitts, PhD[a]

KEYWORDS

- Cough • Swallow • Breathing • Airway • Central pattern generator • Brainstem

KEY POINTS

- Airway protection is the prevention and/or correction of aspiration, and various behaviors, such as cough and swallow, contribute to this process.
- Dysphagia and dystussia (impaired cough) are frequently observed during neurologic diseases in the same patients, leading to increased probability of aspiration and a reduced ability to eject aspirated material from the airways.
- Available evidence suggests that these behaviors are regulated by a common neural control system, which also controls breathing.
- Investigation of this neural control system has been facilitated by computational modeling methods, which allow simulation and prediction of its behavior.
- Future interrogation of this complex control system with computational modeling will promote a greater understanding of pathologic processes that contribute to aspiration syndromes.

Conflict of Interest: D.C. Bolser and T.E. Pitts are partners in Sensory Integrated Solutions, LLC, a startup company that will market devices for dysphagia. D.C. Bolser has consulted with Merck and Co. in the last calendar year. P.W. Davenport is a partner in Aspire Products, LLC, which markets respiratory muscle training devices. K.F. Morris and C. Gestreau have no conflicts to declare.
This work was supported by grants R01 HL103415 (D.C. Bolser, PI), R01 HL109025 (P.W. Davenport, PI), and K99 HL111215 (T.E. Pitts, PI) from the National Institutes of Health.
[a] Department of Physiological Sciences, College of Veterinary Medicine, University of Florida, 1600 SW Archer Rd, Gainesville, FL 32610, USA; [b] Center of Research in Neurobiology and Neurophysiology of Marseille, Aix Marseille Universite, CRN2M-UMR7286, 13344 Cedex 15, Marseille, France; [c] Department of Molecular Pharmacology and Physiology, Morsani College of Medicine, University of South Florida, 12901 Bruce B. Downs Blvd, Tampa, FL, USA
* Corresponding author.
E-mail address: bolser@ufl.edu

Otolaryngol Clin N Am 46 (2013) 957–964
http://dx.doi.org/10.1016/j.otc.2013.09.013
0030-6665/13/$ – see front matter © 2013 Elsevier Inc. All rights reserved.

INTRODUCTION

Airway protection is the prevention and/or correction of aspiration. During swallowing, aspiration is prevented during the pharyngeal phase of swallow by closure of the vocal folds, changes in the breathing pattern, and protection of the laryngeal orifice by appropriate movement of the epiglottis. Another behavior, the expiration reflex, prevents aspiration by producing a rapidly rising expiratory airflow to eject adherent material away from the vocal folds. Other behaviors, such as laryngeal adduction and apnea, also participate in the prevention of aspiration. If aspiration occurs, cough is elicited as a defensive reflex to produce high-velocity airflows that create shear forces to dislodge and eject material from the airway.[1]

Most neuromuscular diseases result in impaired cough (dystussia) and/or impaired swallow function (dysphagia). Cough and swallows are controlled by complex brainstem networks, which, until recently, have been studied in isolation. However, in neurologic disease, both swallow and cough function are frequently impaired. In patients with acute stroke, those with dysphagia and aspiration also have profound dystussia.[2,3] Furthermore, the risk of aspiration due to dysphagia can be predicted by several mechanical features of voluntary cough in patients with stroke and Parkinson disease.[3,4] These impairments of swallow and cough contribute to a high risk of aspiration,[5] which seeds the subglottic airways with pathogen-laden material[6] resulting in a high prevalence of aspiration pneumonia. Mortality rates of aspiration pneumonia can approach 40%.[5] High rates of aspiration also occur in patients following anterior cervical spinal surgery (>40%), in elderly patients in long-term care facilities, in patients with gastrointestinal problems, and in patients with other neurologic disorders such as Parkinson disease.[5]

A specific relationship between cough and dysphagia has been recognized and is termed silent aspiration.[5] In these patients, aspiration and penetration of contrast material are noted during videofluoroscopy, but the aspirated dye does not provoke coughing. Patients with silent aspiration (atussia) have a 13-fold increased risk of developing pneumonia.[7] By definition, this group shows the consequences of impaired cough in combination with dysphagia.

Swallow can be coordinated with breathing such that most swallows occur during expiration,[8,9] although swallowing can be observed during a brief interruption of inspiration, with aspiration prevented by laryngeal adduction. This expiratory phase preference for swallow and breathing is thought to reduce the probability of aspiration as material passes through the pharynx. Until recently, the extent to which this expiratory phase preference actually protects from aspiration was not clear. Cvejic and colleagues[10] investigated laryngeal penetration and aspiration in patients with chronic obstructive pulmonary disease (COPD). Penetration/aspiration scores were significantly worse in COPD patients than in controls, and during deglutition of larger volumes (100 mL), there were fewer swallows restricted to the expiratory phase in COPD patients.[10] The COPD patients had a higher prevalence of swallows at the inspiratory/expiratory phase transition than normals. On follow-up, COPD patients with penetration/aspiration during videofluoroscopy had more serious adverse outcomes. It should be noted that it took larger volumes of barium to demonstrate penetration/aspiration in these COPD patients, although all patients who had predominant swallow occurrence at the inspiration/expiration phase transition were in the penetrator/aspirator group. These findings support a hypothesis that breathing phase preference for swallow is a mechanism that becomes an important contributor to airway protection only if larger volumes are swallowed. With low bolus volumes, breathing phase preference may have relatively little influence on the risk of aspiration in dysphagic individuals.

NEUROPHYSIOLOGY OF SWALLOWING

Swallowing is composed of 3 phases: (1) an oral or preparative phase, (2) a pharyngeal phase, and (3) an esophageal phase.[11] The pharyngeal and esophageal phases are stereotypical and can occur as isolated events or become rhythmic. Full execution of swallowing can include multiple rhythmic pharyngeal phases that precede the esophageal phase.[11] Although the oral and pharyngeal phases of swallow are subject to significant modification by suprapontine mechanisms, the minimal neural circuitry necessary for their production is contained within the brainstem.[11] The extent to which the esophageal phase is controlled by suprapontine mechanisms in not clear.[12] The pharyngeal phase of swallow is most involved in airway protection.

The function of the pharyngeal phase swallow is to move a bolus from the oral cavity through the pharynx to the esophagus. Upper airway muscle activity must be controlled and organized to close the glottis and laryngeal vestibule, move the hyolaryngeal complex superior and anterior, invert the epiglottis, and ultimately protect the subglottic airways. Failure to close the glottal opening during swallow increases the risk of penetration or aspiration. Laryngeal aspiration increases the risk that material will enter the trachea and promote aspiration pneumonia.

The pharyngeal phase of swallow is produced by the coordinated action of a variety of muscles that can be segregated by function: tongue retractors (eg, styloglossus), laryngeal elevators (eg, geniohyoid), laryngeal depressors (eg, sternothyroid), laryngeal adduction (eg, thyroartytenoid), and upper esophageal sphincter opening and closing (cricopharyngeus).[11] Motor activation of these muscles is brief (usually less than 600 ms) and ballistic-like. These muscles can be activated rhythmically, leading to repetitive swallowing.[11]

NEUROPHYSIOLOGY OF COUGH AND BREATHING

The function of cough is to remove fluids, mucus, and/or foreign bodies from the respiratory tract by the generation of high-velocity airflows. These airflows are generated by a complex and sequential cough motor pattern involving 3 phases: inspiration, compression, and expulsion.[13] The inspiratory phase of cough is generated by a large burst of activity in inspiratory muscles, including the diaphragm and inspiratory intercostals.[13,14] The compressive phase of cough is generated by laryngeal adduction that is produced by ballistic-like activity in expiratory laryngeal muscles during rapidly rising expiratory thoracic and abdominal muscle activity.[13] The increased intrathoracic pressure during the compression phase elicits large airflows during the expulsive phase of cough, which is driven by intense motor activation of expiratory thoracic and abdominal muscles.[13]

According to current hypotheses for the neurogenesis of cough and breathing, a single network of neurons mediates both motor tasks.[15,16] The anatomic connectivity of these neurons, in combination with their intrinsic membrane properties, regulates their discharge patterns and accounts for the temporal and spatial distribution of motor drive to respiratory muscle motoneurons. The same network can produce such different behaviors by mechanisms that include alteration of the excitability of key elements, presynaptic modulation, and/or recruitment of previously silent elements. Collectively, these processes represent network reconfiguration. The term respiratory pattern generator describes the configuration of this network when it generates breathing, and the term cough pattern generator describes the configuration that is responsible for cough. The neural network that makes up the swallow pattern generator may overlap somewhat with that for breathing and coughing,[17] but much of it, especially the network that makes up the dorsal swallow group, is considered to be separate.[11]

The authors have proposed[18,19] that cough is coordinated by a distributed brainstem network that includes populations of neurons (or assemblies) that cooperate to exert control over the entire network. They have described these populations of neurons as behavioral control assemblies (BCAs) and also have proposed that BCAs exist for different behaviors that interact to ensure the appropriate expression of airway protective behaviors. These BCAs interact with central pattern generators (CPGs) for various behaviors. A CPG contains elements for controlling the duration of action of each muscle, and regulates the temporal activation patterns between multiple muscles that contribute to a single behavior. In this context, a BCA is a regulatory element that is separate from the CPG, but controls it.[18–20] This hypothesis is grounded in control system theory that invokes elements known as holons.[21] Holons are elements of a larger hierarchical system that exert definable control over the entire organizational apparatus. They also can be controlled by higher-order holons in the control system.[21] According to this hypothesis, both the cough/breathing CPG and the cough BCA can usefully be described as separate holons, which constitute part of a larger regulatory system for respiratory behaviors (**Fig. 1**). It is important to note that the evidence for BCAs is restricted to experiments on coughing. The extent to which BCAs operate to control swallowing has not yet been clearly demonstrated by experimental results. However, placing the control of swallow in context of a holarchical system may stimulate directed investigation into the existence of BCAs in the regulation of this behavior. A simplified representation for this proposed control system is shown in **Fig. 1**, with the BCA regulation of cough and the swallow and cough/breathing pattern generators highlighted. The figure also illustrates that the mechanisms that underlie temporal coordination of these behaviors are not currently understood.

CONTROL HYPOTHESIS FOR COORDINATION OF SWALLOW, BREATHING, AND COUGHING

The exact neural processes by which these behaviors are coordinated are not well understood. The coordinating mechanisms are a property of the brainstem circuits that

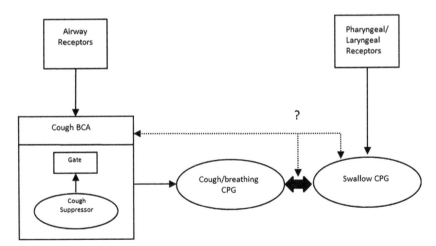

Fig. 1. Schematic representation of proposed interaction between the cough/breathing and swallow cycle pattern generators (CPGs). The cough BCA is shown with gating and cough suppressor subcomponents.[26–28] The large dual arrow indicates reciprocal interactions between the cough/breathing central pattern generators. The dotted line indicates possible relationships between the cough control system and the swallow CPG that underlie temporal coordination.

generate these behaviors, and their expression is manifest in what could loosely be termed as rules that govern how swallow, breathing, and coughing interact. The temporal relationship between swallow and coughing differs from the phase preference that is seen during breathing, and is consistent with phase restriction.[8] Swallowing only occurs during the period of motor quiescence between the end of the active expiratory motor burst and the onset of the next cough inspiration.[8] The reason why there are differences in the relationship between swallow and cough and breathing may relate to the significant differences in mechanics between the behaviors. The large pressures and flows associated with coughing necessitate that swallowing must be prevented from occurring during the inspiratory phase of this behavior, because complete laryngeal adduction would be difficult to achieve. In contrast, lower airflows during breathing are more easily interrupted by the laryngeal adduction required for swallow to occur without aspiration.

COMPUTATIONAL MODELING OF COMPLEX BRAINSTEM CIRCUITS FOR AIRWAY PROTECTION

Given the high complexity of the neural circuits governing these behaviors, the authors have employed computational modeling and simulation to aid in understanding their function. Computational modeling does not replace experimental investigation in animal models and people, but it provides tools to make predictions based on current knowledge. Given that breathing and swallowing are capable of repetitive and rhythmic activation, the authors have hypothesized that their interaction can be explained through loose coupling between 2 different oscillators. Creating oscillatory circuits is a common modeling technique, and coupling oscillators have been used to explain the interaction of brainstem networks for breathing.[22] A detailed synaptic model of the medullary network for breathing and swallow has been developed.[22] This model is supported by in vitro and in vivo recordings of brainstem neurons.[22] **Fig. 2**B is a simulation from a novel network model from **Fig. 2**A. The simulations produce trains of action potentials for each population that can be analyzed with the same tools used for the in vivo parameters, which provided the experimental knowledge base for the model. In simulation, this coupled oscillator circuit was able to produce repetitive breathing, with a swallow occurring during the appropriate period (expiration) of the breathing cycle. The results of this simulation can be used to predict interactions of the control systems for cough and swallow that are not currently known.

To loosely couple the oscillators, excitatory connections between neuronal populations were chosen instead of inhibitory connections, although likely either option is appropriate. In order to inhibit the occurrence of swallow during the inspiratory phase of breathing, inspiratory populations excited the swallow B population in the model (see **Fig. 2**), which in turn suppressed the swallow A population. Note the swallow A population excited the motor neuron populations during swallow production. An additional connection was added from the expiratory populations, at the beginning of the expiratory cycle, to increase the likelihood that swallow would be produced at the end of the expiratory cycle.

The simulation shown in **Fig. 2**B shows swallows (indicated by hypoglossal bursts) occurring during the expiratory phase of breathing. In some instances, 2 swallows were observed in a single simulated expiratory phase. Phrenic activity was ramp-like, as has been shown in previous simulations of the breathing pattern.[16,23] There was no significant coactivation of expiratory motor activity and hypoglossal and phrenic discharge. In animal models, hypoglossal nerve or motoneuron discharge is mainly out of phase with phrenic nerve activity during fictive swallow, but in phase

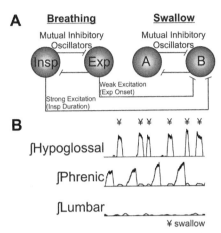

A   Breathing   Swallow

Mutual Inhibitory   Mutual Inhibitory
Oscillators   Oscillators

Insp   Exp   A   B

Weak Excitation
(Exp Onset)
Strong Excitation
(Insp Duration)

B   ¥   ¥¥   ¥   ¥ ¥

∫Hypoglossal

∫Phrenic

∫Lumbar

¥ swallow

Fig. 2. Proposed dual oscillator model for the coupling of breathing and swallow. (*A*) Functional organizational model for the interaction between breathing and swallow. There are 2 neuronal populations for breathing inspiration (Insp) and expiration (Exp), and 2 for swallow. Population (*A*) controls activity for swallow production, and population (*B*) is the interswallow duration population. The oscillators are connected through mutual inhibition with a certain amount of accommodation, which allows for oscillation. To loosely connect the 2 oscillators, the authors entrained them through excitation from the breathing population to the swallow (*B*) population. The Insp population provided excitation throughout the inspiratory duration, which suppressed swallow production during the Insp phase of breathing, and the Exp population provided excitation at the beginning of the expiratory period, which should allow for swallow production at the end of the expiratory period. (*B*) Results from a simulation from the current model producing breathing and swallow. The swallow stimulus elicited swallows (¥) at the appropriate phase of the breathing cycle.

during fictive breathing.[24,25] Therefore, the simulation results meet several qualitative criteria used for identification of swallow in animal models.

The authors' preliminary simulation suggests that temporal coordination between the swallow and breathing CPGs (oscillators) can be approximated without separate intervening circuits that could be categorized as BCAs. However, production of the temporal relationship (or rule set) governing the coexpression of cough and swallow[8] may require more complex neural circuitry than the authors have proposed in **Fig. 2**.

SUMMARY

Airway protective behaviors, such as cough and swallow, are frequently impaired in neurologic disease and contribute to increased risk of aspiration. Emerging evidence supports the concept that impairments of multiple airway-protective behaviors can result from an insult to a single unified control system in the brainstem. The authors' understanding of the brainstem networks that participate in cough, breathing, and swallowing has been facilitated by the use of computational modeling methods. Moving forward, simulation and prediction of the behavior of these networks and how they interact will shed significant light on the regulation of airway protection and how this regulatory system is susceptible to pathologic processes.

REFERENCES

1. Korpas J, Tomori Z. Cough and other respiratory reflexes. Basel (Switzerland), New York: S. Karger; 1979.

2. Smith Hammond CA, Goldstein LB, Zajac DJ, et al. Assessment of aspiration risk in stroke patients with quantification of voluntary cough. Neurology 2001;56(4):502–6.
3. Smith Hammond CA, Goldstein LB, Horner RD, et al. Predicting aspiration in patients with ischemic stroke: comparison of clinical signs and aerodynamic measures of voluntary cough. Chest 2009;135(3):769–77.
4. Pitts T, Troche M, Mann G, et al. Using voluntary cough to detect penetration and aspiration during oropharyngeal swallowing in patients with Parkinson disease. Chest 2010;138(6):1426–31.
5. Smith Hammond CA, Goldstein LB. Cough and aspiration of food and liquids due to oral-pharyngeal dysphagia: ACCP evidence-based clinical practice guidelines. Chest 2006;129(Suppl 1):154S–68S.
6. Scannapieco FA. Role of oral bacteria in respiratory infection. J Periodontol 1999; 70(7):793–802.
7. Daniels SK, Schroeder MF, McClain M, et al. Dysphagia in stroke: development of a standard method to examine swallowing recovery. J Rehabil Res Dev 2006; 43(3):347–56.
8. Pitts T, Rose MJ, Mortensen AN, et al. Coordination of cough and swallow: a meta-behavioral response to aspiration. Respir Physiol Neurobiol 2013. [Epub ahead of print].
9. Martin-Harris B, Brodsky MB, Price CC, et al. Temporal coordination of pharyngeal and laryngeal dynamics with breathing during swallowing: single liquid swallows. J Appl Physiol 2003;94(5):1735.
10. Cvejic L, Harding R, Churchward T, et al. Laryngeal penetration and aspiration in individuals with stable COPD. Respirology 2011;16(2):269–75.
11. Jean A. Brain stem control of swallowing: neuronal network and cellular mechanisms. Physiol Rev 2001;81(2):929–69.
12. Steele CM, Miller AJ. Sensory input pathways and mechanisms in swallowing: a review. Dysphagia 2010;25(4):323–33.
13. Leith DE, Butler JP, Sneddon SL, et al. Cough. In: Macklem PT, Mead J, editors. Handbook of physiology. The respiratory system. Mechanics of breathing, Part I, vol. III. Bethesda (MD): American Physiological Society; 1986. p. 315–36.
14. van Lunteren E, Daniels R, Deal EC Jr, et al. Role of costal and crural diaphragm and parasternal intercostals during coughing in cats. J Appl Physiol 1989;66(1): 135–41.
15. Shannon R, Baekey DM, Morris KF, et al. Functional connectivity among ventrolateral medullary respiratory neurones and responses during fictive cough in the cat. J Physiol 2000;525(Pt 1):207–24.
16. Shannon R, Baekey DM, Morris KF, et al. Ventrolateral medullary respiratory network and a model of cough motor pattern generation. J Appl Physiol 1998; 84(6):2020–35.
17. Gestreau C, Milano S, Bianchi AL, et al. Activity of dorsal respiratory group inspiratory neurons during laryngeal-induced fictive coughing and swallowing in decerebrate cats. Exp Brain Res 1996;108(2):247–56.
18. Bolser DC, Poliacek I, Jakus J, et al. Neurogenesis of cough, other airway defensive behaviors and breathing: a holarchical system? Respir Physiol Neurobiol 2006;152(3):255–65.
19. Bolser DC, Pitts TE, Morris KF. The use of multiscale systems biology approaches to facilitate understanding of complex control systems for airway protection. Curr Opin Pharmacol 2011;11(3):272–7.
20. Bolser DC, Davenport PW. Codeine and cough: an ineffective gold standard. Curr Opin Allergy Clin Immunol 2007;7(1):32–6.

21. Koestler A. The ghost in the machine. New York: The Macmillan Company; 1967.
22. Lindsey BG, Rybak IA, Smith JC. Computational models and emergent properties of respiratory neural networks. Compr Physiol 2012;2(3):1619–70.
23. Rybak IA, O'Connor R, Ross A, et al. Reconfiguration of the pontomedullary respiratory network: a computational modeling study with coordinated in vivo experiments. J Neurophysiol 2008;100(4):1770–99.
24. Gestreau C, Dutschmann M, Obled S, et al. Activation of XII motoneurons and premotor neurons during various oropharyngeal behaviors. Respir Physiol Neurobiol 2005;147(2–3):159–76.
25. Roda F, Gestreau C, Bianchi AL. Discharge patterns of hypoglossal motoneurons during fictive breathing, coughing, and swallowing. J Neurophysiol 2002;87(4):1703–11.
26. Bolser DC, Hey JA, Chapman RW. Influence of central antitussive drugs on the cough motor pattern. J Appl Physiol 1999;86(3):1017–24.
27. Poliacek I, Corrie LW, Wang C, et al. Microinjection of DLH into the region of the caudal ventral respiratory column in the cat: evidence for an endogenous cough-suppressant mechanism. J Appl Physiol 2007;102(3):1014–21.
28. Poliacek I, Wang C, Corrie LW, et al. Microinjection of codeine into the region of the caudal ventral respiratory column suppresses cough in anesthetized cats. J Appl Physiol 2010;108(4):858–65.

Clinical Assessment

Causes of Dysphagia Among Different Age Groups
A Systematic Review of the Literature

Dylan F. Roden, MD, MPH, Kenneth W. Altman, MD, PhD*

KEYWORDS

- Dysphagia • Epidemiology • Prevalence • Incidence • Age • Odynophagia
- Deglutition disorders • Interdisciplinary

KEY POINTS

- The causes and associations of dysphagia with different disease states are different among different age groups.
- Dysphagia is increasingly seen by clinicians based on increasing prevalence of gastroesophageal reflux disease, a growing population more than 65 years old, and a longer life expectancy.
- Infancy and early childhood dysphagia are associated with neurodevelopmental delay.
- Childhood through young adult dysphagia is more commonly related to acute infectious processes.
- Dysphagia in middle age is associated with gastroesophageal and immunologic causes.
- The age group older than 60 years is more affected by oncologic and neurologic causes of dysphagia.
- Older age groups have more prominent dysphagia related to stroke, neurodegenerative disease, and dementia.
- Although these generalizations may be of help to the primary assessment of nonsevere dysphagia, neoplastic causes should always be considered.
- A thorough dysphagia assessment should be always be used in the presence of multiple symptoms, severe dysphagia, and failure to respond to initial treatment.

This article was presented as a poster at the Combined Section Meetings of the Triological Society, Phoenix, AZ, January 23–25, 2013.
Financial Disclosures: There was no financial support for this research or work. There are no disclosures.
Conflicts of Interest: None.
Department of Otolaryngology–Head & Neck Surgery, Mount Sinai School of Medicine, One Gustave L. Levy Place, New York, NY 10029, USA
* Corresponding author. Department of Otolaryngology–Head & Neck Surgery, Mount Sinai School of Medicine, One Gustave L. Levy Place, Box 1189, New York, NY 10029.
E-mail address: kenneth.altman@mountsinai.org

Otolaryngol Clin N Am 46 (2013) 965–987
http://dx.doi.org/10.1016/j.otc.2013.08.008
0030-6665/13/$ – see front matter © 2013 Elsevier Inc. All rights reserved.

Abbreviations: Causes of Dysphagia	
AC	Adenocarcinoma
ALS	Amyotrophic lateral sclerosis
CI	Confidence interval
DES	Diffuse esophageal spasm
EE	Eosinophilic esophagitis
EGD	Esophagogastroduodenoscopy
GEJ	Gastroesophageal junction
GERD	Gastroesophageal reflux disease
GI	Gastrointestinal
HTGM	Heterotopic gastric mucosa
MS	Multiple sclerosis
NSMD	Nonspecific motility disorder
PEG	Percutaneous endoscopic gastrostomy
PPI	Proton Pump Inhibitor
RR	Relative Risk
SCC	Squamous Cell Carcinoma
SIR	Standardized incidence ratio
SS	Systemic Sclerosis
TBI	Traumatic brain injury
UES	Upper Esophageal Sphincter

INTRODUCTION

Dysphagia is an increasingly common problem, but it is poorly understood by most clinicians. It most commonly affects the elderly population, in which oropharyngeal dysphagia is associated with muscle atrophy, cognitive decline, and increased aspiration risk in as many as 35% of patients older than 75 years.[1] Dysphagia is prevalent in both the unhealthy and the community-dwelling elderly population, with concomitant increased risks for malnutrition and aspiration pneumonia.[2] Although the world population is expected to have 1 billion people older than 65 years by 2020, this number is forecasted to grow to 2 billion by 2050, with a resulting dramatic impact on health care.[3]

In addition to the elderly population, a growing awareness of dysphagia in other age groups is appreciated, and associated with a different spectrum of diseases, such as gastroesophageal or laryngopharyngeal reflux. It is therefore imperative that specialists as well as primary care physicians recognize dysphagia, understand likely contributing causes based on age and comorbid diseases, and have the ability to prioritize proper evaluation and treatment plans. However, there is little in the existing literature that connects the causes and associations with dysphagia across all age groups.

Dysphagia may be delineated as mechanical/obstructive causes in young patients, and neurologic/muscular causes in elderly patients. Hoy and colleagues[4] assessed 100 consecutive patients presenting to an outpatient tertiary care swallowing center over a 15-month period. The mean age at presentation was 62 years, and 27% of the identified causes of dysphagia were reflux disease, 14% with postradiation dysphagia, and 11% with cricopharyngeus muscle dysfunction.

Dysphagia in infancy is associated anecdotally with neurodevelopmental delay; in childhood and adolescence it is associated with acute and chronic upper respiratory and tonsil disease; in middle age it is associated predominantly with reflux; and in the elderly it is associated with neurodegenerative disease. We hypothesize that there are different comorbid disease associations with dysphagia based on age, and performed a systematic review of the existing literature to evaluate this hypothesis.

METHODS

A literature review of the PubMed database from July 2002 to July 2012 was performed to identify all articles published on the prevalence of dysphagia. Terms for inclusion were dysphagia and related words (dysphagia, odynophagia, globus, deglutition, failure to thrive) linked with an "or" statement, as well as epidemiologic words (prevalence, incidence, etiology, co-morbidity, comorbidity) linked with an "or" statement, and these two searches were linked with an "and" statement. The search only returned articles that satisfied the search criteria based on the content of the title and abstract of the article.

Exclusion criteria were articles published in languages other than English, articles that were published before July 2002, and articles published on the treatment of dysphagia rather than defining prevalence. Review articles permitted identification of additional references for analysis.

RESULTS

The initial search returned 2511 articles. After applying the exclusion criteria, 133 articles remained. An additional 56 articles were identified as pertinent references on analysis of review articles, and added to the 133 articles already identified, combined for a total of 189 articles. This process is shown in the Prisma diagram in **Fig. 1**. The population ranged in age from neonates to individuals more than 100 years old, and included a total of 1,013,392 subjects. **Fig. 2** is a graph of all the references organized chronologically by the average age of patients studied. It shows that roughly two-thirds of the published literature on dysphagia represents adults older than 50 years.

Prevalence of Dysphagia in the General Population

The reports of dysphagia prevalence vary depending on assessment tool and average age of population studied. Results representative of the general population are

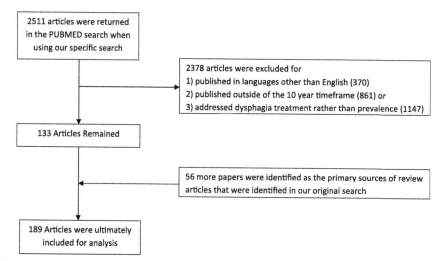

Fig. 1. How the systematic literature review yielded the final 189 articles that were included for analysis.

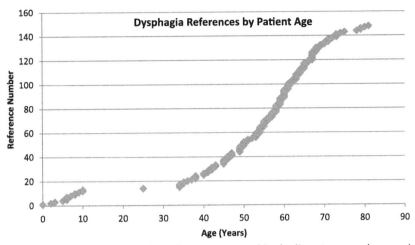

Fig. 2. Scatter plot representing the references returned in the literature search, organized by the average age of the patients studied along the x-axis. Each point symbolizes 1 single reference. This graph shows that about two-thirds of the dysphagia literature is written about adults more than 50 years old.

summarized in **Table 1**.[5–16] We identified 5 studies that attempted to identify the prevalence of dysphagia through the use of a questionnaire distributed to a random sample of the population. The prevalence ranged from 1.7% to 11.3%, although all of these studies were done in an attempt to identify the prevalence of gastroesophageal reflux disease (GERD) and its associated symptoms.[5–9] None of these studies were conducted in the United States, and the symptom of dysphagia was more common in the presence of other heartburn-related symptoms. The dysphagia prevalence in elderly adults ranged from 11.4% to 16%, and in unhealthy older patients it was higher at 54% to 55.2%.[10–14]

Causes of Dysphagia in Different Age Groups

All 189 articles were reviewed and organized based on mean or median age of patients studied. **Table 2** shows the different causes of dysphagia separated by the age of patients, and stratified by decade.[7–193] This table shows that there are distinct causes or associations with dysphagia depending on patient age. The causes of dysphagia in infancy, childhood, and adolescence include congenital causes, acute infectious causes, injury, and neurodevelopmental delay. In the middle-aged population, gastroesophageal and immunologic causes of dysphagia manifest, whereas in the elderly population neurologic and oncologic causes are observed.

NEUROLOGIC CAUSES OF DYSPHAGIA

Most of the epidemiologic dysphagia literature is written on the neurologic causes of dysphagia (61 articles; 10,300 patients). Parkinson disease, stroke, and various causes of dementia are the most frequently published neurologic causes. Some meta-analyses exist that enhanced our systematic review. Alagiakrishnan and colleagues[17] (2012) analyzed 19 articles relating to dementia, and reported a dysphagia prevalence range of 13% to 57%. Kalf and colleagues[18] (2011) performed a meta-analysis of the prevalence of dysphagia in Parkinson disease, identifying 10 articles reporting subjective dysphagia statistics, and determined a pooled prevalence of 35%

Table 1
Dysphagia in the general population

Country	Age of Patients Studied (y)	n	Evaluation Method	Dysphagia Prevalence
China	18–70	2789	Feeling of food stuck in chest or throat >1/mo	1.7
China	>18	2209	Feeling of food stuck in chest or throat	3.5
Japan	>40	82,894	Did you suffer from dysphagia in the last month?	6.9
Australia	>15	2973	Do you have dysphagia rarely or more than rarely?	10.9
Germany	20–91	268	Do you have dysphagia?	11.3
USA	>18 (in doctor's office)	947	Do you have dysphagia several times a month or more?	22.6
Australia	>18	672	Have you ever had dysphagia?	16
United Kingdom	>69 (healthy)	637	Sydney Oropharyngeal Dysphagia Questionnaire	11.4
United States	>65 (healthy)	107	Do you have difficulties with swallowing?	15
Netherlands	>87 (mixed health)	130	Cough with meals? Food stuck? Food spill? Swallowing more than once to get 1 bite down	16
Michigan	>60 (unhealthy)	189	Clinical examination, fluoroscopic examination, FEES	54
Spain	>70 (with pneumonia)	134	Clinical bedside assessment with water swallow	55.2

This table summarizes a group of studies designed to define the prevalence of dysphagia in the general population. The definition of dysphagia and the age of the population studied were not consistent in all studies, and thus these parameters were included in the table.
    Data from Refs.[5–16]

(95% confidence interval [CI], 28–41). They also reviewed 4 articles reporting objective dysphagia statistics in the Parkinson population, and determined a pooled prevalence of 82% (95% CI, 77–87). Martino and colleagues[19] (2005) summarized 24 articles on dysphagia in patients who had strokes. The reported prevalence of dysphagia was lowest with water swallow screening tests (37%–45%), higher with clinical testing (51%–55%), and highest with instrumental testing (64%–78%), implying that the method of testing affects the reported dysphagia rates. Another stroke review article published by Flowers and colleagues[20] (2011) analyzed 17 articles and stratified dysphagia risk based on stroke location. The incidence of dysphagia according to stroke region was:

- 0% in the cerebellum
- 6% in the midbrain

Table 2
Causes of dysphagia across all age groups

0–9 y	10–19 y	20–29 y	30–39 y	40–49 y	50–59 y	60–69 y	70–79 y	80–89 y
EE	TBI	Neck infection	EE	EE	EE	Stroke	Stroke	Alzheimer
Systemic sclerosis			Inflammatory myopathy	Sjögren syndrome	Inflammatory myopathy	Parkinson disease	Parkinson disease	Frontotemporal dementia
TBI			MS	HTGM	HTGM	ALS	Alzheimer	
Thyroglossal duct cyst			Thyroglossal duct cyst	Nasopharyngeal cancer	Systemic sclerosis	Lymphocytic esophagitis	Anaplastic thyroid cancer	
Prematurity			HTGM	Achalasia	Achalasia	HTGM	Achalasia	
Mitochondrial cytopathy				Acute supraglottitis	DES	Inclusion body myositis	DES	
Cerebral palsy				MS	MS	Esophageal SCC	Stricture	
Cardiac surgery				Cervical dystonia	NSMD	Anaplastic thyroid cancer	Antipsychotic exposure	
				Nutcracker esophagus	Stroke	Esophageal AC		
				Lymphocytic Esophagitis	Lymphocytic esophagus	GEJ AC		
				Hyperdynamic UES	Head and neck cancer	Head and neck cancer		
				GERD	GERD	Laryngectomy		
				Esophagitis	Esophagitis	Schatzki ring		
				Reflux surgery	Reflux surgery	Alzheimer		
				Mental health disorder	Type 1 diabetes	Zenker diverticulum		
				Tetraplegia	Food impaction	Cardiac surgery		
					Mucositis	Stricture		
					Cervical spine surgery	Cervical spine surgery		
					Cerebral palsy	Frontotemporal dementia		
					Mental health disorder	Mental health disorder		
					Radiation			
					Chemoradiation			
					Thyroid disease			

Abbreviations: AC, adenocarcinoma; ALS, amyotrophic lateral sclerosis; DES, diffuse esophageal spasm; EE, eosinophilic esophagitis; GEJ, gastroesophageal junction; HTGM, heterotopic gastric mucosa; MS, multiple sclerosis; NSMD, nonspecific motility disorder; TBI, traumatic brain injury.
This table lists the most commonly published causes of dysphagia in each age group, stratified by decade. Many more causes of dysphagia manifest in the elderly populations, and dysphagia may represent severe diseases such as neurodegenerative processes or cancer.

- 43% in the pons
- 40% in the medial medulla
- 57% in the lateral medulla

They intended to develop a neuroanatomical model of dysphagia for the brain but were limited to the infratentorial region because of limitations in the quality of the literature.

Performing an analysis of the original articles identified in these review articles, as well as incorporating more recent publications, it is evident that subjective measurements, such as questionnaires, under-report the prevalence of dysphagia compared with more objective measures that incorporate a clinical assessment or an imaging modality. This under-reporting is particularly apparent in the neurodegenerative disease population, such as[17,18,21–42]:

- Parkinson disease (15%–52% subjective, 41%–87% objective)
- Alzheimer disease (7% subjective, 13%–29% objective)
- Frontotemporal dementia (19%–26% subjective, 57% objective)

The enormous variability in dysphagia reporting in patients who have had strokes (25%–81%) is caused by differences in assessment as well as stroke location.[19,20,43–68] Other neurologic diseases commonly associated with dysphagia include[69–77]:

- Multiple sclerosis (24%–34%)
- ALS (86%)
- Cervical dystonia (2%–36%), and
- Cerebral palsy (6% adult, 99% pediatric)

Table 3 summarizes the causes of dysphagia encountered in this literature review.[17–193]

IMMUNOLOGIC CAUSES OF DYSPHAGIA

Thirty-one articles were published on immunologic causes of dysphagia, representing 338,071 patients. Most of these articles (21 of 31) are about EE.[78–99] Other disease processes that were analyzed include lymphocytic esophagitis (2 articles), inflammatory myopathies (5 articles), systemic sclerosis (2 articles), and Sjögren syndrome (1 article).[100–108]

Sixteen articles, including 1 review article, were published on EE in the adult population; an additional 5 articles were published on EE in the pediatric population. A review article concluded that the average prevalence of EE in the general population was 0.03%, and 2.8% in the symptomatic population with dysphagia.[78] Ronkainen and colleagues[79] performed esophagogastroduodenoscopy (EGDs) on a randomly selected sample of 1000 people in northern Sweden and diagnosed EE in 0.4%. When retrospectively reviewing esophageal biopsies, investigators in both China and the United States came to similar conclusions, finding evidence of EE in 0.34% to 0.5% of specimens.[80,81] In studies of EE in patients undergoing endoscopy for any indication, the prevalence ranged from 1.0% to 6.5%.[82–85] When studying only patients whose indication for endoscopy was dysphagia, EE was even more common, being present in 12% to 15% of patients.[86,87] Among patients with EE, dysphagia is more common in adults than in children; $70.5 \pm 23.7\%$ versus $32.6 \pm 8.5\%$ respectively.[78–99]

Two articles were published on lymphocytic esophagitis, a rare condition (0.09% of all EGD biopsies), but one that is commonly associated with dysphagia (53%–67%).[99,100] Five articles were written about dysphagia in patients with inflammatory myopathy.[101–105] The different subsets of inflammatory myopathies seem to have

Table 3
Causes discussed in the dysphagia literature. The dysphagia prevalences associated with these comorbid conditions are shown, as well as the average age at which these diseases present

Cause	Qualifier	Dysphagia Prevalence (%)	Average Age (y)
Stroke	—	25–81	56–79
Alzheimer disease	—	7–29	68–79
Parkinson disease	—	15–87	61–75
Frontotemporal dementia	—	19–57	61–80
Multiple sclerosis	—	24–34	34–50
ALS	—	86	65
EE	Pediatric	21–40	6–10
EE	Adult	33–100	34–50
Systemic sclerosis	Pediatric	39	6
Systemic sclerosis	Adult	74	54
Sjögren syndrome	—	65	47
Inflammatory myopathy	—	18–86	34–68
Reflux disease	—	6–50	40–51
Stricture	—	83	65
HTGM	—	21–39.4	37–60
Motility disorder	DES, NSMD, achalasia, etc	76–94	49–71
Zenker diverticulum	—	86	67
Head and neck cancer	Pretreatment	9.2–67	49–64
Head and neck cancer	Posttreatment	23–100	49–64
Esophageal SCC	—	62–93	65
Esophageal AC	—	53–79	63
Anaplastic thyroid cancer	—	40	69
Mucositis	—	29.10	57
Cervical spine surgery	Anterior approach	0–21.3	54–57
Cervical spine surgery	Posterior approach	0.9–1.87	54–61
Reflux surgery	Nissen	22–52	47–58
Reflux surgery	Anterior 90	4.8–34	47–53
Pediatric cardiac surgery	—	18–22	0–5
Mental health illness	—	9–42	46–68
Neck infection	—	44	25
Supraglottitis	—	80	49
Pediatric head trauma	—	3.8–5.3	6–10
Acute tetraplegia	—	41	49
Thyroglossal duct cyst	Pediatric presentation	10.60	7
Thyroglossal duct cyst	Adult presentation	20.30	36
Thyroid disease	—	39	51

Abbreviation: HTGM, heterotopic gastric mucosa.
Data from Refs.[7,8,17–73,78–99,101–108,110–121,123,125–128,130–152,154,156–168,170–187,191]

varying prevalences of dysphagia; 65% to 86% in inclusion body myositis, 30% to 60% in polymyositis, and 18% to 20% in dermatomyositis.[101,102] Mustafa and Dahbour[103] pooled patients with different inflammatory myopathies and reported a combined dysphagia prevalence of 40%. As with most autoimmune processes, episodic flares are common, as suggested by a 94% affirmative response rate to the question, "Have you ever had dysphagia?"[101] Azuma and colleagues[104] showed that patients with inflammatory myopathy have a higher likelihood of developing malignancy (standardized incidence ratio [SIR], 13.8). Gastric cancer was the most common malignancy and merits a full dysphagia work-up in these patients.

Systemic sclerosis is a disease with a bimodal age distribution. In the adult article, 74% of people experienced upper gastrointestinal (GI) symptoms, although it did not specify which symptoms.[106] In the pediatric article, 39% of juvenile patients with SS had dysphagia.[107] Dysphagia in Sjögren syndrome was reported in 65% of patients.[108]

GASTROESOPHAGEAL CAUSES OF DYSPHAGIA

Sixteen articles were written on gastroesophageal causes of dysphagia, analyzing 547,156 patients. Although most articles focused on a patient population with 1 specific disease, 2 studies were broader in scope, attempting to diagnose a myriad of patients presenting with the common complaint of dysphagia. When analyzing a national endoscopy database for all patients whose indication for endoscopy was dysphagia, 40.8% of patients had a stricture, 22.1% showed evidence of esophagitis, 13.3% had Schatzki ring, 2.2% had acute food impaction, and 0.9% had malignancy.[109] Tsuboi and colleagues[110] reviewed 24 years of data for all patients undergoing esophageal manometry and 12.1% of patients had nonspecific motility disorder, 6.9% had nutcracker esophagus, 4.6% had diffuse esophageal spasm, and 3.1% had achalasia, whereas most (73.4%) had normal motility.

Reflux and related complications, motility disorders, and HTGM were among the most common gastroesophageal causes of dysphagia published in the recent literature. There were 5 articles written on the prevalence of HTGM. In EGDs conducted for any indication, the diagnosis of HTGM was made in 0.18% to 13.8% of patients (mean, 4.7%).[111–115] The prevalence of dysphagia was 21.0% to 39.4% and the severity of dysphagia correlated with larger patch size.

Three articles were written on GERD and its related complications such as erosive esophagitis and stricture. In a study that reviewed patients undergoing endoscopy for any reason, the prevalence of reflux esophagitis was 12.3%.[112] In patients with GERD-like symptoms having endoscopy, reflux esophagitis was diagnosed in 22.8%.[116] Dysphagia affects about 37% of patients with GERD, and may be even more prevalent in older adults with GERD.[117,118] In patients diagnosed with stricture, 83% of them reported symptoms of dysphagia.[119]

There were an additional 3 articles written on motility disorders. Diffuse esophageal spasm was diagnosed in 4% of manometries in one study; however, 76% of those patients complained of dysphagia.[120] Dysphagia was a presenting symptom in 94% of patients who were later diagnosed with achalasia.[121] In a manometry article attempting to determine the cause of globus, a hyperdynamic upper esophageal sphincter was diagnosed in 60% of patients.[122]

Zenker diverticulum is commonly associated with difficulty swallowing, with a reported dysphagia prevalence of 86%.[123] Food impaction in the esophagus is also commonly associated with dysphagia, and one article showed seasonal variation in those cases associated with atopy; impaction was more common in the summer and fall compared with winter and spring.[124]

CONGENITAL CAUSES OF DYSPHAGIA

Prematurity is the most frequent cause of difficulty feeding in newborns. In a national database review in Taiwan, 50% to 91.7% of low birth weight infants (<2500 g) had feeding problems in their first 5 years of life as measured by need for hospital readmission or outpatient appointment requests for feeding trouble. There are a multitude of factors that contribute to difficulty feeding in low birth weight newborns, but the conclusion of this study was that feeding resources and parent education materials were underused despite the well-established problems experienced by this patient population.

OTHER CAUSES

There are several other categories that contribute to the long list of possible dysphagia causes. Oncologic, endocrine, psychiatric, infectious disease, surgical complications, injuries, and congenital causes have all been described, and are included in **Table 3**. Although it is apparent that oncologic causes of pharyngeal obstruction, and infectious pharyngitis/tonsillitis, result in dysphagia, there was a paucity of literature focusing on these comorbid conditions.

ONCOLOGIC
Head and Neck Cancer

This literature contributed 26 articles representing 3165 patients.[125–150] These studies investigated dysphagia in patients at initial diagnosis as well as long-term dysphagia and percutaneous endoscopic gastrostomy (PEG) tube dependence in patients with varying lengths of follow-up after head and neck cancer treatment with different modalities.

Other Cancers

Other oncologic causes included esophageal, gastric, and lung cancer, and were described in 5 articles representing 2080 patients.[151–155]
   Other possible causes of dysphagia:

- There were 17 articles representing 12,213 patients addressing dysphagia complications from reflux, cardiac, cerebellopontine angle, and cervical spine surgeries.[156–172]
- Altered mental status from psychiatric illnesses and side effects of neuroleptic medications contribute to dysphagia in this patient population, as described in 8 studies representing 273 patients.[173–180]
- There were 2 articles representing 481 patients published on infectious causes (deep space neck infections and acute supraglottitis).[181,182]
- Traumatic brain injuries and tetraplegia are associated with dysphagia as described in 4 articles representing 3069 patients.[183–186]
- Congenital causes vary from prematurity (the most frequent cause of difficulty feeding in newborns) to thyroglossal duct and laryngeal cysts to mitochondrial cytopathies, as described in 4 articles representing 2275 patients.[187–190]
- Endocrine causes were outlined in 3 studies representing 360 patients, and described thyroid disease as well as neuropathy from long-standing diabetes mellitus.[191–193]

DISCUSSION

This review highlights some of the most serious limitations in the dysphagia literature. The definition of dysphagia and the criteria used to make this diagnosis are not widely agreed on. In some studies dysphagia is defined as difficulty swallowing, whereas others describe dysphagia as a specific sensation of food being stuck in the chest. The time course and frequency of symptoms leading to a diagnosis of dysphagia vary depending on author and country of publication. These differences result in significant variability in the reporting of dysphagia prevalence from study to study in patients with the same disease. The instrumentation used to objectively measure dysphagia is also inconsistent. Although some investigators use swallowing speed or swallowing time to identify patients with dysphagia, others use radiographic imaging modalities, others use water swallow tests, and still others use videofluoroscopy. The most common assessment method is the simple question, "Do you have trouble swallowing?" It would be helpful to have a more universal definition of dysphagia, and a reliable assessment method, so that different studies could be compared more directly.

This review shows that most articles concerning dysphagia pertain to neurologic causes. The prevalence of dysphagia in patients with neurodegenerative diseases is very high, which also highlights how many of these patients would not be diagnosed with dysphagia without a formal dysphagia evaluation involving an objective measurement, such as an imaging modality. Asking these patients a simple question about problems swallowing does not capture all of the patients that are having difficulty. A dysphagia screen should be implemented and repeated as a patient's neurologic disease becomes more advanced. This finding has serious potential implications because there is a significant increased risk of pneumonia in patients with dysphagia (RR, 3.17; 95% CI, 2.07–4.87) and even greater risk of pneumonia in patients with aspiration (RR, 11.56; 95% CI, 3.36–39.77).[19] In contrast, it is unclear when a patient's dysphagia becomes a health concern. One study diagnosed 22% of older healthy adults with dysphagia based on swallowing speed.[30] This dysphagia is probably not concerning for most of those patients. Perhaps both dysphagia and aspiration scores should be calculated. It may be helpful to evaluate multiple measurements of dysphagia on a longitudinal group of high-risk patients to see which screening modality is the strongest predictor of dysphagia-related complications.

Immunologic and gastroesophageal causes of dysphagia typically affect young, otherwise healthy people. Reflux is a major culprit, but recently EE and HTGM are increasingly recognized as contributors as well. From 1999 to 2009 there was a large increase in the prevalence of EE, from 1.6% to 11.2%, with a concurrent decrease in the prevalence of GERD from 39.3% to 24.1% at a single academic center in the United States.[194] The frequency of biopsy with endoscopy increased over this same time period from 36.7% to 68.7%. EE and HTGM should be considered in addition to other common problems, such as reflux, when an isolated complaint of dysphagia presents in a young, healthy person.

Dysphagia in patients with head and neck cancers after treatment is a serious and persistent complication (**Table 4**). One of the attractive features of chemoradiotherapy was the possibility of avoiding surgery, and thus offering a patient an organ-preserving therapy. However, there is a large body of evidence to suggest that these treatment protocols do not reduce the prevalence of chronic dysphagia or gastrostomy tube dependence.[144] There are currently no large patient studies comparing dysphagia outcome across the many different treatment modalities. Although the reasons for this are complicated, the dogma that chemoradiation is superior to surgery in terms of preventing dysphagia may not be accurate.

Dysphagia and aspiration can have grave consequences. In patients receiving treatment of head and neck cancer, the presence of aspiration can often go unnoticed, with some reporting 45% of aspirations to be clinically silent.[133] Sensory innervation to the

Table 4
Posttreatment dysphagia prevalences in patients with head and neck cancers

Treatment Modality	Months' Follow-up (range)	n	Dysphagia Prevalence	Aspiration Prevalence	1+ Year PEG Dependence	Pharyngeal Stricture Requiring Dilation
CRT	29 (12–152)	23	—	43.5	—	—
CRT	2 (1–10)	63	84.2	49	—	—
CRT	11	57	95	58	—	—
CRT	17	55	91	36	—	5.5
CRT	3	36	56	—	—	—
CRT	(1–3)	29	—	65	—	—
CRT	(6–12)	29	—	62	—	—
CRT	2 (1–4)	10	—	90	—	—
CRT	17 (12–30)	10	—	70	60	30
CRT	4	18	—	81	—	—
CRT	4	11	—	11	—	—
CRT	12	18	—	60	78	17
CRT	12	11	—	11	18	0
CRT	32 (12–73)	122	—	25.4	24.6	17.2
CRT	12	83	—	26.5	21.7	20.5
CRT	23.1 ± 18.5	27	—	—	47	—
RT	29 (12–152)	5	—	20	—	—
RT	56 (12–119)	50	76	24	—	—
Surgery plus RT	29 (12–152)	40	—	39	—	—
Surgery plus RT	34	53	85	40	—	—
Surgery plus RT	28	25	40	—	—	—
RT plus surgery	28	8	75	—	—	—
Surgery	29 (12–152)	40	—	40	—	—
Mix	29 (12–152)	74	97	39	24	—
Mix	(2–72)	81	23	—	—	—
Mix	28.5 (2–65)	87	50.6	—	—	—
Mix	11	25	100	60	—	24
Mix	26 (15–82)	25	92	64	32	—
Mix	12	35	48	—	40	—

These articles quantify the prevalence of dysphagia in patients with head and neck cancers after various treatment modalities. The table is organized by treatment modality. There were different methods used to evaluate patients for the presence of dysphagia as well as differences in length of follow-up. PEG dependence at 1-year follow-up was a useful comparison point across studies when these data were available.
Data from Refs.[127,128,132,134–141,143–145,150]

larynx and pharynx is often adversely affected by cytotoxic treatments, as shown by the absence of a gag reflex in 78% of patients receiving neck irradiation of 60 Gy for nasopharyngeal cancer.[141] Many of the deaths during and after head and neck cancer treatment are attributable to aspiration pneumonia, regardless of treatment modality.[128,132,135] Preventive measures against aspiration pneumonia are imperative in these high-risk patients.

Anecdotally, the most common clinical findings are not well represented in the dysphagia epidemiology literature. These etiologies include nasopharyngitis and chronic tonsillitis in the pediatric population, as well as reflux in the adult population. Nevertheless, this review provides a framework in order to target specific populations with dysphagia, and can assist providers in addressing the health care needs of their patients.

SUMMARY

Dysphagia has many different etiologies and can affect a person of any age. A universal definition and assessment tool would be useful in formalizing dysphagia evaluation. Dysphagia screening and repeat objective testing in patients with neurodegenerative disease may be worthwhile in order to reduce the risk of aspiration pneumonia. Consider EGD with biopsy to evaluate for EE or HTGM in young, otherwise healthy patients with dysphagia refractory to PPIs. Although this article does not represent an exhaustive list of all possible dysphagia causes, it can serve as a guide to aid in the diagnosis of dysphagia based on age.

REFERENCES

1. Barczi SR, Sullivan PA, Robbins J. How should dysphagia care of older adults differ? Establishing optimal practice patterns. Semin Speech Lang 2000;21: 347–61.
2. Sura L, Madhavan A, Carnaby G, et al. Dysphagia in the elderly: management and nutritional considerations. Clin Interv Aging 2012;7:287–98.
3. Ageing and life course. WHO 2013. World Health Organization; 2013. Available at: http://www.who.int/ageing/en/. Accessed on September 9, 2012.
4. Hoy M, Domer A, Plowman EK, et al. Causes of dysphagia in a tertiary care swallowing center. Ann Otol Rhinol Laryngol 2012;122:335–8.
5. Yamagishi H, Koike T, Ohara S, et al. Prevalence of gastroesophageal reflux symptoms in a large unselected general population in Japan. World J Gastroenterol 2008;14(9):1358–64.
6. Bollschweiler E, Knoppe K, Wolfgarten E, et al. Prevalence of dysphagia in patients with gastroesophageal reflux in Germany. Dysphagia 2008;23(2): 172–6.
7. Wang JH, Luo JY, Dong L, et al. Epidemiology of gastroesophageal reflux disease: a general population-based study in Xi'an of northwest China. World J Gastroenterol 2004;10(11):1647–51.
8. Wong WM, Lai KC, Lam KF, et al. Prevalence, clinical spectrum and health care utilization of gastro-oesophageal reflux disease in a Chinese population: a population-based study. Aliment Pharmacol Ther 2003;18(6):595–604.
9. Watson DI, Lally CJ. Prevalence of symptoms and use of medication for gastroesophageal reflux in an Australian community. World J Surg 2009; 33(1):88–94.
10. Holland G, Jayasekeran V, Pendleton N, et al. Prevalence and symptom profiling of oropharyngeal dysphagia in a community dwelling of an elderly population: a self-reporting questionnaire survey. Dis Esophagus 2011;24(7):476–80.
11. Chen PH, Golub JS, Hapner ER, et al. Prevalence of perceived dysphagia and quality-of-life impairment in a geriatric population. Dysphagia 2009; 24(1):1–6.
12. Bloem BR, Lagaay AM, van Beek W, et al. Prevalence of subjective dysphagia in community residents aged over 87. BMJ 1990;300(6726):721–2.

13. Langmore SE, Terpenning MS, Schork A, et al. Predictors of aspiration pneumonia: how important is dysphagia? Dysphagia 1998;13(2):69–81.
14. Cabre M, Serra-Prat M, Palomera E, et al. Prevalence and prognostic implications of dysphagia in elderly patients with pneumonia. Age Ageing 2010; 39(1):39–45.
15. Wilkins T, Gillies RA, Thomas AM, et al. The prevalence of dysphagia in primary care patients: a HamesNet Research Network study. J Am Board Fam Med 2007;20(2):144–50.
16. Eslick GD, Talley NJ. Dysphagia: epidemiology, risk factors and impact on quality of life–a population-based study. Aliment Pharmacol Ther 2008;27(10):971–9.
17. Alagiakrishnan K, Bhanji RA, Kurian M. Evaluation and management of oropharyngeal dysphagia in different types of dementia: a systematic review. Arch Gerontol Geriatr 2013;56(1):1–9.
18. Kalf JG, de Swart BJ, Bloem BR, et al. Prevalence of oropharyngeal dysphagia in Parkinson's disease: a meta-analysis. Parkinsonism Relat Disord 2012;18(4): 311–5.
19. Martino R, Foley N, Bhogal S, et al. Dysphagia after stroke: incidence, diagnosis, and pulmonary complications. Stroke 2005;36(12):2756–63.
20. Flowers HL, Skoretz SA, Streiner DL, et al. MRI-based neuroanatomical predictors of dysphagia after acute ischemic stroke: a systematic review and meta-analysis. Cerebrovasc Dis 2011;32(1):1–10.
21. Shinagawa S, Adachi H, Toyota Y, et al. Characteristics of eating and swallowing problems in patients who have dementia with Lewy bodies. Int Psychogeriatr 2009;21(3):520–5.
22. Priefer BA, Robbins J. Eating changes in mild-stage Alzheimer's disease: a pilot study. Dysphagia 1997;12(4):212–21.
23. Horner J, Alberts MJ, Dawson DV, et al. Swallowing in Alzheimer's disease. Alzheimer Dis Assoc Disord 1994;8(3):177–89.
24. Suh MK, Kim H, Na DL. Dysphagia in patients with dementia: Alzheimer versus vascular. Alzheimer Dis Assoc Disord 2009;23(2):178–84.
25. Ikeda M, Brown J, Holland AJ, et al. Changes in appetite, food preference, and eating habits in frontotemporal dementia and Alzheimer's disease. J Neurol Neurosurg Psychiatr 2002;73(4):371–6.
26. Langmore SE, Olney RK, Lomen-Hoerth C, et al. Dysphagia in patients with frontotemporal lobar dementia. Arch Neurol 2007;64(1):58–62.
27. Tian H, Abouzaid S, Sabbagh MN, et al. Health care utilization and costs among patients with AD with and without dysphagia. Alzheimer Dis Assoc Disord 2013; 27:138–44.
28. Edwards LL, Quigley EM, Pfeiffer RF. Gastrointestinal dysfunction in Parkinson's disease: frequency and pathophysiology. Neurology 1992;42:726–32.
29. Hartelius L, Svensson P. Speech and swallowing symptoms associated with Parkinson's disease and multiple sclerosis: a survey. Folia Phoniatr Logop 1994;46:9–17.
30. Clarke CE, Gullaksen E, Macdonald S, et al. Referral criteria for speech and language therapy assessment of dysphagia caused by idiopathic Parkinson's disease. Acta Neurol Scand 1998;97:27–35.
31. Siddiqui MF, Rast S, Lynn MJ, et al. Autonomic dysfunction in Parkinson's disease: a comprehensive symptom survey. Parkinsonism Relat Disord 2002;8: 277–84.
32. Verbaan D, Marinus J, Visser M, et al. Patient-reported autonomic symptoms in Parkinson disease. Neurology 2007;69:333–41.

33. Martinez-Martin P, Schapira AH, Stocchi F, et al. Prevalence of nonmotor symptoms in Parkinson's disease in an international setting; study using nonmotor symptoms questionnaire in 545 patients. Mov Disord 2007;22:1623–9.
34. Cheon SM, Ha MS, Park MJ, et al. Nonmotor symptoms of Parkinson's disease: prevalence and awareness of patients and families. Parkinsonism Relat Disord 2008;14:286–90.
35. Miller N, Allcock L, Hildreth AJ, et al. Swallowing problems in Parkinson disease: frequency and clinical correlates. J Neurol Neurosurg Psychiatr 2009;80: 1047–9.
36. Barone P, Antonini A, Colosimo C, et al. The PRIAMO study: a multicenter assessment of nonmotor symptoms and their impact on quality of life in Parkinson's disease. Mov Disord 2009;24:1641–9.
37. Walker RW, Dunn JR, Gray WK. Self-reported dysphagia and its correlates within a prevalent population of people with Parkinson's disease. Dysphagia 2011;26:92–6.
38. Nilsson H, Ekberg O, Olsson R, et al. Quantitative assessment of oral and pharyngeal function in Parkinson's disease. Dysphagia 1996;11:144–50.
39. Coates C, Bakheit AM. Dysphagia in Parkinson's disease. Eur Neurol 1997;38: 49–52.
40. Muller J, Wenning GK, Verny M, et al. Progression of dysarthria and dysphagia in postmortem-confirmed parkinsonian disorders. Arch Neurol 2001;58:259–64.
41. Perez-Lloret S, Nègre-Pagès L, Ojero-Senard A, et al, COPARK Study Group. Oro-buccal symptoms (dysphagia, dysarthria, and sialorrhea) in patients with Parkinson's disease: preliminary analysis from the French COPARK cohort. Eur J Neurol 2012;19(1):28–37.
42. Sung HY, Kim JS, Lee KS, et al. The prevalence and patterns of pharyngoesophageal dysmotility in patients with early stage Parkinson's disease. Mov Disord 2010;25(14):2361–8.
43. Barer DH. The natural history and functional consequences of dysphagia after hemispheric stroke. J Neurol Neurosurg Psychiatr 1989;52:236–41.
44. DePippo KL, Holas MA, Reding MJ. The Burke dysphagia screening test: validation of its use in patients with stroke. Arch Phys Med Rehabil 1994;75:1284–6.
45. Gordon C, Hewer RL, Wade DT. Dysphagia in acute stroke. BMJ 1987;295: 411–4.
46. Gottlieb D, Kipnis M, Sister E, et al. Validation of the 50 ml^3 drinking test for evaluation of post-stroke dysphagia. Disabil Rehabil 1996;18:529–32.
47. Hinds NP, Wiles CM. Assessment of swallowing and referral to speech and language therapists in acute stroke. QJM 1998;91:829–35.
48. Kidd D, Lawson J, Nesbitt R, et al. Aspiration in acute stroke: a clinical study with videofluoroscopy. QJM 1993;86:825–9.
49. Lim SH, Lieu PK, Phua SY, et al. Accuracy of bedside clinical methods compared with fiberoptic endoscopic examination of swallowing (FEES) in determining the risk of aspiration in acute stroke patients. Dysphagia 2001;16: 1–6.
50. Odderson IR, Keaton JC, McKenna BS. Swallow management in patients on an acute stroke pathway: quality is cost effective. Arch Phys Med Rehabil 1995;76: 1130–3.
51. Wade DT, Hewer RL. Motor loss and swallowing difficulty after stroke: frequency, recovery, and prognosis. Acta Neurol Scand 1987;76:50–4.
52. Chua KS, Kong KH. Functional outcome in brainstem stroke patients after rehabilitation. Arch Phys Med Rehabil 1996;77:194–7.

53. Daniels SK, Brailey K, Priestly DH, et al. Aspiration in patients with acute stroke. Arch Phys Med Rehabil 1998;79:14–9.
54. Hamdy S, Aziz Q, Rothwell JC, et al. Explaining oropharyngeal dysphagia after unilateral hemispheric stroke. Lancet 1997;350:686–92.
55. Hamdy S, Aziz Q, Rothwell JC, et al. Recovery of swallowing after dysphagic stroke relates to functional reorganization in the intact motor cortex. Gastroenterology 1998;115:1104–12.
56. Kim H, Chung CS, Lee KH, et al. Aspiration subsequent to a pure medullary infarction: lesion sites, clinical variables, and outcome. Arch Neurol 2000;57:478–83.
57. Mann G, Hankey GJ, Cameron D. Swallowing function after stroke: prognosis and prognostic factors at 6 months. Stroke 1999;30:744–8.
58. Meng NH, Wang TG, Lien IN. Dysphagia in patients with brainstem stroke: incidence and outcome. Am J Phys Med Rehabil 2000;79:170–5.
59. Parker C, Power M, Hamdy S, et al. Awareness of dysphagia by patients following stroke predicts swallowing performance. Dysphagia 2004;19:28–35.
60. Sala R, Munto MJ, de la Calle J, et al. Swallowing changes in cerebrovascular accidents: incidence, natural history, and repercussions on the nutritional status, morbidity, and mortality. Rev Neurol 1998;27:759–66.
61. Schelp AO, Cola PC, Gatto AR, et al. Incidence of oropharyngeal dysphagia associated with stroke in a regional hospital in Sao Paulo State – Brazil. Arq Neuropsiquiatr 2004;62:503–6 [in Portuguese].
62. Sharma JC, Fletcher S, Vassallo M, et al. What influences outcome of stroke–pyrexia or dysphagia? Int J Clin Pract 2001;55:17–20.
63. Smithard DG, O'Neill PA, Park C, et al. Complications and outcome after stroke: does dysphagia matter? Stroke 1996;27:1200–4.
64. Teasell R, Foley N, Fisher J, et al. The incidence, management, and complications of dysphagia in patients with medullary strokes admitted to a rehabilitation unit. Dysphagia 2002;17:115–20.
65. Suntrup S, Warnecke T, Kemmling A, et al. Dysphagia in patients with acute striatocapsular hemorrhage. J Neurol 2012;259(1):93–9.
66. Falsetti P, Acciai C, Palilla R, et al. Oropharyngeal dysphagia after stroke: incidence, diagnosis, and clinical predictors in patients admitted to a neurorehabilitation unit. J Stroke Cerebrovasc Dis 2009;18(5):329–35.
67. Warnecke T, Teismann I, Meimann W, et al. Assessment of aspiration risk in acute ischaemic stroke–evaluation of the simple swallowing provocation test. J Neurol Neurosurg Psychiatr 2008;79(3):312–4.
68. Teasell R, Foley N, Doherty T, et al. Clinical characteristics of patients with brainstem strokes admitted to a rehabilitation unit. Arch Phys Med Rehabil 2002;83(7):1013–6.
69. De Pauw A, Dejaeger E, D'hooghe B, et al. Dysphagia in multiple sclerosis. Clin Neurol Neurosurg 2002;104(4):345–51.
70. Calcagno P, Ruoppolo G, Grasso MG, et al. Dysphagia in multiple sclerosis – prevalence and prognostic factors. Acta Neurol Scand 2002;105(1):40–3.
71. Danesh-Sani SA, Rahimdoost A, Soltani M, et al. Clinical assessment of orofacial manifestations in 500 patients with multiple sclerosis. J Oral Maxillofac Surg 2013;71:290–4.
72. Poorjavad M, Derakhshandeh F, Etemadifar M, et al. Oropharyngeal dysphagia in multiple sclerosis. Mult Scler 2010;16(3):362–5.
73. Chen A, Garrett CG. Otolaryngologic presentations of amyotrophic lateral sclerosis. Otolaryngol Head Neck Surg 2005;132(3):500–4.

74. Camargo CH, Teive HA, Becker N, et al. Cervical dystonia: clinical and therapeutic features in 85 patients. Arq Neuropsiquiatr 2008;66(1):15–21.
75. Ertekin C, Aydogdu I, Seçil Y, et al. Oropharyngeal swallowing in craniocervical dystonia. J Neurol Neurosurg Psychiatr 2002;73(4):406–11.
76. Henderson CM, Rosasco M, Robinson LM, et al. Functional impairment severity is associated with health status among older persons with intellectual disability and cerebral palsy. J Intellect Disabil Res 2009;53(11):887–97.
77. Calis EA, Veugelers R, Sheppard JJ, et al. Dysphagia in children with severe generalized cerebral palsy and intellectual disability. Dev Med Child Neurol 2008;50(8):625–30.
78. Sealock RJ, Rendon G, El-Serag HB. Systematic review: the epidemiology of eosinophilic oesophagitis in adults. Aliment Pharmacol Ther 2010;32(6):712–9.
79. Ronkainen J, Talley NJ, Aro P, et al. Prevalence of oesophageal eosinophils and eosinophilic oesophagitis in adults: the population-based Kalixanda study. Gut 2007;56:615–20.
80. Shi YN, Sun SJ, Xiong LS, et al. Prevalence, clinical manifestations and endoscopic features of eosinophilic esophagitis: a pathological review in China. J Dig Dis 2012;13(6):304–9.
81. Kapel RC, Miller JK, Torres C, et al. Eosinophilic esophagitis: a prevalent disease in the United States that affects all age groups. Gastroenterology 2008; 134(5):1316–21.
82. Almansa C, Krishna M, Buchner AM, et al. Seasonal distribution in newly diagnosed cases of eosinophilic esophagitis in adults. Am J Gastroenterol 2009;104: 828–33.
83. Veerappan GR, Perry JL, Duncan TJ, et al. Prevalence of eosinophilic esophagitis in an adult population undergoing upper endoscopy: a prospective study. Clin Gastroenterol Hepatol 2009;7:420–6.
84. Kanakala V, Lamb CA, Haigh C, et al. The diagnosis of primary eosinophilic oesophagitis in adults: missed or misinterpreted? Eur J Gastroenterol Hepatol 2010;22(7):848–55.
85. Sorser SA, Barawi M, Hagglund K, et al. Eosinophilic esophagitis in children and adolescents: epidemiology, clinical presentation and seasonal variation. J Gastroenterol 2013;48(1):81–5.
86. Prasad GA, Talley NJ, Romero Y, et al. Prevalence and predictive factors of eosinophilic esophagitis in patients presenting with dysphagia: a prospective study. Am J Gastroenterol 2007;102:2627–32.
87. Mackenzie SH, Go M, Chadwick B, et al. Eosinophilic oesophagitis in patients presenting with dysphagia – a prospective analysis. Aliment Pharmacol Ther 2008;28:1140–6.
88. Straumann A, Simon HU. Eosinophilic esophagitis: escalating epidemiology? J Allergy Clin Immunol 2005;115:418–9.
89. Kerlin P, Jones D, Remedios M, et al. Prevalence of eosinophilic esophagitis in adults with food bolus obstruction of the esophagus. J Clin Gastroenterol 2007; 41:356–61.
90. Ramakrishnan R, Chong H. Eosinophilic oesophagitis in adults. Histopathology 2008;52:897–900.
91. Foroutan M, Norouzi A, Molaei M, et al. Eosinophilic esophagitis in patients with refractory gastroesophageal reflux disease. Dig Dis Sci 2010;55:28–31.
92. Joo MK, Park JJ, Kim SH, et al. Prevalence and endoscopic features of eosinophilic esophagitis in patients with esophageal or upper gastrointestinal symptoms. J Dig Dis 2012;13(6):296–303.

93. Ricker J, McNear S, Cassidy T, et al. Routine screening for eosinophilic esophagitis in patients presenting with dysphagia. Therap Adv Gastroenterol 2011; 4(1):27–35.
94. García-Compeán D, González González JA, Marrufo García CA, et al. Prevalence of eosinophilic esophagitis in patients with refractory gastroesophageal reflux disease symptoms: a prospective study. Dig Liver Dis 2011;43(3):204–8.
95. Cohen MC, Rao P, Thomson M, et al. Eosinophils in the oesophageal mucosa: clinical, pathological and epidemiological relevance in children: a cohort study. BMJ Open 2012;2(1):e000493.
96. Mukkada VA, Haas A, Maune NC, et al. Feeding dysfunction in children with eosinophilic gastrointestinal diseases. Pediatrics 2010;126(3):e672–7.
97. Eroglu Y, Lu H, Terry A, et al. Pediatric eosinophilic esophagitis: single-center experience in northwestern USA. Pediatr Int 2009;51(5):612–6.
98. Aceves SS, Newbury RO, Dohil R, et al. Distinguishing eosinophilic esophagitis in pediatric patients: clinical, endoscopic, and histologic features of an emerging disorder. J Clin Gastroenterol 2007;41(3):252–6.
99. Haque S, Genta RM. Lymphocytic oesophagitis: clinicopathological aspects of an emerging condition. Gut 2012;61(8):1108–14.
100. Cohen S, Saxena A, Waljee AK, et al. Lymphocytic esophagitis: a diagnosis of increasing frequency. J Clin Gastroenterol 2012;46(10):828–32.
101. Mulcahy KP, Langdon PC, Mastaglia F. Dysphagia in inflammatory myopathy: self-report, incidence, and prevalence. Dysphagia 2012;27(1):64–9. http://dx.doi.org/10.1007/s00455-011-9338-0.
102. Cox FM, Verschuuren JJ, Verbist BM, et al. Detecting dysphagia in inclusion body myositis. J Neurol 2009;256(12):2009–13.
103. Mustafa KN, Dahbour SS. Clinical characteristics and outcomes of patients with idiopathic inflammatory myopathies from Jordan 1996-2009. Clin Rheumatol 2010;29(12):1381–5.
104. Azuma K, Yamada H, Ohkubo M, et al. Incidence and predictive factors for malignancies in 136 Japanese patients with dermatomyositis, polymyositis and clinically amyopathic dermatomyositis. Mod Rheumatol 2011;21(2):178–83.
105. Claire Langdon P, Mulcahy K, Shepherd KL, et al. Pharyngeal dysphagia in inflammatory muscle diseases resulting from impaired suprahyoid musculature. Dysphagia 2012;27(3):408–17.
106. Wielosz E, Borys O, Zychowska I, et al. Gastrointestinal involvement in patients with systemic sclerosis. Pol Arch Med Wewn 2010;120(4):132–6.
107. Russo RA, Katsicas MM. Clinical characteristics of children with juvenile systemic sclerosis: follow-up of 23 patients in a single tertiary center. Pediatr Rheumatol Online J 2007;5:6.
108. Mandl T, Ekberg O, Wollmer P, et al. Dysphagia and dysmotility of the pharynx and oesophagus in patients with primary Sjögren's syndrome. Scand J Rheumatol 2007;36(5):394–401.
109. Krishnamurthy C, Hilden K, Peterson KA, et al. Endoscopic findings in patients presenting with dysphagia: analysis of a national endoscopy database. Dysphagia 2012;27(1):101–5.
110. Tsuboi K, Hoshino M, Srinivasan A, et al. Insights gained from symptom evaluation of esophageal motility disorders: a review of 4,215 patients. Digestion 2012;85(3):236–42.
111. Neumann WL, Luján GM, Genta RM. Gastric heterotopia in the proximal oesophagus ("inlet patch"): association with adenocarcinomas arising in Barrett mucosa. Dig Liver Dis 2012;44(4):292–6.

112. Hori K, Kim Y, Sakurai J, et al. Non-erosive reflux disease rather than cervical inlet patch involves globus. J Gastroenterol 2010;45(11):1138–45.

113. Alagozlu H, Simsek Z, Unal S, et al. Is there an association between *Helicobacter pylori* in the inlet patch and globus sensation? World J Gastroenterol 2010;16(1):42–7.

114. Poyrazoglu OK, Bahcecioglu IH, Dagli AF, et al. Heterotopic gastric mucosa (inlet patch): endoscopic prevalence, histopathological, demographical and clinical characteristics. Int J Clin Pract 2009;63(2):287–91.

115. Baudet JS, Alarcón-Fernández O, Sánchez Del Río A, et al. Heterotopic gastric mucosa: a significant clinical entity. Scand J Gastroenterol 2006;41(12): 1398–404.

116. Lin M, Gerson LB, Lascar R, et al. Features of gastroesophageal reflux disease in women. Am J Gastroenterol 2004;99(8):1442–7.

117. Pilotto A, Franceschi M, Leandro G, et al. Clinical features of reflux esophagitis in older people: a study of 840 consecutive patients. J Am Geriatr Soc 2006; 54(10):1537–42.

118. Vakil NB, Traxler B, Levine D. Dysphagia in patients with erosive esophagitis: prevalence, severity, and response to proton pump inhibitor treatment. Clin Gastroenterol Hepatol 2004;2(8):665–8.

119. Ruigómez A, García Rodríguez LA, Wallander MA, et al. Esophageal stricture: incidence, treatment patterns, and recurrence rate. Am J Gastroenterol 2006; 101(12):2685–92.

120. Almansa C, Heckman MG, DeVault KR, et al. Esophageal spasm: demographic, clinical, radiographic, and manometric features in 108 patients. Dis Esophagus 2012;25(3):214–21.

121. Fisichella PM, Raz D, Palazzo F, et al. Clinical, radiological, and manometric profile in 145 patients with untreated achalasia. World J Surg 2008;32(9):1974–9.

122. Kwiatek MA, Mirza F, Kahrilas PJ, et al. Hyperdynamic upper esophageal sphincter pressure: a manometric observation in patients reporting globus sensation. Am J Gastroenterol 2009;104(2):289–98.

123. Valenza V, Perotti G, Di Giuda D, et al. Scintigraphic evaluation of Zenker's diverticulum. Eur J Nucl Med Mol Imaging 2003;30(12):1657–64.

124. Larsson H, Bergquist H, Bove M. The incidence of esophageal bolus impaction: is there a seasonal variation? Otolaryngol Head Neck Surg 2011;144(2):186–90.

125. Kubrak C, Olson K, Jha N, et al. Nutrition impact symptoms: key determinants of reduced dietary intake, weight loss, and reduced functional capacity of patients with head and neck cancer before treatment. Head Neck 2010;32(3):290–300.

126. Nguyen NP, Vos P, Moltz CC, et al. Analysis of the factors influencing dysphagia severity upon diagnosis of head and neck cancer. Br J Radiol 2008;81(969): 706–10.

127. García-Peris P, Parón L, Velasco C, et al. Long-term prevalence of oropharyngeal dysphagia in head and neck cancer patients: impact on quality of life. Clin Nutr 2007;26(6):710–7.

128. Nguyen NP, Frank C, Moltz CC, et al. Aspiration rate following chemoradiation for head and neck cancer: an underreported occurrence. Radiother Oncol 2006;80(3):302–6.

129. Platteaux N, Dirix P, Dejaeger E, et al. Dysphagia in head and neck cancer patients treated with chemoradiotherapy. Dysphagia 2010;25(2):139–52.

130. Pauloski BR, Rademaker AW, Logemann JA, et al. Pretreatment swallowing function in patients with head and neck cancer. Head Neck 2000;22(5): 474–82.

131. Stenson KM, MacCracken E, List M, et al. Swallowing function in patients with head and neck cancer prior to treatment. Arch Otolaryngol Head Neck Surg 2000;126(3):371–7.
132. Eisbruch A, Lyden T, Bradford CR, et al. Objective assessment of swallowing dysfunction and aspiration after radiation concurrent with chemotherapy for head-and-neck cancer. Int J Radiat Oncol Biol Phys 2002;53(1):23–8.
133. Rosen A, Rhee TH, Kaufman R. Prediction of aspiration in patients with newly diagnosed untreated advanced head and neck cancer. Arch Otolaryngol Head Neck Surg 2001;127(8):975–9.
134. Feng FY, Kim HM, Lyden TH, et al. Intensity-modulated radiotherapy of head and neck cancer aiming to reduce dysphagia: early dose-effect relationships for the swallowing structures. Int J Radiat Oncol Biol Phys 2007;68(5):1289–98.
135. Nguyen NP, Moltz CC, Frank C, et al. Dysphagia following chemoradiation for locally advanced head and neck cancer. Ann Oncol 2004;15(3):383–8.
136. Levendag PC, Teguh DN, Voet P, et al. Dysphagia disorders in patients with cancer of the oropharynx are significantly affected by the radiation therapy dose to the superior and middle constrictor muscle: a dose-effect relationship. Radiother Oncol 2007;85(1):64–73.
137. Smith RV, Kotz T, Beitler JJ, et al. Long-term swallowing problems after organ preservation therapy with concomitant radiation therapy and intravenous hydroxyurea: initial results. Arch Otolaryngol Head Neck Surg 2000;126(3):384–9.
138. Nguyen NP, Moltz CC, Frank C, et al. Long-term aspiration following treatment for head and neck cancer. Oncology 2008;74(1–2):25–30.
139. Nguyen NP, Moltz CC, Frank C, et al. Evolution of chronic dysphagia following treatment for head and neck cancer. Oral Oncol 2006;42(4):374–80.
140. Caudell JJ, Schaner PE, Meredith RF, et al. Factors associated with long-term dysphagia after definitive radiotherapy for locally advanced head-and-neck cancer. Int J Radiat Oncol Biol Phys 2008;73(2):410–5.
141. Hughes PJ, Scott PM, Kew J, et al. Dysphagia in treated nasopharyngeal cancer. Head Neck 2000;22(4):393–7.
142. de Cássia Braga Ribeiro K, Kowalski LP, Latorre Mdo R. Perioperative complications, comorbidities, and survival in oral or oropharyngeal cancer. Arch Otolaryngol Head Neck Surg 2003;129(2):219–28.
143. Nguyen NP, Moltz CC, Frank C, et al. Dysphagia severity following chemoradiation and postoperative radiation for head and neck cancer. Eur J Radiol 2006;59(3):453–9.
144. Shiley SG, Hargunani CA, Skoner JM, et al. Swallowing function after chemoradiation for advanced stage oropharyngeal cancer. Otolaryngol Head Neck Surg 2006;134(3):455–9.
145. Maurer J, Hipp M, Schäfer C, et al. Impact on quality of life after radio(chemo) therapy of head and neck cancer. Strahlenther Onkol 2011;187(11):744–9.
146. Caudell JJ, Schaner PE, Desmond RA, et al. Dosimetric factors associated with long-term dysphagia after definitive radiotherapy for squamous cell carcinoma of the head and neck. Int J Radiat Oncol Biol Phys 2010;76(2):403–9.
147. Smith RV, Goldman SY, Beitler JJ, et al. Decreased short- and long-term swallowing problems with altered radiotherapy dosing used in an organ-sparing protocol for advanced pharyngeal carcinoma. Arch Otolaryngol Head Neck Surg 2004;130(7):831–6.
148. Bieri S, Bentzen SM, Huguenin P, et al. Early morbidity after radiotherapy with or without chemotherapy in advanced head and neck cancer. Experience from four nonrandomized studies. Strahlenther Onkol 2003;179(6):390–5.

149. Maclean J, Cotton S, Perry A. Post-laryngectomy: it's hard to swallow: an Australian study of prevalence and self-reports of swallowing function after a total laryngectomy. Dysphagia 2009;24(2):172–9.
150. Vu KN, Day TA, Gillespie MB, et al. Proximal esophageal stenosis in head and neck cancer patients after total laryngectomy and radiation. ORL J Otorhinolaryngol Relat Spec 2008;70(4):229–35.
151. Gibbs JF, Rajput A, Chadha KS, et al. The changing profile of esophageal cancer presentation and its implication for diagnosis. J Natl Med Assoc 2007;99(6): 620–6.
152. Smithers BM, Fahey PP, Corish T, et al. Symptoms, investigations and management of patients with cancer of the oesophagus and gastro-oesophageal junction in Australia. Med J Aust 2010;193(10):572–7.
153. Lövgren M, Tishelman C, Sprangers M, et al. Symptoms and problems with functioning among women and men with inoperable lung cancer–a longitudinal study. Lung Cancer 2008;60(1):113–24.
154. Nishimura N, Nakano K, Ueda K, et al. Prospective evaluation of incidence and severity of oral mucositis induced by conventional chemotherapy in solid tumors and malignant lymphomas. Support Care Cancer 2012;20(9):2053–9.
155. Langendijk JA, Aaronson NK, de Jong JM, et al. Quality of life after curative radiotherapy in stage I non-small-cell lung cancer. Int J Radiat Oncol Biol Phys 2002;53(4):847–53.
156. Fehlings MG, Smith JS, Kopjar B, et al. Perioperative and delayed complications associated with the surgical treatment of cervical spondylotic myelopathy based on 302 patients from the AOSpine North America Cervical Spondylotic Myelopathy Study. J Neurosurg Spine 2012;16(5):425–32.
157. Street JT, Lenehan BJ, DiPaola CP, et al. Morbidity and mortality of major adult spinal surgery. A prospective cohort analysis of 942 consecutive patients. Spine J 2012;12(1):22–34.
158. Kalb S, Reis MT, Cowperthwaite MC, et al. Dysphagia after anterior cervical spine surgery: incidence and risk factors. World Neurosurg 2012;77(1):183–7.
159. Shamji MF, Cook C, Pietrobon R, et al. Impact of surgical approach on complications and resource utilization of cervical spine fusion: a nationwide perspective to the surgical treatment of diffuse cervical spondylosis. Spine J 2009;9(1): 31–8.
160. Lee MJ, Bazaz R, Furey CG, et al. Risk factors for dysphagia after anterior cervical spine surgery: a two-year prospective cohort study. Spine J 2007;7(2): 141–7.
161. Riley LH 3rd, Vaccaro AR, Dettori JR, et al. Postoperative dysphagia in anterior cervical spine surgery. Spine (Phila Pa 1976) 2010;35(Suppl 9):S76–85.
162. Smith-Hammond CA, New KC, Pietrobon R, et al. Prospective analysis of incidence and risk factors of dysphagia in spine surgery patients: comparison of anterior cervical, posterior cervical, and lumbar procedures. Spine (Phila Pa 1976) 2004;29(13):1441–6.
163. Bazaz R, Lee MJ, Yoo JU. Incidence of dysphagia after anterior cervical spine surgery: a prospective study. Spine (Phila Pa 1976) 2002;27(22):2453–8.
164. Cai W, Watson DI, Lally CJ, et al. Ten-year clinical outcome of a prospective randomized clinical trial of laparoscopic Nissen versus anterior 180° partial fundoplication. Br J Surg 2008;95(12):1501–5.
165. Mark LA, Okrainec A, Ferri LE, et al. Comparison of patient-centered outcomes after laparoscopic Nissen fundoplication for gastroesophageal reflux disease or paraesophageal hernia. Surg Endosc 2008;22(2):343–7.

166. Lindeboom MY, Ringers J, Straathof JW, et al. The effect of laparoscopic partial fundoplication on dysphagia, esophageal and lower esophageal sphincter motility. Dis Esophagus 2007;20(1):63–8.

167. Spence GM, Watson DI, Jamiesion GG, et al. Single center prospective random-ized trial of laparoscopic Nissen versus anterior 90 degrees fundoplication. J Gastrointest Surg 2006;10(5):698–705.

168. Watson DI, Jamieson GG, Lally C, et al, International Society for Diseases of the Esophagus–Australasian Section. Multicenter, prospective, double-blind, ran-domized trial of laparoscopic Nissen vs anterior 90 degrees partial fundoplica-tion. Arch Surg 2004;139(11):1160–7.

169. Barker J, Martino R, Reichardt B, et al. Incidence and impact of dysphagia in patients receiving prolonged endotracheal intubation after cardiac surgery. Can J Surg 2009;52(2):119–24.

170. Kohr LM, Dargan M, Hague A, et al. The incidence of dysphagia in pediatric pa-tients after open heart procedures with transesophageal echocardiography. Ann Thorac Surg 2003;76(5):1450–6.

171. Maurer I, Latal B, Geissmann H, et al. Prevalence and predictors of later feeding disorders in children who underwent neonatal cardiac surgery for congenital heart disease. Cardiol Young 2011;21(3):303–9.

172. Starmer HM, Best SR, Agrawal Y, et al. Prevalence, characteristics, and man-agement of swallowing disorders following cerebellopontine angle surgery. Oto-laryngol Head Neck Surg 2012;146(3):419–25.

173. Regan J, Sowman R, Walsh I. Prevalence of dysphagia in acute and community mental health settings. Dysphagia 2006;21(2):95–101.

174. Rudolph JL, Gardner KF, Gramigna GD, et al. Antipsychotics and oropharyn-geal dysphagia in hospitalized older patients. J Clin Psychopharmacol 2008; 28(5):532–5.

175. Aldridge KJ, Taylor NF. Dysphagia is a common and serious problem for adults with mental illness: a systematic review. Dysphagia 2012;27(1):124–37. http://dx.doi.org/10.1007/s00455-011-9378-5.

176. Avidan B, Sonnenberg A, Giblovich H, et al. Reflux symptoms are associated with psychiatric disease. Aliment Pharmacol Ther 2001;15(12):1907–12.

177. Feve A, Angelard B, Lacau St Guily J. Laryngeal tardive dyskinesia. J Neurol 1995;242(7):455–9.

178. Fioritti A, Giaccotto L, Melega V. Choking incidents among psychiatric patients: retrospective analysis of thirty-one cases from the West Bologna psychiatric wards. Can J Psychiatry 1997;42(5):515–20.

179. Hussar AE, Bragg DG. The effect of chlorpromazine on the swallowing function in chronic schizophrenic patients. Am J Psychiatry 1969;126(4):570–3.

180. Nagamine T. Serum substance P levels in patients with chronic schizophrenia treated with typical or atypical antipsychotics. Neuropsychiatr Dis Treat 2008; 4(1):289–94.

181. Bizaki AJ, Numminen J, Vasama JP, et al. Acute supraglottitis in adults in Finland: review and analysis of 308 cases. Laryngoscope 2011;121(10): 2107–13. http://dx.doi.org/10.1002/lary.22147.

182. Bakir S, Tanriverdi MH, Gün R, et al. Deep neck space infections: a retrospective review of 173 cases. Am J Otol 2012;33(1):56–63.

183. Shem K, Castillo K, Wong S, et al. Dysphagia in individuals with tetraplegia: inci-dence and risk factors. J Spinal Cord Med 2011;34(1):85–92.

184. Morgan AT. Dysphagia in childhood traumatic brain injury: a reflection on the ev-idence and its implications for practice. Dev Neurorehabil 2010;13(3):192–203.

185. Morgan AT, Mageandran SD, Mei C. Incidence and clinical presentation of dysarthria and dysphagia in the acute setting following paediatric traumatic brain injury. Child Care Health Dev 2010;36(1):44–53.
186. Morgan A, Ward E, Murdoch B, et al. Incidence, characteristics, and predictive factors for dysphagia after pediatric traumatic brain injury. J Head Trauma Rehabil 2003;18(3):239–51.
187. Ren W, Zhi K, Zhao L, et al. Presentations and management of thyroglossal duct cyst in children versus adults: a review of 106 cases. Oral Surg Oral Med Oral Pathol Oral Radiol Endod 2011;111(2):e1–6.
188. Howe TH, Hsu CH, Tsai MW. Prevalence of feeding related issues/difficulties in Taiwanese children with history of prematurity, 2003-2006. Res Dev Disabil 2010;31(2):510–6.
189. Jeyakumar A, Williamson ME, Brickman TM, et al. Otolaryngologic manifestations of mitochondrial cytopathies. Am J Otol 2009;30(3):162–5.
190. Prowse S, Knight L. Congenital cysts of the infant larynx. Int J Pediatr Otorhinolaryngol 2012;76(5):708–11.
191. Banks CA, Ayers CM, Hornig JD, et al. Thyroid disease and compressive symptoms. Laryngoscope 2012;122(1):13–6.
192. Nagaiah G, Hossain A, Mooney CJ, et al. Anaplastic thyroid cancer: a review of epidemiology, pathogenesis, and treatment. J Oncol 2011;2011:542358.
193. Rosztóczy A, Róka R, Várkonyi TT, et al. Regional differences in the manifestation of gastrointestinal motor disorders in type 1 diabetic patients with autonomic neuropathy. Z Gastroenterol 2004;42(11):1295–300.
194. Kidambi T, Toto E, Ho N, et al. Temporal trends in the relative prevalence of dysphagia etiologies from 1999–2009. World J Gastroenterol 2012;18(32):4335–41.

Oropharyngeal Dysphagia
Screening and Assessment

Renée Speyer, PhD[a,b],*

KEYWORDS

- Oropharyngeal dysphagia • Screening • Assessment • Quality of life
- Diagnostic performance • Reliability • Methodology

KEY POINTS

- Bedside screening is an essential first step in the management of patients at risk for dysphagia. If patients fail the screening further assessment is required.
- Assessment may relate to different aspects of swallowing. Abnormalities in swallowing are not necessarily correlated and may show dissimilar changes after treatment. Therefore, including several evaluation techniques when studying swallowing problems may be useful.
- There are a great variety of screening and assessment tools for dysphagia available; use of a particular tool must be justified based on its reliability and validity and its discriminative and evaluative purpose.
- There is an urgent need for evidence-based clinical guidelines for screening and assessment of patients with oropharyngeal dysphagia.

INTRODUCTION

Because the human aerodigestive tract caters to the combined functions of breathing, vocalizing, and swallowing, the large supralaryngeal space created by the low larynx positioning in adults increases a risk of aspiration or choking. Any dysfunction in this system may lead to dysphagia.[1] Dysphagia is associated with high morbidity and mortality rates. It can lead to dehydration, malnutrition, or aspiration pneumonia and may have major effects on social and psychological well-being.[2] Early and reliable screening for symptoms of dysphagia in subject populations at risk is an effective

Funding Sources: N/A.

Conflict of Interest: Nil.

[a] Discipline of Speech Pathology, School of Public Health, Tropical Medicine and Rehabilitation Sciences, James Cook University, 1 Discovery Drive, Townsville, Queensland 4811, Australia; [b] Department of Otorhinolaryngology and Head and Neck Surgery, Leiden University Medical Center, Albinusdreef 2, Leiden, 2333 ZA, The Netherlands

* Discipline of Speech Pathology, School of Public Health, Tropical Medicine and Rehabilitation Sciences, James Cook University, Townsville, Queensland 4811, Australia.

E-mail addresses: renee.speyer@jcu.edu.au; r.speyer@online.nl

Otolaryngol Clin N Am 46 (2013) 989–1008

http://dx.doi.org/10.1016/j.otc.2013.08.004
0030-6665/13/$ – see front matter © 2013 Elsevier Inc. All rights reserved.

Abbreviations	
FEES	Fiberoptic endoscopic evaluation of swallowing
FHS	Functional health status
HRQOL	Health-related quality of life
Se	Sensitivity
Sp	Specificity
VFS	Videofluoroscopy

and vital first step in appropriate dysphagia management.[3] Those patients that fail the initial screening need to be referred for further clinical assessment. Apart from video-fluoroscopic (VFS) and fiberoptic endoscopic evaluation of swallowing (FEES), a variety of assessment tools and patient self-evaluation questionnaires are found in the literature. This article provides an overview of bedside screening and assessment tools for patients with oropharyngeal dysphagia with emphasis on diagnostic performance and methodology.

BEDSIDE SCREENING
An Overview

It is generally agreed that the first step in the management of patients at risk for oropharyngeal dysphagia is bedside screening.[4] Bedside screening aims at identifying patients at risk for aspiration or unsafe swallowing as a step before further clinical assessment. Screening tools need to meet several criteria: easy administration, few time-consuming procedures, noninvasive methods avoiding distress to patients, and well-defined noncomplex training of health allied practitioners. Above all, screening methods need to be valid and reliable. In 2009, Bours and colleagues[5] published a systematic review on the psychometric characteristics of bedside screening tests for detecting dysphagia in adult patients with neurologic disorders using either VFS or FEES as a reference test. Meanwhile, Kertscher and colleagues[6] have carried out an updated review of the literature including recent literature up to December 2012. In both reviews, criteria on validity, generalizability, and reliability were adapted from the Dutch Cochrane Center (**Table 1**) and used to assess the methodologic quality of the included studies on diagnostic tests. An overview of studies with an overall sufficient methodologic quality is presented in **Table 2**. Next, diagnostic performance was determined by calculating prevalence, sensitivity, specificity, positive and negative predictive value, and likelihood ratio of a negative or positive test. Sufficient diagnostic performance was defined as high sensitivity ($\geq$70%) and moderate specificity ($\geq$60%). Studies showing sufficient methodologic quality and describing bedside screening tests having sufficient diagnostic performance are summarized in **Table 3**. The list of different types of bedside screening includes trial swallow tests using different aliquots of water, various viscosities and/or volumes, or combining the results of pulse oximetry. Furthermore, data are available on the application of oxygen desaturation using a single water swallow, the screening for clinical features during an oropharyngeal examination, and the implementation of a standardized form on clinical identifiers to detect unsafe swallow. The feasibility of the screening tests in terms of complexity and time required to execute the screening proved to be sufficient for all 10 studies. Further details on the studies that were included in the review, especially on other psychometric characteristics, such as likelihood ratios of screening tools, can be found in the original articles and in the systematic reviews by Bours and colleagues[5] and Kertscher and colleagues.[6]

Table 1
Criteria for methodologic quality assessment of studies (according to the Dutch Cochrane Center)

Number	Quality Criteria[a]	Domain
1	Were the reference test and the index test interpreted independently (blinded)?	Validity
2	Was the reference test applied to all patients who received the index test?	
3	Was the index test applied independent of relevant information on clinical data of the patient regarding the target condition?	
4	Was the period between the reference test and the index test short enough to be reasonably sure that the target condition did not change between the two tests? (within 24 h in acute stroke, and within 7 d in order neurologic diseases)	
5	Was the selection of the study population valid?	
6	Are data presented in enough detail to calculate appropriate test characteristic?	
7	Was the study population appropriate to evaluate the proposed use of the index test?	Generalizability
8	Was the index test described in detail so it could be reproduced?	Reliability
9	Were satisfactory definitions used for normal/abnormal reference test results and normal/abnormal index test results?	

[a] Scoring of criteria: +, if item has been addressed; −, if item has been violated; ?, if no information is available.

Data from Methodological Quality Assessment in Diagnostic Studies. Available at: http://www.cochrane.nl.

Selection of Bedside Screening

Summarizing all studies, both cited literature reviews conclude that no statistical pooling proved possible because of the heterogeneity of the bedside screening tests, the differences in implementation of tests, and diversity in end points either in the reference or in the index test. Only a few tests met the criteria for sufficient methodologic quality and diagnostic performance. Still, when deciding which type of bedside screening to implement in a clinical setting several factors need to be considered. First of all, the criteria used to describe study quality may sometimes be open to discussion and different interpretation.[22,23] Furthermore, the psychometric characteristics of a diagnostic test need to be taken into account. In both literature reviews[5,6] sufficient diagnostic performance was defined as high sensitivity and moderate specificity: sensitivity greater than or equal to 70% and specificity greater than or equal to 60%. These fixed cutoff points, however, could be argued. Apart from the fact that cutoff points may be somewhat arbitrary, possibly excluding screening tests by only failing a few percentages, different bedside tests may aim at different goals in distinct clinical settings. For example, the 3-oz water swallow test by Suiter and Leder[19] did meet the original methodologic quality standards but failed the criteria on psychometric characteristics. Although the sensitivity was very high (97%) the specificity was only 49%, suggesting an optimal patient safety by missing hardly any patients at risk for aspiration, but meanwhile having many false-negatives. Failing the screening protocol indicates the need for further assessment, but not all work settings may be

Table 2
Studies with sufficient methodologic quality[a]: type of bedside screening plus diagnostic performance[b]

References (N = 16)	Type of Bedside Screening	Diagnostic Performance
Chong et al,[7] 2003	Trial swallow using water	+
	Trial swallow using water in combination with oxygen desaturation	+
	Trial swallow using different viscosities in combination with oxygen desaturation	+
	Oxygen desaturation	−
Clavé et al,[8] 2008	Trial swallow using different viscosities	+
	Trial swallow using different viscosities in combination with oxygen desaturation	+
Daniels et al,[9] 1997	Trial swallow using water	−
	Clinical features	+
Leder & Espinosa,[10] 2002	Standardized form with clinical features	−
Lim et al,[11] 2001	Trial swallow using water	+
	Trial swallow using different viscosities in combination with oxygen desaturation	+
	Oxygen desaturation	+
Logemann et al,[12] 1999	Trial swallow using various viscosities	−
	Clinical features	−
	Standardized form with clinical features	−
Mann,[13] 2002	Standardized form with clinical features	+
Mari et al,[14] 1997	Trial swallow using water	−
Martino et al,[15] 2009	Trial swallow using water	+
McCullough et al,[16] 2001	Trial swallow using different viscosities	+
	Clinical features	−
	History components	−
Smith et al,[17] 2000	Trial swallow using different viscosities	+
	Trial swallow using different viscosities in combination with oxygen desaturation	+
	Oxygen desaturation	−
Smithard et al,[18] 1998	Trial swallow using water	+
Suiter & Leder,[19] 2008	Trial swallow using water	−
Trapl et al,[20] 2007	Trial swallow using different viscosities	+
Wakasugi et al,[21] 2008	Cough elicitation	−

[a] Methodologic quality is considered to be sufficient if no more than one criteria (see **Table 1**) has been allocated a minus or a question mark.
[b] Diagnostic performance is considered to be sufficient (+) when minimum criteria of specificity $\geq 60\%$ and sensitivity $\geq 70\%$ are met; other studies are indicated by a minus (−).
Data from Refs.[7–21]; Bours GJ, Speyer R, Lemmens J, et al. Bedside screening methods for dysphagia in neurologic patients: a systematic review. J Adv Nurs 2009;65(3):487; and Kertscher B, Speyer R, Palmieri M, et al. Bedside screening to detect oropharyngeal dysphagia in patients with neurologic disorders: an updated systematic review. 2013 Sep 13. [Epub ahead of print].

able to deal with so many requests for follow-up. Another choice to be made is the type of boluses used in the screening test. Clavé and colleagues[8] introduce the volume-viscosity swallowing test, a trial swallow protocol including three different viscosities and volumes. The test results may provide direct indications for choices on

Table 3
Overview of studies with sufficient methodologic quality and bedside screening with sufficient diagnostic performance (specificity ≥60% and sensitivity ≥70%)

Type of Bedside Screening	References (N = 11)	Description Bedside Screening	End Point Bedside Screening	Psychometric Characteristics	
				Sensitivity	Specificity
Trial swallow using water	Chong et al,[7] 2003	5 × 10 mL of water	Coughing, choking, or voice change	79	63
	Lim et al,[11] 2001	5 × 10 mL of water	Coughing, choking, or voice change	85	75
	Martino et al,[15] 2009	Toronto Bedside Swallowing Screening Test 1st step: screening for abnormalities (eg, breathiness, gurgles, hoarseness, whisper quality of voice, and tongue moments); 2nd step: 10 × 1 tsp. of water	Failure at any item (of 1st or 2nd step)	91 (all patients) 96 (acute patients) 80 (rehabilitation patients)	67 (all patients) 64 (acute patients) 68 (rehabilitation patients)
	Smithard et al,[18] 1998	1st step: 3 × 5 mL of water; 2nd step: 60 mL of water (in 2 min)	Coughing, choking, and/or wet voice: present in two out of three trials (1st step) or any swallow (2nd step) Assessment by physician	70	66

(continued on next page)

Table 3
(continued)

Type of Bedside Screening	References (N = 11)	Description Bedside Screening	End Point Bedside Screening	Psychometric Characteristics	
				Sensitivity	Specificity
Trial swallow using different viscosities	McCullough et al,[16] 2001	*4 sections*: history, oral motor (speech and praxis), voice, and trial swallows *Protocol trial swallows* Thin liquid (2 × 5 mL); Thick liquid (2 × 5 mL); Puree (2 × 5 mL); Solid (2 × 0.25 of a cookie)	Subjective overall judgment of likelihood of aspiration	78 (trial swallows)	63 (trial swallows)
	Smith et al,[17] 2000	Variety of quantities and consistencies	Subjective assessment of aspiration	80	68
	Trapl et al,[20] 2007	Gugging Swallowing Screen *1st step*: Indirect swallowing test (saliva test); *2nd step*: Direct swallowing test; Semisolid (one-third to one-half tsp., 5 × 0.50 tsp. of thickened water); Thin liquid (3, 5 10, 20, 50 mL of water); Solid (5 × small piece of dry bread)	Risk of aspiration on Gugging Swallowing Screen	100	63
	Clavé et al,[8] 2008	*Volume-Viscosity Swallowing Test* Nectar (5, 10, and 20 mL); Water (5, 10, and 20 mL); Pudding (5, 10, and 20 mL)	Penetration Piecemeal deglutition (multiple swallows per bolus)	84 88	65 87

Trial swallow using water in combination with oxygen desaturation	Chong et al,[7] 2003	*Water test* 5 × 10 mL of water *Pulse oximetry* (during fiberoptic endoscopic evaluation of swallowing) 3 to 5 spoons of 8 mL honey, nectar, thin and paste consistency	Coughing, choking, or voice change or ≥2% desaturation	94	63
Trial swallow using different viscosities in combination with oxygen desaturation	Chong et al,[7] 2003	*Water test* 5 × 10 mL of water *Pulse oximetry* (during fiberoptic endoscopic evaluation of swallowing) 3 to 5 spoons of 8 mL honey, nectar, thin and paste consistency	Coughing, choking, or voice change or ≥2% desaturation	94	63
	Clavé et al,[8] 2008	*Volume-Viscosity Swallowing Test* Nectar (5, 10, and 20 mL); Water (5, 10, and 20 mL); Pudding (5, 10, and 20 mL) *Finger pulse oximetry* (during Volume-Viscosity Swallowing Test)	Impaired safety (eg, voice change including wet voice, cough, or decrease in oxygen saturation ≥3%)	88	65
	Lim et al,[11] 2001	*Water test* 5 × 10 mL of water *Pulse oximetry* 10 mL of water	Coughing, choking, or voice change or ≥2% desaturation	98	70

(continued on next page)

Table 3
(continued)

Type of Bedside Screening	References (N = 11)	Description Bedside Screening	End Point Bedside Screening	Psychometric Characteristics	
				Sensitivity	Specificity
	Smith et al,[17] 2000	*Swallow test* Various quantities and viscosities *Pulse oximetry* (during videofluoroscopy) 3, 5, 10, and 20 mL thick liquid; Same quantities dilute liquid; 5 mL yoghurt; 5 ml solid (bread)	Subjective assessment of aspiration and ≥2% desaturation	73	76
Oxygen desaturation	Lim et al,[11] 2001	Oxygen desaturation test (10 mL of water)	≥2% desaturation	77	83
Clinical features	Daniels et al,[9] 1997	Oropharyngeal examination including examination of gag reflex, volitional cough, speech, and voice	Feature/end point: dysphonia (present/absent)	73	72
Standardized form with clinical features	Mann,[13] 2002	Clinical assessment including oral-motor-sensory examination (voice, speech, and language function)	Feature/end point: dysphagia (definite/probable/possible)	73	89
		Swallow test: 5 and 20 mL of water, thickened fluid	Feature/end point: aspiration (definite/probable/possible)	93	63

Data from Refs.[7–9,11,13,15–18,20], Bours GJ, Speyer R, Lemmens J, et al. Bedside screening methods for dysphagia in neurologic patients: a systematic review. J Adv Nurs 2009;65(3):483–7; and Kertscher B, Speyer R, Palmieri M, et al. Bedside screening to detect oropharyngeal dysphagia in patients with neurologic disorders: an updated systematic review. 2013 Sep 13. [Epub ahead of print].

oral intake after screening with regard to advised viscosities and volumes unlike, for example, the 3-oz water swallow test by Suiter and Leder[19] or the Toronto Bedside Swallowing Screening Test by Martino.[15] These two screening tools focus on identifying aspiration or dysphagia after which, in case of failing the screening protocol, further assessment is required. The concept of screening may differ from study to study and the distinction between what is considered to be screening and what is considered to be assessment may become an underlying issue.

Differences between screening protocols may not always have major implications for patients' well-being, but the consequences for health care professionals within their work settings may be substantial. In general, it is accepted that a screening tool needs to be valid, reliable, and feasible. Other requirements resulting from the implementation of a chosen screening protocol may affect the number of health care professionals involved, changes in workload and time pressure, or need for training of staff in screening procedures to improve outcome reliability. Furthermore, the availability of follow-up assessments, such as FEES or VFS, must be addressed and the need for trained personnel in performing these gold standard assessments. Future cost-effectiveness studies are required to measure the effects of bedside screening for oropharyngeal dysphagia in relation to increased health care costs because of the complications as a result of aspiration.

ASSESSMENT
Gold Standards

After screening for oropharyngeal dysphagia and failing the test protocol, further assessment is usually required. In the literature, VFS and FEES are taken as the gold standards for further assessment. Either one is used to assess the swallow physiology and functioning and to define the success or failure of swallowing therapy, frequently along with a variety of clinical evaluations, such as dysphagia severity ratings or dietary status.[24] As in bedside screening, protocols may differ in chosen cut-off points for aspiration or penetration, number of trial swallows, or bolus consistencies and volumes offered to the patient during assessment. No guidelines or consensus exist on protocols in either of the gold standards. Different types of variables may be measured using visuoperceptual ratings, although there are little data available on intrasubject or intersubject variability, or using one of many software applications to derive complementary objective measurements,[25,26] including spatial or temporal variables (**Table 4**).

Clinical Assessment

Another step after screening is clinical examination or assessment by a dysphagia therapist. Although in many countries swallowing assessment and treatment are provided by speech and language pathologists, there are exceptions. Other disciplines, such as occupational therapists, dieticians, nurses, or physiotherapists, also can be involved, or can even be the main health caretaker in a patient's dysphagia treatment. Many different definitions and descriptions of clinical assessments can be found in the literature. Miller,[33] for example, distinguishes in the process of clinical examination for dysphagia, the subjective description of the swallowing problem or patients' complaints, the medical history taking, the expert's clinical observations during interview and examination process, including the evaluation of a patient's mental status, and finally the physical examination. The clinical examination may fulfill multiple purposes: to identify possible causes of dysphagia and to assess swallowing safety or risk of aspiration; to decide on oral versus alternative feeding routes; to clarify the need for

Table 4
Screening and assessment of oropharyngeal dysphagia

Method	Description	Main Purposes	Health Caretakers
Bedside screening	Types: Trial swallow using water Trial swallow using different viscosities Trial swallow using water in combination with oxygen desaturation Trial swallow using different viscosities in combination with oxygen desaturation Oxygen desaturation Clinical features Standardized form with clinical features	To detect patients at risk for oropharyngeal dysphagia First step of decision-making process in patients at risk for oropharyngeal dysphagia Failure indicates need for further assessment	Usually, nurses or other health caretakers (eg, speech pathologist)
Gold standard	Videofluoroscopy of swallowing act (VFS) Visuoperceptual evaluation by experts Quantitative evaluation using software applications[25,26] Variables[27] Visuoperceptual variables: Penetration Aspiration Scale,[28] piecemeal deglutition Spatial variables: Quantification of changes in spatial dimensions (eg, hyoid movement) Temporal variables: timing and duration of changes in anatomic configuration (eg, duration of velopharyngeal junction) Fiberoptic Endoscopic Evaluation of Swallowing (FEES) Variables Mainly visuoperceptual variables	To detect and quantify abnormalities in swallowing function/physiology and/or anatomic structures Is considered to be the gold standard in diagnosing presence of (silent) aspiration, thus in determining safety of swallowing Although considered to be the gold standard, no consensus/guidelines about protocols for either FEES nor VFS	Usually, physician (eg, radiologist, neurologist, gastroenterologist, laryngologist) plus dysphagia therapist

Clinical assessment	Including, eg, Medical/patient history (eg, pneumonia, weight loss) Assessment of cognition and communication Evaluation of the oral, laryngeal, and pharyngeal anatomy, physiology, and function (including cranial nerve examination) Oral intake/nutritional status (eg, Functional Oral Intake Scale,[29] Mini Nutritional Assessment[30]) Mealtime observations Intervention trial (bolus modification, postural adjustments and/or swallow maneuvers)[1]	To detect and quantify abnormalities in swallowing function/physiology and/or anatomic structures To clarify the need for further assessment (eg, gold standard, supplementary methods) Assessment outcome may provide direct information for intervention/treatment by dysphagia therapist	Dysphagia therapist, usually a speech pathologist
Patient self-evaluation	Functional health status questionnaires (eg, 10-item Eating Assessment Tool,[39] Sydney Swallow Questionnaire[40]) Health-related quality of life questionnaires (see **Table 5**)	To describe the functional health status as experienced by the patient To describe the impact of oropharyngeal dysphagia on quality of life as experienced by the patient	Patient Patient
Supplementary methods	Examples: 1. Cough reflex testing 2. Cervical suscultation 3. Oxygen desaturation 4. FEESST[31] 5. Esophagography 6. Video manometry 7. EMG and sEMG 8. Esophageal Ph monitoring 9. Gastroesophageal/laryngopharyngeal reflux questionnaires	Corresponding main purposes: 1. To determine presence/absence of cough reflex 2. To detect (audible) residue in airways 3. To quantify reduced oxygen saturation of arterial blood 4. To quantify motor and sensory deficiencies during FEES 5. To visualize/detect abnormalities in esophageal function and/or anatomy	Depending on supplementary method: physician, dysphagia therapist, and/or researcher

(continued on next page)

Table 4
(continued)

Method	Description	Main Purposes	Health Caretakers
	10. Scintigraphy 11. Endoscopic ultrasound 12. Other imaging techniques: eg, computed tomography, magnetic resonance imaging, functional magnetic resonance imaging, positron emission tomography 13. Oral motor pressure measurements 14. Respiratory indicators (eg, sustained fever, rhonchi, sputum Gram stain, or sputum culture)	6. To assess oropharyngeal/esophageal motility, pressures and coordination during swallow (optional: combined with FEES/VFS) 7. To detect electrical potential activity within muscles (EMG) or muscle strength using surface electrodes (sEMG; eg, submental muscle placement) 8. To diagnose and quantify gastroesophageal reflux disease by measuring esophageal pH 9. To describe the functional health status and impact of gastroesophageal/laryngopharyngeal reflux as experienced by the patient 10. To visualize and track (radionuclide) bolus movement and residue/aspiration by use of a gamma camera 11. To study the oral aspects of bolus preparation and transfer (soft tissue visualization) 12. To visualize abnormalities in swallowing function/physiology and/or anatomic structures (different pros and cons per technique) 13. To quantify oral motor muscle pressure/strength[32] 14. To identify indicators associated with pneumonia[32]	

Abbreviations: EMG, electromyography; FEES, fiberoptic endoscopic evaluation of swallowing; FEESST, fiberoptic endoscopic evaluation of swallowing with sensory testing; VFS, videofluoroscopy.

further assessment (eg, FEES or VFS); and to establish baseline or pretreatment clinical data to be compared with follow-up assessment after intervention or during the course of progressive diseases. Other authors provide similar overviews on swallowing examination, but with different focus on issues relevant to specific subject populations. For example, in dysphagic patients with head and neck oncology the effects of irradiation and chemotherapy may be highly relevant in the diagnostic and prognostic management of the swallowing disorder, whereas in patients suffering from progressive neurologic diseases palliative care ethical questions, such as the maintaining of artificial feeding, may need to be addressed. Furthermore, clinical assessment may refer to a huge variety of assessment questionnaires and tools describing different aspects of oropharyngeal dysphagia. In the absence of systematic literature reviews it is hard to provide a complete overview.

Most clinical handbooks on dysphagia seem to agree on the relevance of the following elements in the assessment of dysphagia: the medical and patient history taking; the assessment of cognition and communication abilities; the evaluation of the oral, laryngeal, and pharyngeal physiology, anatomy, and functioning with special focus on the cranial nerve examination; and the oral intake assessment.[34–37] Medical and patient history may refer to medical chart reviewing to retrieve information on such factors as diseases associated with dysphagia; respiratory impairment or use of medication; the occurrence of (possibly recurrent) pneumonia; or sudden weight loss. The dietary level and the nutritional status can be reviewed by such instruments as the Functional Oral Intake Scale by Crary and colleagues[29] or the Mini Nutritional Assessment by Guigoz,[30] in addition to mealtime observations and trial swallows providing patients with liquid and food boluses of different consistencies and volumes possibly in combination with postural adjustments and swallow maneuvers.[1] **Table 4** presents examples of commonly used assessment procedures for dysphagia in clinical practice. However, little information has been published on the validity and reliability of this process of clinical assessment for dysphagia.

Patient Self-Evaluation

Patient self-evaluation (see **Table 4**) is covered by self-administered questionnaires. Two different concepts need to be distinguished: functional health status (FHS) versus health-related quality of life (HRQOL). FHS refers to the influence of a given disease, oropharyngeal dysphagia, on particular functional aspects, whereas HRQOL is the unique personal perception of someone's health, taking into account social, functional, and psychological issues.[38] Even though FHS and HRQOL are considered two distinct concepts, many inventories combine them, making it hard to distinguish between disease-related functioning and disease-related quality-of-life as experienced by the patient.

In general, self-administered FHS inventories aim at quantifying the symptomatic severity of oropharyngeal dysphagia as experienced by the patient. Several examples are found in the literature, such as the Eating Assessment Tool (EAT-10)[39] or the Sydney Swallow Questionnaire (SSQ).[40] The first questionnaire, the EAT-10, is a clinical instrument for documenting the initial dysphagia severity and monitoring a patient's treatment response. Ten symptom-specific items using five-point scales (0–4: no problem to severe problem) result in a total score ranging between zero and 40. Based on normative data, an EAT-10 score of three or higher is considered to be abnormal, thus distinguishing between normal and abnormal swallow behavior.[39] The SSQ contains 17 items recorded as visual analogue scales. Wallace and colleagues[40] ascribe strong face, content, and construct validity and test-retest reliability to the SSQ. Although many FHS questionnaires can be found in the literature, restricted data are available on the measurement properties of these health status questionnaires.

Table 5
Questionnaires on HRQoL in oropharyngeal dysphagia

References (N = 5)	HRQoL Questionnaire	Abbreviation	Domains (N_items)	Total Number of Items[a] (including one single item)	Single Items (N_items)	Rating Scale	Range of Total Score[b]
Chen et al,[42] 2001	MD Anderson Dysphagia Inventory	MDADI	Physical (8) Functional (5) Emotional (6)	20 (including one single item)	Global assessment (1)	5-point scale	20–100
Ekberg et al,[43] 2002	European Dysphagia Group Questionnaire[c]	EDGQ	Background data (3) Eating habits (5) Personal feelings and importance (8) Seeking help (8) Medical status (4)	28	NA	Mostly dichotomous scale (plus "Don't know" option)	NA
McHorney et al,[2] 2002 McHorney et al,[44,45] 2000	SWAL-QOL	SWAL-QOL	Burden (2) Eating duration (2) Eating desire (3) Symptom frequency (14) Food selection (2) Communication (2) Fear (4) Mental health (5) Social functioning (5) Fatigue (3) Sleep (2)	44	Food and liquid intake (3) Global health (1)	5-point scale	0–100
Silbergleit et al,[46] 2012	Dysphagia Handicap Index	DHI	Physical (9) Functional (9) Emotional (7)	25	Severity (1)	3-point scale	0–100
Woisard et al,[47] 2006	Deglutition Handicap Index	DHI	Physical (10) Functional (10) Emotional (10)	30	NA	5-point scale	0–120

[a] Total scores based on total number of items excluding single items, except for the MDADI (one single item included in the total score).
[b] In case of MDADI and SWAL-QOL low scores indicate low functioning and high scores high functioning, whereas in case of the Deglutition Handicap Index and the Dysphagia Handicap Index low scores indicate high functioning and high scores low functioning.
[c] Interview (in contrast to all other self-administered questionnaires).

Adapted from Timmerman AA, Speyer R, Heijnen BJ, et al. Psychometric characteristics of health-related quality of life questionnaires in oropharyngeal dysphagia. In press; with permission.

More recently, quality-of-life questionnaires too have become part of the assessment protocol for swallowing disorders, taking a patient's well-being into consideration when judging the effects of a therapy.[24] **Table 5** provides an overview of questionnaires describing mainly HRQOL in oropharyngeal dysphagia as retrieved by systematic literature search.[41] One of the earliest published questionnaires, the SWAL-QOL by McHorney and colleagues,[2,44,45] is still considered the gold standard and exhibits good internal-consistency reliability and short-term reproducibility. However, because of the rather large number of 11 subscales and 44 items, this questionnaire is not always considered to be the best choice for daily clinical practice with a lot of time pressure. In that light other questionnaires have been developed. Before being able to choose which instruments should be used, measurement properties of these questionnaires need to be determined and compared with quality criteria, such as those defined by Terwee and colleagues.[48] **Table 6** provides an overview of definitions of measurement properties of health status questionnaires based on a classification according to Terwee and colleagues.[48]

Supplementary Methods

Apart from the previously mentioned methods, several other evaluation techniques are available for assessment of dysphagia (see **Table 4**). Although some of these methods are well-known and commonly used, other techniques are less frequently applied and

Table 6	
Definitions of measurement properties of health status questionnaire	
Measurement Property[a]/Domain	**Definition**
Content validity	The extent to which the measurement incorporates the construct or domain of the phenomenon under study.
Internal consistency	The extent to which items in a (sub)scale are intercorrelated, thus measuring the same construct.
Criterion validity	The extent to which the measurement correlates with an external criterion (gold standard) of the phenomenon under study.
Construct validity	The extent to which a measurement corresponds to theoretical concepts (constructs) concerning the phenomenon under study.
Reproducibility	Synonym: repeatability. The degree to which repeated measurements in stable persons (test-retest) provide similar answers.
Agreement	The extent to which the scores on repeated measures are close to each other (absolute measurement error).
Reliability	The extent to which patients can be distinguished from each other, despite measurement errors (relative measurement error).
Responsiveness	The ability of a questionnaire to detect clinically important changes over time in the construct to be measured.
Floor or ceiling effect	The number of respondents who achieved the lowest or highest possible score.
Interpretability	The degree to which qualitative meaning, clinical or commonly understood connotations, can be assigned to an instrument's quantitative scores or change in scores.

[a] Classification according to Terwee and colleagues.
Adapted from Refs.[48–52]

restricted only to experimental settings. **Table 4** presents a quick glance at the variety in supplementary methods; it is beyond the scope of this article to describe the advantages and disadvantages of each method in more detail. Furthermore, the list of supplementary methods in **Table 4** is not complete because improved methods have replaced older techniques (eg, the present use of VFS recordings instead of a single radiograph image of the swallow act) and newly developed methods continue to be presented. The latter include the introduction of dual-axis swallowing accelerometry as a tool for noninvasive analysis of swallowing function[53] and the use of acoustic analysis or airflow measurement of voluntary cough to help in detecting dysphagia.[54,55] Choices of supplementary methods may be influenced by factors related to workplace setting, research, clinician's preference and expertise, and criteria on reliability and validity.

SUMMARY

Because patients do not necessarily show abnormalities or changes after treatment intervention in all aspects of swallowing, it may be useful to include several evaluation techniques when studying swallowing problems. For example, objectified findings on VFS or endoscopic recordings of swallowing may not be consistent with a patient's own judgment of therapy outcome.[24] It is clear from the literature that many different screening and clinical assessment or instrumental examination tools are being used in daily practice. Pettigrew and O'Toole[56] described an international concern for clinician disagreement in the profession of speech and language therapy regarding the variability in conducting clinical examinations and clinical decision-making in dysphagia. Clinicians not only use a wide range of assessment tools; they also make different choices about outcome parameters, rating procedures, or protocols. Even for the gold standards, FEES and VFS, no agreement exists on the number of swallow trials, the bolus consistencies, or volumes to be used.[1]

Apart from the great diversity in screening and assessment of dysphagia, methodologic problems in research and clinical practice are common and need to be considered. These problems include inadequate randomization during patient allocation to different intervention groups; lack of blinding assessors to moment of measurement (eg, pretreatment vs posttreatment); and failure to apply the intention-to-treat principle to all participating patients. In addition, the frequent use of unvalidated or unreliable instruments or questionnaires may generate data that cannot be interpreted adequately and, therefore, result in data that actually do not contribute to formal patient examination.[24] In light of these methodologic problems and the heterogeneity of study designs reported in the literature, statistical pooling of outcome data usually remains a hazardous challenge.[1] To improve the quality of clinical measurements, the reliability and validity of health questionnaires need to be determined and compared with criteria on measurement properties (eg, Terwee and colleagues[48]). Furthermore, information on interrater and intrarater reliability should be provided when describing visuoperceptual evaluation of videorecordings (eg, FEES or VFS) or perceptual assessment of voice samples. Despite great variety in screening and assessment tools for dysphagia, the use of an instrument can only be justified by its sufficient reliability and validity and the discriminative and evaluative purposes of the assessment.[57]

The lack of consensus, protocols, and guidelines for screening and assessment of oropharyngeal dysphagia is striking, both in the literature and in daily clinical practice. There is an urgent need for standardization in terminology, specified protocols for different examination tools, and well-defined clinical pathways for distinct patient populations with oropharyngeal dysphagia. Recent international initiatives seem promising, such as the foundation of the International Dysphagia Diet Standardisation

Initiative, a clinical expert group that aims at the development of global standardized terminology and definitions for texture modified foods and thickened liquids. Furthermore, a growing number of associations of clinical professionals are involved in evidence-based guideline development including aspects of screening and assessment (eg, the European Society for Swallowing Disorders; the European Society for Clinical Nutrition and Metabolism). Despite international increased awareness of oropharyngeal dysphagia and its impact on a patient's well-being or need for early screening and assessment, future implementation of newly developed guidelines in clinical practice and in the education of professionals will prove essential when evaluating the final outcome of initiatives on standardization and guideline development in the field of oropharyngeal dysphagia.

REFERENCES

1. Speyer R. Behavioural treatment of oropharyngeal dysphagia: bolus modification and management, sensory and motor behavioural techniques, postural adjustments, and swallow manoeuvres. In: Ekberg O, editor. Dysphagia: diagnosis and treatment. Berlin: Springer-Verlag; 2012. p. 477–91.
2. McHorney CA, Robbins J, Lomax K, et al. The SWAL-QOL and SWAL-CARE outcomes tool for oropharyngeal dysphagia in adults: III. Documentation of reliability and validity. Dysphagia 2002;17:97–114.
3. Perry L, Love CP. Screening for dysphagia and aspiration in acute stroke: a systematic review. Dysphagia 2001;16:7–18.
4. Takizawa C, Altman KW, Derex L, et al. Clinical pathway of stroke patients - Opinion paper on dysphagia treatment pathway (under review).
5. Bours GJ, Speyer R, Lemmens J, et al. Bedside screening methods for dysphagia in neurologic patients: a systematic review. J Adv Nurs 2009;65(3):477–93.
6. Kertscher B, Speyer R, Palmieri M, et al. Bedside screening to detect oropharyngeal dysphagia in patients with neurological disorders: an updated systematic review. In press.
7. Chong MS, Lieu PK, Sitoh YY, et al. Bedside clinical methods useful as screening test for aspiration in elderly patients with recent and previous strokes. Ann Acad Med Singap 2003;32(6):790–4.
8. Clavé P, Arreola V, Romea M, et al. Accuracy of the volume-viscosity swallow test for clinical screening of oropharyngeal dysphagia and aspiration. Clin Nutr 2008; 27:806–15.
9. Daniels SK, McAdam CP, Brailey K. Clinical assessment of swallowing and prediction of dysphagia severity. Am J Speech Lang Pathol 1997;6(4):17–24.
10. Leder SB, Espinosa JF. Aspiration risk after acute stroke: comparison of clinical examination and fiberoptic endoscopic evaluation of swallowing. Dysphagia 2002;17(3):214–8.
11. Lim SH, Lieu PK, Phua SY, et al. Accuracy of bedside clinical methods compared with fiberoptic endoscopic examination of swallowing (FEES) in determining the risk of aspiration in acute stroke patients. Dysphagia 2001;16(1):1–6.
12. Logemann JA, Veis S, Colangelo L. A screening procedure for oropharyngeal dysphagia. Dysphagia 1999;14(1):44–51.
13. Mann GD. MASA: the Mann assessment of swallowing ability. Dysphagia series. New York: Singular Thomson Learning; 2002.
14. Mari F, Matei M, Ceravolo MG, et al. Predictive value of clinical indices in detecting aspiration in patients with neurological disorders. J Neurol Neurosurg Psychiatry 1997;63(4):456–60.

15. Martino R, Silver F, Teasell R, et al. The Toronto Bedside Swallowing Screening Test (TOR-BSST) development and validation of a dysphagia screening tool for patients with stroke. Stroke 2009;40:555–61.
16. McCullough GH, Wertz RT, Rosenbek JC. Sensitivity and specificity of clinical/bedside examination signs for detecting aspiration in adults subsequent to stroke. J Commun Disord 2001;34:55–72.
17. Smith HA, Lee SH, O'Neill PA, et al. The combination of bedside swallowing assessment and oxygen saturation monitoring of swallowing in acute stroke: a safe and humane screening tool. Age Ageing 2000;29(6):495–9.
18. Smithard DG, O'Neill PA, Park C, et al. Can bedside assessment reliably exclude aspiration following acute stroke? Age Ageing 1998;27(2):99–106.
19. Suiter DM, Leder SB. Clinical utility of the 3-ounce water swallowing test. Dysphagia 2008;23:244–50.
20. Trapl M, Enderle P, Nowotny M, et al. Dysphagia bedside screening for acute stroke patients. The Gugging swallowing screen. Stroke 2007;38:2948–52.
21. Wakasugi Y, Tohara H, Hattori F, et al. Screening test for silent aspiration at the bedside. Dysphagia 2008;23:364–70.
22. Steele C, Cichero JA. Screening for aspiration risk [letters to the editor]. J Trauma Acute Care Surg 2012;73(1):292–3.
23. Leder SB, Suiter DM, Warner HL, et al. Re: screening for aspiration risk [letters to the editor]. J Trauma Acute Care Surg 2012;73(1):293.
24. Speyer R, Baijens L, Heijnen M, et al. Effects of therapy in oropharyngeal dysphagia by speech and language therapists: a systematic review. Dysphagia 2010;25:40–65.
25. Clavé P, De Kraa M, Arreola V, et al. The effect of bolus viscosity on swallowing function in neurogenic dysphagia. Aliment Pharmacol Ther 2006;24:1385–94.
26. Rofes L, Arreola V, Cabré M, et al. Diagnosis and management of oropharyngeal dysphagia and its nutritional and respiratory complications in the elderly. Gastroenterol Res Pract 2011;13. http://dx.doi.org/10.1155/2011/818979.
27. Baijens LW, Speyer R, Lima Passos V, et al. Swallowing in Parkinson patients versus healthy controls: reliability of measurements in videofluoroscopy. Gastroenterol Res Pract 2011;9. http://dx.doi.org/10.1155/2011/380682.
28. Rosenbek JC, Robbins JA, Roecker EB, et al. A penetration-aspiration scale. Dysphagia 1996;11:93–8.
29. Crary MA, Carnaby Mann GD, Groher ME. Initial psychometric assessment of a functional oral intake scale for dysphagia in stroke patients. Arch Phys Med Rehabil 2005;86:1516–20.
30. Guigoz G. The mini nutritional assessment (MNA) review of the literature – what does it tell us? J Nutr Health Aging 2006;10(6):466–87.
31. Aviv JE, Kim T, Sacco RL, et al. FEESST: a new bedside endoscopic test of the motor and sensory components of swallowing. Ann Otol Rhinol Laryngol 1998;107:378–87.
32. Robbins J, Kays SA, Gangnon RE, et al. The effects of lingual exercise in stroke patients with dysphagia. Arch Phys Med Rehabil 2007;88(2):150–8.
33. Miller RM. Clinical examination for dysphagia. In: Groher ME, editor. Dysphagia: diagnosis and management. Newton (MA): Butterworth-Heinemann; 1997. p. 169–89.
34. Daniels SK, Huckabee ML. Dysphagia following stroke. San Diego (CA): Plural Publishing; 2008.
35. Goodrich SJ, Walker AI. Clinical swallow evaluation. In: Leonard R, Kendall K, editors. Dysphagia assessment and treatment planning: a team approach. San Diego (CA): Plural Publishing; 2008. p. 103–36.

36. Groher ME. Clinical evaluation of adults. In: Groher ME, Crary MA, editors. Dysphagia: clinical management in adults and children. Maryland Heights (MI): Mosby Elsevier; 2010. p. 162–90.
37. Murry T, Carrau RL. Evaluation of dysphagia. In: Clinical management of swallowing disorders: Evaluation of dysphagia. San Diego (CA): Plural Publishing; 2006. p. 97–136.
38. Ferrans CE, Zerwic JJ, Wilbur JE, et al. Conceptual model of health-related quality of life. J Nurs Scholarsh 2005;4:336–42.
39. Belafsky PC, Mouadeb DA, Rees CJ, et al. Validity and reliability of the Eating Assessment Tool (EAT-10). Ann Otol Rhinol Laryngol 2008;117(12):919–24.
40. Wallace KL, Middleton S, Cook IJ. Development and validation of a self-report symptom inventory to assess the severity of oral-pharyngeal dysphagia. Gastroenterology 2000;118(4):678–87.
41. Timmerman AA, Speyer R, Heijnen BJ, et al. Psychometric characteristics of health-related quality of life questionnaires in oropharyngeal dysphagia (under review).
42. Chen AY, Frankowski R, Bishop-Leone J, et al. The development and validation of a dysphagia-specific quality-of-life questionnaire for patients with head and neck cancer: the MD Anderson Dysphagia Inventory. Arch Otolaryngol Head Neck Surg 2001;127:870–6.
43. Ekberg O, Hamdy S, Woisard V, et al. Social and psychological burden of dysphagia: its impact on diagnosis and treatment. Dysphagia 2002;17:139–46.
44. McHorney CA, Bricker DE, Kramer AE, et al. The SWAL-QOL outcomes tool for oropharyngeal dysphagia in adults: I. Conceptual foundation and item development. Dysphagia 2000;15:115–21.
45. Mchorney CA, Bricker DE, Robbins JA, et al. The SWAL-QOL outcomes tool for oropharyngeal dysphagia in adults: II. Item reduction and preliminary scaling. Dysphagia 2000;15:122–33.
46. Silbergleit AK, Schultz L, Jacobson BH, et al. The dysphagia handicap index: development and validation. Dysphagia 2012;27:46–52.
47. Woisard V, Andrieux MP, Puech M. Validation of a self assessment questionnaire for swallowing disorders (Deglutition Handicap Index). Rev Laryngol Otol Rhinol (Bord) 2006;127(5):315–25.
48. Terwee CB, Bot SD, de Boer MR, et al. Quality criteria were proposed for measurement properties of health status questionnaires. J Clin Epidemiol 2007;60:34–42.
49. Last JM, editor. A dictionary of epidemiology. Oxford (United Kingdom): Oxford University Press; 2001.
50. Mokkink LB, Terwee CB, Patrick DL, et al. COSMIN checklist manual. 2012. Available at: www.cosmin.nl. Accessed March 5, 2013.
51. Everitt BS. Medical statistics from A to Z: a guide for clinicians and medical students. Cambridge (United Kingdom): Cambridge University Press; 2006.
52. McHorney CA, Tarlov AR. Individual-patient monitoring in clinical practice: are available health status surveys adequate? Qual Life Res 1995;4(4):293–307.
53. Lee J, Sejdić E, Steele CM, et al. Effects of liquid stimuli on dual-axis swallowing accelerometry signals in a healthy population. Biomed Eng Online 2010;9:7. Available at: http://www.biomedical-engineering-online.com/content/9/1/7.
54. Smith Hammond CA, Goldstein LB, Horner RD, et al. Predicting aspiration in patients with ischemic stroke: comparison of clinical signs and aerodynamic measures of voluntary cough. Chest 2009;135(3):769–77.
55. Pitts T, Troche M, Mann G, et al. Using voluntary cough to detect penetration and aspiration during oropharyngeal swallowing in patients with Parkinson disease. Chest 2010;138(6):1426–31.

56. Pettigrew CM, O'Toole C. Dysphagia evaluation practices of speech and language therapist in Ireland: clinical assessment and instrumental examination decision-making. Dysphagia 2007;22:235–44.

57. Speyer R, Pilz W, Kruis van der J, et al. Reliability and validity of student peer assessment in medical education: a systematic review. Med Teach 2011;33: e572–85.

The Modified Barium Swallow and the Functional Endoscopic Evaluation of Swallowing

Susan Brady, MS, CCC-SLP, BRS-S[a],*, Joseph Donzelli, MD[b]

KEYWORDS

- Deglutition • Dysphagia • Endoscopy • Fluoroscopy • Swallow

KEY POINTS

- It is important for physicians and clinicians to have a basic understanding of the protocols for both the modified barium swallow (MBS) and functional endoscopic evaluation of swallowing (FEES), including indications for use, advantages, and disadvantages.
- The MBS and FEES are valuable swallowing diagnostic tools and show good agreement with diagnostic findings as related to tracheal aspiration, laryngeal penetration, pharyngeal residue, diet level, and compensatory swallow safety strategies.
- The determination of which procedure is needed to evaluate swallowing function is driven by specific patient characteristics and the field of view necessary to evaluate the suspected dysphagia.
- Both the MBS and FEES should be considered the gold standard for evaluating the swallow.

NATURE OF THE PROBLEM

Dysphagia can be a symptom of several different underlying medical conditions or diseases (**Fig. 1**). The swallowing disorder may result from either a specific anatomic (ie, tumor or genetic malformation) or physiologic/functional issue (ie, sensation loss, coordination, or muscle paralysis). Regardless of the underlying medical condition, in order to effectively treat swallowing disorders such as providing appropriate dietary recommendations, behavior management strategies, and rehabilitation exercises, the health care team first need to correctly identify the specific biomechanical aspects of the swallowing function through the appropriate use and interpretation of a diagnostic

Financial Disclosures: The authors have no relevant financial disclosures regarding this topic.
[a] Departments of Speech-Language Pathology and Clinical Education, Swallowing Center, Marianjoy Rehabilitation Hospital, 26 West 171 Roosevelt Road, Wheaton, IL 60187, USA;
[b] Department of Otolaryngology, Midwest ENT, Springbrook Medical Center, 1247 Rickert Drive, Naperville, IL 60540, USA
* Corresponding author.
E-mail address: sbrady@marianjoy.org

Otolaryngol Clin N Am 46 (2013) 1009–1022
http://dx.doi.org/10.1016/j.otc.2013.08.001
0030-6665/13/$ – see front matter © 2013 Elsevier Inc. All rights reserved.

Abbreviations	
FEES	Fiber-optic endoscopic examination of the swallow
MBS	Modified barium swallow
SLP	Speech language pathologist

swallow procedure. The purpose of a diagnostic swallow procedure is to assess dysphagia and when appropriate make recommendations for diet level, swallow safety strategies, and swallowing rehabilitation interventions.[1]

The 2 most common diagnostic swallowing procedures available are the modified barium swallow (MBS) and the functional endoscopic evaluation of swallowing (FEES). Both procedures have been validated and have published evidence-based guidelines developed in accordance with the scientific evidence available in the literature for the performance and interpretation of these examinations.[2,3] The MBS has been available since the 1950s and incorporates the use of a radiograph along with barium in order to evaluate the physiology of the swallow function.[4] The MBS is known by several different names, such as the videofluoroscopic swallow study, cookie swallow, pharyngogram with videorecording, or video pharyngogram.[5]

The FEES, compared with the MBS, is a newer procedure and evaluates swallow function using nasal endoscopy.[6,7] The FEES is also known as the fiber-optic endoscopic evaluation of swallowing[6] or the videoendoscopic evaluation of the swallow.[7] The challenge for physicians and clinicians is to determine when the MBS or the FEES is the preferred swallowing test. This article describes both procedures, compares and contrasts the MBS and FEES, and discusses clinical indications for each procedure in order to assist the health care provider with this decision-making process.

MBS PROCEDURE
Key Points of Procedure

The MBS allows for the identification of normal and abnormal anatomy and physiology of the swallow as viewed by radiograph. The MBS also evaluates the integrity of airway protection before, during, and after the swallow. The MBS is used to evaluate the effectiveness of bolus modifications, postural changes, and swallowing maneuvers to improve swallowing safety and efficiency.[2] The potential variations to the MBS protocol along with equipment needs and radiation considerations are reviewed in this section.

Technique Summary

The MBS examination involves the use of barium and fluoroscopy to assess the oral and pharyngeal phase of the swallow. The fluoroscopic images allow for the motion-picture radiograph of the dynamic swallow function.[8] The assessment of the esophagus is usually not a major component of the MBS; however, a screening of the esophageal phase of the swallow during the MBS may be conducted.[5] The MBS is usually recorded for the availability of further review and analysis. Traditionally, the MBS is completed in the radiology department with a radiologist, radiology technician, and a swallowing clinician (usually a speech language pathologist [SLP]).

MBS Protocol Summary

The standard MBS protocol developed by Logemann[9] has been the basis for the development of many subsequent protocols. Although in clinical practice there are many variations in the standard clinical protocol for the MBS, **Table 1** summarizes

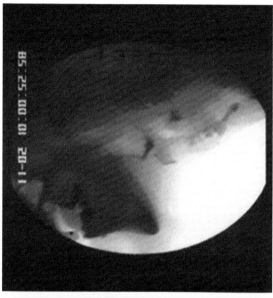
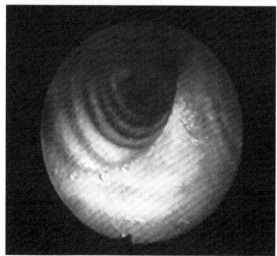

Fig. 1. View of aspiration on FEES versus MBS.

Table 1
MBS protocol and potential variations

MBS Protocol	Potential Variations
Type of barium	Specific type of barium used during the MBS (eg, Varibar [E-Z – EM Inc., Melville, NY])
Ratio of food to barium mixtures	Specific recipes used for mixing barium suspension with food and liquid
Bolus consistencies	Honey thick liquids, nectar thick liquids, thin liquids, pureed, ground, chopped, bread/cookie, raw vegetable
Bolus size	1 mL, 3 mL, 5 mL, small cup sip, uncontrolled large sip, consecutive swallows, 30 mL
Method of bolus presentation	Clinician administered vs patient self-feeding; liquids by spoon, cup, and straw
Sequence of bolus presentation	Variation in the specific consistency to begin protocol (ie, thin vs nectar thick vs pudding)
Number of bolus presentations for each specific bolus	Many protocols range from 1 to 3 presentations for each bolus
Evaluation of bolus modifications, postural changes, and swallowing maneuvers to improve swallow efficiency and safety	Interventions such as sour boluses, chin tuck, head turn, oral holding, supraglottic swallow, supersupraglottic swallow, throat clear, multiple swallows, Mendelsohn maneuver
Esophageal screen	Debate regarding if esophageal screen should be routinely performed within the MBS protocol and how it should be conducted

the details of most MBS protocols as well as the potential variations. The challenge in clinical practice is to determine when it is necessary to perform a standardized protocol versus performing a tailor-made study designed to match typical eating behaviors.[10] In addition, when designing an MBS protocol for clinical practice, the examiner must take into account how to obtain as much information about the swallow function with the minimum amount of radiation exposure. If advancing a patient to test a particular bolus consistency or size is determined not safe for the patient, then it is often deferred during the MBS protocol.

Equipment

The basic fluoroscopic unit required for completion of the MBS consists of a constant radiograph source, a radiograph detector, a monitor, and recording system. The constant radiograph source of the fluoroscopy system is the radiograph tube powered by a moderately complex generator, which provides the radiograph beam. The energy and quantity of radiographs are modulated by a feedback mechanism within the unit, and the appropriate amount of radiographs is produced based on the thickness and density of the tissue/body part. During the MBS, the patient must be correctly centered in order for the feedback system of the radiograph machine to function properly. Placed between the patient who is receiving the MBS and the radiograph tube is a collimator, which can be adjusted to limit the size and shape of the radiograph beam. The radiograph detector of the fluoroscopy system is the image intensifier, which is an electronic cylinder that converts radiograph energy into light. This step is required in order for the radiograph to be visualized by the camera for viewing on a monitor and be available for recording.[5] Specialized chairs have been made for the MBS examinations to fit into the space between the table and the image intensifier tower. Furthermore, mobile fluoroscopic units (C-arm systems) have fluoroscopic capability and may also be used for MBS. When using a C-arm system, a regular chair or wheelchair may be used for the patient.

Radiation

The amount of radiation exposure is dependent on time exposure, distance from the radiograph tube, and shielding. Radiation dose during the MBS is lower than a routine chest computed tomography (CT) and it would take more than 40 MBS examinations in a year to exceed the annual radiation exposure dose limits.[11] Using a recording device assists with reducing the amount of radiation time that the patient and health care team may be exposed to by reducing the number of swallows required during the MBS. During the MBS, the patient must remain close to the radiograph tube in order to obtain the radiograph images; however, because of radiation scatter, health care team members should distance themselves as far as possible from the radiograph tube. This distance may be accomplished by allowing the patient to feed themselves whenever possible. Shielding protocols should be followed in order to reduce radiation exposure. For patients (especially children), a lap shield can be used to protect reproductive organs from radiation. Health care team members conducting the MBS, if they are not behind a lead glass shield, should also wear a thyroid collar, full lead apron, and protective eye goggles.[5]

FEES PROCEDURE

Key Points of Procedure

The FEES examination allows for an evaluation of the anatomic structures, secretion levels, swallowing ability, and sensory ability. The use of topical anesthesia, sensory testing, assessment of secretion level, swallowing ability, use of blue food coloring, and pediatric considerations are discussed in this section.

Technique Summary

The FEES examination requires a flexible laryngoscope with a halogen or xenon light source. The endoscopist can visualize the image directly through the eyepiece or by using a chip camera attached to the laryngoscope. When using a chip camera, the image can then be viewed on a monitor and recorded for further analysis. A complete FEES examination includes an assessment of the anatomic structures at rest and in movement, the accumulated oropharyngeal secretion level, and bolus flow of various foods and liquids while swallowing. If difficulty with swallowing is observed, then there are several therapeutic interventions that may be performed during the FEES in order to evaluate the effectiveness of the intervention.[1]

Assessment of Anatomy

The FEES not only identifies the signs and symptoms of dysphagia, it is also capable of providing a view of the anatomy and physiology of the swallow.[2] A common physiologic abnormality observed during the FEES is the presence of reduced vocal fold mobility. This reduction in vocal fold mobility has been associated with increased incidence of aspiration.[12]

Topical Anesthesia

The use of a topical anesthesia during the FEES is part of some protocols. Although some physicians and clinicians choose to use a topical anesthesia during the FEES, a systematic review of the literature[13] found no evidence to support reduce pain or discomfort when using a topical treatment before nasal endoscopy. In addition, for nonphysicians performing the FEES, the administration of a topical anesthesia varies by state laws, and clinicians should be aware of local rules and regulations.[2]

Sensory Testing

Understanding the relationship between sensory input, airway protection, and swallowing ability is an important clinical component of the FEES.[14] During the FEES, sensation may be either directly assessed with light touching of the endoscope to the pharyngeal/laryngeal structures or indirectly assessed based on the patient's response to the presence of pharyngeal residue, laryngeal penetration, or aspiration.[2,14] Further, there are specialized endoscopes with an instrument channel that allows for the delivery of calibrated puffs of air to the mucosa of the larynx. The addition of the puffs of air during the examination is known as the fiber-optic endoscopic evaluation of swallowing with sensory testing (FEESST) and was first described by Aviv and colleagues.[15] During the FEESST, sensation is inferred by monitoring the laryngeal adductor reflex, which is elicited after the delivery of the puffs of air. The degree of sensory deficit is inferred by the amount of calibrated puffs of air required to elicit the laryngeal adductor reflex.[15] The utilization of FEESST is not a required element for the FEES.

Secretion Level

Suspected or observed difficulty swallowing saliva or secretions is a clinical indication for the performance of the FEES. Before any bolus presentation, the clinical protocol involves an observation of secretions, including describing the amount and location.[2] Evaluation of secretion levels with a reliable measure is imperative, because clinicians should be able to use this information in order to quickly differentiate between safe levels of accumulated secretions and those that are dangerously high. Furthermore, by being able to quickly discern the secretion levels, the examiner is potentially able to provide better and more appropriate treatment, thus reducing the incidence or complication of aspiration pneumonia and its associated health care costs.[16] Various secretion scales are available in the literature, and **Table 2** provides an example of a

Table 2 Secretion severity scale	
Secretion Level	**Description**
Level 1: functional level	No endolaryngeal secretions present. The accumulation/pooling of pharyngeal secretions may range from none/minimal to >25% in the pyriform sinuses or vallecular space
Level 2: severe level	Endolaryngeal secretions are present. Laryngeal penetration of secretions above the level of the true vocal cords; intermittent laryngeal penetration of secretions on inhalation; but no aspiration of secretions observed
Level 3: profound level	Secretions present at or below the level of the vocal cords

Adapted from Donzelli J, Brady S, Wesling M, et al. Predictive value of accumulated oropharyngeal secretions for aspiration during video nasal endoscopic evaluation of the swallow. Ann Otol Rhinol Laryngol 2003;112(5):470; with permission.

3-point secretion scale developed by Donzelli and colleagues,[17] which measures the presence, amount, and location of oropharyngeal secretions. With this 3-point secretion scale, the score that the patient receives is the point of maximum secretions present (no transition score is available). A higher score indicates more secretions. The 3-point secretion scale also distinguishes between laryngeal penetration and aspiration of secretions. The predictive validity of the 3-point secretion scale in relation to aspiration revealed that this scale is correlated to aspiration (Spearman ρ .516, $P<.0001$) and to diet outcome recommendations (Spearman ρ .72, $P<.0001$), with patients receiving a higher secretion level being more likely to aspirate and also to receive a lower diet level or be nil by mouth.[17]

Use of Blue Food Coloring

Some FEES protocols involve using food coloring (eg, FD&C Blue No. 1) mixed with the food and liquid in order to enhance the visualization of the bolus so that the examiner may discern the bolus from surrounding oropharyngeal mucosa, secretion, and for the detection of laryngeal penetration or aspiration. The amount of blue dye added to the food and liquid used during the FEES is small (1–2 mL). Although some physicians and clinicians choose to use blue dye during the FEES, some potential risks are related to increased gastrointestinal permeability. Some adverse events have been reported using blue dye with enteral feedings; however, there have been no reports of adverse events with using blue dye during the FEES.[2,18] Patients who may be at increased risk for increased gastrointestinal permeability for absorbing blue dye may include those who have had sepsis, burns, trauma, shock, renal failure, celiac sprue, and inflammatory bowel disease.[18] Furthermore, a study by Leder and colleagues[19] found that the FEES maintained both a high intrarater and interrater reliability in detecting the critical features of pharyngeal dysphagia and aspiration using either blue dye or non–blue-dyed foods. For examiners who choose not to use food coloring, it is recommended that foods that are highly reflective are used during the FEES procedure.[18,19]

Swallow Function and Bolus Flow During FEES

When presenting a bolus, the FEES procedure is described as having a preswallow and postswallow segment, which is divided by the whiteout segment. The whiteout segment occurs during the height of the pharyngeal phase of the swallow as a result of the light that is emitted from the endoscope. A view of the hyopharynx is not possible during the whiteout period; therefore, events that may occur during this period are inferred. Laryngeal penetration and aspiration can be observed in the preswallow segment for those patients who show airway invasion before the initiation of the pharyngeal swallow and in the postswallow segment for those patients who show airway invasion during and after the swallow. Pharyngeal residue is the material from the bolus that is left over in the pharynx after the swallow and is viewed in the postswallow segment. With normal swallow physiology, minimal to no pharyngeal residue should be observed.[9]

COMPARISON OF THE MBS VERSUS THE FEES
Key Points of MBS Versus FEES

Some investigators have stated that the MBS is the gold standard to evaluate swallow function; however, recent research has supported both the MBS and FEES are valuable procedures for evaluating dysphagia. Both the MBS and the FEES are considered the most comprehensive tests available to evaluate the swallow function.[20] The MBS and FEES show good agreement with diagnostic findings related to laryngeal penetration, aspiration, pharyngeal residue, compensatory swallow safety strategies recommendations, and diet recommendations.[21,22] The decision for which diagnostic swallow procedure is needed is usually driven by specific patient characteristics and the field of view necessary to most completely reveal the pathophysiology of the suspected dysphagia for that individual patient.[1] Additional considerations, such as equipment and personnel available at the facility, may also be a determining factor.

Clinical Indicators

From a clinical perspective, some patients may benefit from 1 diagnostic procedure over the other. Although both the MBS and the FEES can be used to evaluate swallow function with many disorders, occasionally the suspected or known swallow dysfunction or characteristic may lend itself to select 1 swallow examination over the other. **Table 3** summarizes common findings and specific patient characteristics that may direct the physician or clinician to select 1 procedure over the other. **Table 3** should not be considered either exhaustive or prescriptive, rather a general outline of which type of patients may benefit from 1 examination over the other. Both the MBS and the FEES are able to assess swallow function with these patient characteristics and

Table 3
Common findings and specific patient characteristics: MBS versus FEES

Characteristic: Suspected Dysfunction	MBS	FEES
Aspiration	X	X
Laryngeal penetration	X	X
Pharyngeal residue	X	X
Reduced hyolaryngeal excursion	X	—
Swallow response delay	X	X
Upper esophageal dysfunction	X	—
Oral phase dysfunction	X	—
Agitated or confused patient	X	—
Patients with excessive or uncontrolled head movement	X	—
Dysphonia and dysphagia	—	X
Odynophagia	—	X
Wet vocal quality and dysphagia	—	X
Poor oral care or secretion management	—	X
Intensive care unit patient	—	X
Postoral-endotracheal intubation	—	X
Progressive neurologic disease	X (assess oral, pharyngeal, and esophageal phases of swallow)	X (assess for fatigue)
Tracheostomy	X	X
Cervical spine surgery	X (assess postoperative prevertebral soft tissue wall edema and hyolaryngeal elevation)	X (assess vocal fold dysfunction commonly associated with cervical spine surgery)

each individual patient must be evaluated on a case-by-case basis to determine the optimal swallow test to use. The MBS and the FEES can also be used to complement each other with patients who require a series of swallow examinations by alternating between the 2 procedures in order to capture different information about the swallow function.

An additional clinical indication to consider is that when the evaluation of the internal anatomy and management of oropharyngeal secretions is needed to fully evaluate the pathophysiology of the dysphagia, then the FEES is preferred over the MBS.[17] If questions are present regarding oral phase impairments, which cannot be adequately answered during the clinical examination, the need for further evaluation of hyolaryngeal elevation, or a suspicion of esophageal dysfunction contributing to the dysphagia, then the MBS is the preferred procedure.[1] Furthermore, for patients with a tracheostomy tube in place, the additional component of subglottal viewing through the tracheostoma performed by a physician during the FEES[23–25] may also provide additional diagnostic information regarding the presence of aspiration. Please see **Fig. 2** for subglottal viewing with the tracheostomy tube removed.

Clinical Outcomes

Aspiration rates

A randomized clinical trial completed by Aviv[20] compared pneumonia outcome rates between 2 groups of patients. For dysphagia management (ie, diet recommendations, behavioral strategies), patients were randomly assigned to either the MBS group or the FEES with sensory testing group. In the MBS group, 18.41% developed pneumonia, and in the FEES with sensory testing group, 12% developed pneumonia. Results revealed that the aspiration pneumonia rates were similar between each group, suggesting that both diagnostic procedures are acceptable for use to manage dysphagia.[20]

Financial comparison

A follow-up study by Aviv and colleagues[26] also revealed that the FEES was more cost effective than the MBS. In the United States, there are customarily 3 charge codes associated with the MBS: the radiation room charge, the physician/professional

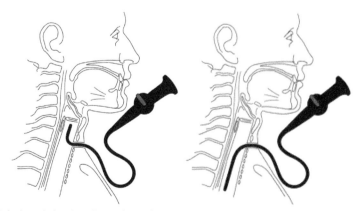

Fig. 2. Subglottal viewing through tracheostoma site. (*From* Donzelli J, Brady S, Wesling M, et al. Predictive value of accumulated oropharyngeal secretions for aspiration during video nasal endoscopic evaluation of the swallow. Ann Otol Rhinol Laryngol 2003;112(5):1747–8; with permission.)

interpretation charge, and the SLP charge. With the FEES, usually only 1 charge code is affiliated with this procedure and either the physician or the clinician may use it. Because reimbursement for health care services may change, this information may be different in the future.

Compensatory Strategies/Swallowing Interventions During the MBS and FEES

The introduction of compensatory strategies and swallowing interventions (eg, postures, maneuvers, bolus modifications, and sensory enhancements) is possible during both the MBS and FEES.[2,3] **Table 4** summarizes the various strategies and interventions available for use during the MBS and FEES as well as the clinical indication for it use. It is important for the examiner to be observant during the MBS and FEES in order to determine the appropriate intervention to attempt and evaluate if the desired effect of the intervention was achieved. Although the examiner can use many of the compensatory strategies during either the MBS or FEES, some strategies are better used with

Table 4 Compensatory strategies used during the MBS and FEES			
Compensatory Strategy	**Rationale/Indication**	**MBS**	**FEES**
Chin tuck posture	Premature spillage, laryngeal penetration, aspiration, pharyngeal residue	X	—
Head rotation posture	Unilateral pharyngeal weakness to close off weaker side (turn head to weaker side); enhance opening of UES	X	X
Head tilt posture	Unilateral pharyngeal weakness. Tilt head to stronger side (ear to shoulder) to use gravity to divert bolus down the stronger side	X	X
Throat clear	Clearing penetrated or aspirated material	X	X[a]
Mendelsohn maneuver	Used to increase vertical and anterior laryngeal motion and increase UES opening	X[a]	X
Effortful swallow	Improve tongue base motion, reduce pharyngeal residue	X	X
Ice chips	Dried secretions	—	X
Breath-holding (supraglottic and supersupraglottic swallow)	Increase airway protection/glottal closure	X	X[a]
Multiple swallows	Used to eliminate or reduce oral and pharyngeal residue by completing a second dry swallow	X	X
Liquid wash or alternating liquids and solids	Used to eliminate or reduce oral and pharyngeal solid bolus residue	X	X
Oral hold	Used with liquid boluses to reduce premature spillage and reduce swallow response delay	X	X
Bolus modifications	Includes viscosity, volume, and sensory (eg, sour boluses) modifications to improve the safety and efficiency of the swallow	X	X

Abbreviation: UES, upper esophageal sphincter.
[a] Indicates the preferred examination to use/view the effectiveness of the compensatory strategy.

1 examination over the other. For example, even although a breath-hold can be used during both the MBS and FEES for increased airway protection, it is only possible during the FEES to see if the patient is accurately performing the voluntary airway closure during the breath-hold maneuver.[27] Conversely, the use of the Mendelsohn maneuver is better visualized during the MBS compared with the FEES because of the tissue apposition with the objective lens at the height of the swallow.[2] It is important for the examiner to recognize the potential advantage to use some compensatory strategies at the same time (eg, chin tuck with head turn).

Logistics of MBS Versus FEES

There are advantages and disadvantages to both the MBS and FEES. **Table 5** provides a comparative summary of each examination. Also, each examination has unique equipment needs that need to be taken into consideration and are outlined in **Table 6**.

Factors Affecting MBS or FEES Results

It is important for the examiner to be cognizant of the fact that the instrumental swallowing assessment, whether it is the MBS or FEES, is only a snapshot picture of the patient's swallow function. Many factors may influence swallow function in either a positive or negative manner. In addition, it is not unusual for a person with dysphagia to show variable swallowing performance, which may be related to the time of day, medication timing, distraction, or other unknown factors. One common question that arises is the contribution that a nasogastric (NG) tube may have on swallow function. In most cases, the presence of an NG tube should not have any adverse contribution to the swallow function.[28] A study by Fattal and colleagues[28] showed no differences in aspiration status within the same person for purees and liquids between the conditions of no NG tube present, a small-bore NG tube, or a large-bore NG tube. However, in clinical practice, these investigators have observed on occasion that removing the NG tube did result in improved swallow function and reports by the

Table 5 Advantages and disadvantages		
	MBS	**FEES**
Advantages	Noninvasive Evaluates oral, pharyngeal, and esophageal phases of the swallow Visualization of cervical hardware after spinal surgery or cervical osteophytes Evaluation of hyolaryngeal elevation	Provides direct view of anatomy structures to evaluate laryngeal and pharyngeal structures May be performed at bedside Uses real food and liquid Examination can last throughout a meal to evaluate for fatigue if needed
Disadvantages	Radiation exposure so examination time may be limited Fluoroscopy unit is turned off between bolus presentations so possible to miss salient event if not imaging between swallows Examination usually requires transportation to radiology department or mobile unit	Whiteout period during height of swallow Examiner must make inferences regarding laryngeal penetration or aspiration during the swallow Time and expense involved with decontamination of endoscope

Table 6		
MBS versus FEES: equipment and materials		
	MBS	**FEES**
Equipment	Fluoroscopy radiograph unit	Nasal-laryngoscope
	Recording/storage device	Endoscope caddy
	Barium	Light source
	Specialized barium, such as Varibar, is	Recording/storage device
	available, which was specifically	Disinfection/infection control
	developed for swallow studies with	materials (eg, Cidex OPA solution;
	various consistencies (thin, nectar	endosheaths)
	thick, honey thick, and pudding)	Food and liquid (may or may not use
		blue food coloring)

patient of increased comfort. Furthermore, the presence of an NG tube does not necessarily prohibit the performance of the FEES examination if the patient has a patent nasal airway (so the endoscope can be inserted on the other side from the NG tube). Some patients may be more comfortable with the temporary removal of the NG tube during the FEES procedure. The examiners should not expect to see any significant differences in swallow function with the NG tube in place; however, the potential impact that the NG tube may have on the person's swallow should be evaluated for each individual patient.

Pediatric Considerations

It is not unusual for a pediatric patient to require several swallowing examinations over their lifetime. Even although the MBS and FEES are both appropriate for use with the pediatric population, the overall lifetime exposure to radiation when completing the MBS is a concern for these young patients. During the MBS, many fluoroscopes have a pediatric setting in order to reduce the amount of radiation exposure and should be used when conducting the swallow examination. There are also additional factors to consider for the pediatric patient when completing the FEES, including use of a smaller-diameter endoscope, use of videos and other distraction devices, and allowing the child to sit on a parent's lap during the examination. The FEES procedure for infants in neonatal intensive care units is often the preferred procedure, because transportation to the radiology department to evaluate the infant's swallow is not needed. Older children may benefit from a previsit to either the MBS or FEES procedure room, where they can see and touch the equipment that will be used during their swallow examination, in order to reduce anxiety. With both the MBS and FEES, compensatory swallow safety strategies are available and may be introduced with the pediatric population during the swallowing examination.

SUMMARY

It is important for the physician and clinician to have a basic understanding of the protocols for both the MBS and FEES, including indications for use, advantages, and disadvantages of each procedure. The MBS and FEES are both valuable swallowing diagnostic tools and show good agreement with diagnostic findings as related to tracheal aspiration, laryngeal penetration, pharyngeal residue, diet level, and compensatory swallow safety strategies. The determination of which procedure is needed to evaluate swallowing function is usually driven by specific patient characteristics and the field of view necessary to most completely evaluate the suspected dysphagia for that individual patient. Additional factors, such as equipment and personnel available at the facility, may also be a determining factor. Both the MBS and FEES should be considered the gold standard for evaluating the swallow.

REFERENCES

1. Leder SB, Murray JT. Fiberoptic endoscopic evaluation of swallowing. Phys Med Rehabil Clin N Am 2008;19(4):787–801.
2. American Speech-Language-Hearing Association. Role of the speech-language pathologist in the performance and interpretation of endoscopic evaluation of swallowing: guidelines. 2004. Available at: http://www.asha.org/members/deskref-journals/deskref/default. Accessed April 8, 2013.
3. American Speech-Language Hearing Association. Guidelines for speech-language pathologists performing videofluoroscopic swallowing studies. 2002. Available at: http://www.asha.org/policy/GL2004-00050.htm. Accessed April 8, 2013.
4. Logemann JA. Evaluation and treatment of swallowing disorders. 2nd edition. Austin (TX): PRO-ED; 1998.
5. Gayler BW. Fluoroscopic equipment for video swallowing studies: current state of technology and future trends. Perspectives (Dysphagia) 2007;16(1):2–7.
6. Langmore SE, Schatz K, Olson N. Fiberoptic endoscopic examination of swallowing safety: a new procedure. Dysphagia 1988;2(4):216–9.
7. Bastian RW. Videoendoscopic evaluation of patients with dysphagia: an adjunct to the modified barium swallow. Otolaryngol Head Neck Surg 1991;104(3):339–50.
8. McCullough G. Significant aspiration for VFSS: a tool to tailor treatment. Perspectives (Dysphagia) 2007;16(2):1–10.
9. Logemann JA. Manual for the videofluoroscopic study of swallowing. Austin (TX): PRO-ED; 1993.
10. Steele CM. Food for thought: physiological implications for the design of the videofluoroscopic swallowing studies. Perspectives (Dysphagia) 2006;15(1):24–8.
11. Kim HM, Choi KY, Kim TW. Patients' radiation dose during videofluoroscopic swallowing studies according to underlying characteristics. Dysphagia 2013;28(2):153–8.
12. Leder SB, Ross DA. Incidence of vocal fold immobility in patients with dysphagia. Dysphagia 2005;20(2):163–9.
13. Burton MJ, Altman KW, Rosenfeld RM. Extracts from The Cochrane Library: topical anaesthetic or vasoconstrictor preparations for flexible fibre-optic nasal pharyngoscopy and laryngoscopy. Otolaryngol Head Neck Surg 2012;146(5):694–7.
14. Langmore SE. Laryngeal sensation: a touchy subject. Dysphagia 1998;13(2):93–4.
15. Aviv JE, Kim T, Sacco RL, et al. FEESST: a new bedside endoscopic test of the motor and sensory components of swallowing. Ann Otol Rhinol Laryngol 1998;107:378–87.
16. Langmore SE, Terpenning MS, Schork A, et al. Predictors of aspiration pneumonia: how important is dysphagia? Dysphagia 1998;13(2):69–81.
17. Donzelli J, Brady S, Wesling M, et al. Predictive value of accumulated oropharyngeal secretions for aspiration during video nasal endoscopic evaluation of the swallow. Ann Otol Rhinol Laryngol 2003;112(5):469–75.

18. Brady S. The use of blue dye and glucose oxidase reagent strips for detection of pulmonary aspiration: efficacy and safety update. Perspectives (Dysphagia) 2005;14(4):8–13.

19. Leder SB, Acton LM, Lisitano HL, et al. Fiberoptic endoscopic evaluation of swallowing (FEES) with and without blue-dyed food. Dysphagia 2005;20(2):157–62.

20. Aviv JE. Prospective, randomized outcome study of endoscopy versus modified barium swallow in patients with dysphagia. Laryngoscope 2000;110(4):563–74.

21. Langmore SE, Schatz K, Olson N. Endoscopic and videofluoroscopic evaluations of swallowing and aspiration. Ann Otol Rhinol Laryngol 1991;100(8):678–81.

22. Rao N, Brady SL, Chaudhuri G, et al. Gold-standard? Analysis of the videofluoroscopic and fiberoptic endoscopic swallow examinations. J Appl Res Clin Exp Ther 2003;3(1):89–96.

23. Brady SL, Wesling M, Donzelli J. Pilot data on swallow function in nondysphagic patients requiring a tracheostomy tube. Int J Otolaryngol 2009;2009:610849.

24. Donzelli J, Brady S, Wesling M, et al. Effects of the removal of the tracheostomy tube on swallowing during the fiberoptic endoscopic exam of the swallow (FEES). Dysphagia 2005;20(4):283–9.

25. Donzelli J, Brady S, Wesling M, et al. Simultaneous modified Evans blue dye procedure and video nasal endoscopic evaluation of the swallow. Laryngoscope 2001;111(10):1746–50.

26. Aviv JE, Sataloff RT, Cohen M, et al. Cost-effectiveness of two types of dysphagia care in head and neck cancer: a preliminary report. Ear Nose Throat J 2001; 80(8):553–6.

27. Donzelli J, Brady S. The effects of breath-holding on vocal fold adduction: implications for safe swallowing. Arch Otolaryngol Head Neck Surg 2004;130(2):208–10.

28. Fattal M, Suiter DM, Warner HL, et al. Effect of presence/absence of a nasogastric tube in the same person on incidence of aspiration. Otolaryngol Head Neck Surg 2011;145(5):796–800.

Normal Esophageal Physiology and Laryngopharyngeal Reflux

Dhyanesh Patel, MD[a], Michael F. Vaezi, MD, PhD, MSc (Epi)[b],*

KEYWORDS

- Esophagus • Anatomy • Physiology • Laryngopharyngeal reflux
- Proton pump inhibitor • pH monitoring • Management

KEY POINTS

- Esophagus is a muscular tube with active peristalsis, which helps propel bolus into the stomach.
- Lower and upper esophageal sphincters act to prevent esophageal and laryngeal exposure to gastroduodenal contents.
- Dysfunction of esophageal peristalsis and/or LES and UES often results in symptoms of dysphagia, chest pain, and chronic pulmonary and laryngeal symptoms.
- Common clinical manifestations of LPR include dysphonia/hoarseness, cough, globus pharyngeus, throat clearing, and dysphagia.
- Laryngoscopic findings are often nonspecific for reflux-induced laryngitis and have high interrater variability.
- In the absence of risk factors for malignancy, empiric 2-month trial of PPI is considered a reasonable approach in patients suspected of having LPR.
- PPI therapy should be tapered in all patients with initial empiric therapy.
- Surgery is not recommended in patients whose symptoms do not respond to PPI unless regurgitation is an accompanying symptom.
- In nonresponders to empiric PPI therapy, other causes for chronic laryngeal inflammation should be entertained.

INTRODUCTION

Esophagus is a complex muscular tube connecting the pharynx to the stomach, which acts as a channel for the transport of food and prevents reflux of gastroduodenal contents. It is the only internal organ that traverses three body cavities. A thorough

Disclosures: Dr Vaezi has received research funding in the past from Takeda pharmaceutical but no COI with this project.
[a] Department of Internal Medicine, Vanderbilt University Medical Center, Nashville, TN, USA;
[b] Division of Gastroenterology, Hepatology and Nutrition, Center for Swallowing and Esophageal Disorders, Vanderbilt University Medical Center, Nashville, TN, USA
* Corresponding author.
E-mail address: Michael.vaezi@vanderbilt.edu

Abbreviations: Esophageal Physiology	
EER	Extraesophageal reflux
GERD	Gastroesophageal reflux disease
LES	Lower esophageal sphincter
LPR	Laryngopharyngeal reflux
PPI	Proton pump inhibitor
TLESR	Transient lower esophageal sphincter relaxation
UES	Upper esophageal sphincter

understanding of this anatomy and physiology is essential in understanding esophageal disease states.

ANATOMY

The proximal margin of the tubular esophagus is the upper esophageal sphincter (UES), the functional unit correlating anatomically with the junction of the inferior pharyngeal constrictor and cricopharyngeus.[1] Although UES function is controlled by numerous muscles based on electromyographic signals,[2,3] most studies indicate that the primary muscular element that generates tone in the sphincter at rest is the cricopharyngeus.[2–5] It is innervated by the pharyngeal plexus and the recurrent laryngeal nerve. The esophagus extends distally 18 to 26 cm within the posterior mediastinum as a hollow muscular tube to the lower esophageal sphincter (LES) (**Fig. 1**). The LES is a 2- to 4-cm long focus of tonically contracted thickened circular smooth muscle that lies within the diaphragmatic hiatus[6] and is the major antireflux barrier protecting the esophagus from reflux of the gastric contents.[7] The LES is innervated by parasympathetic (vagal) and sympathetic (splanchnic) nerves.[8]

The esophageal wall is morphologically distinct compared with the rest of the gastrointestinal tract, because it has no serosa. It is comprised of four layers: (1) mucosa, (2) submucosa, (3) muscularis propria, and (4) the adventitia. The proximal 5% to 33% is skeletal muscle, the middle 35% to 40% mixed muscle, and the distal 50% to 60% smooth muscle.[9] The muscles are arranged into inner circular and outer longitudinal layers. The smooth muscle portions of the esophageal body are innervated by the vagus nerve, which controls peristalsis under physiologic conditions. Neural innervation of the esophagus is from the myenteric or Auerbach plexus, located between the two muscle layers, and Meissner plexus located in the submucosa.[7] The myenteric plexus is responsible for esophageal peristalsis, whereas the Meissner complex is the site of afferent sensory input (**Fig. 2**). Excitatory stimulation from acetylcholine mediates contraction of the longitudinal and circular muscle layers. Inhibitory neurons predominately affect the circular muscle layer by nitric oxide. Excitatory stimulation from acetylcholine has its largest effect proximally, whereas inhibitory effect of nitric oxide is seen distally.[10]

PHYSIOLOGY

Functionally, the UES, the esophageal body, and the LES act in coordinated manner to allow normal swallowing. Swallowing begins when a food bolus is propelled into the pharynx from the mouth. This oropharyngeal phase of swallowing is voluntary, whereas the esophageal phase that follows is involuntary. In rapid sequence and with precise coordination the larynx is elevated and the epiglottis seals the airway.

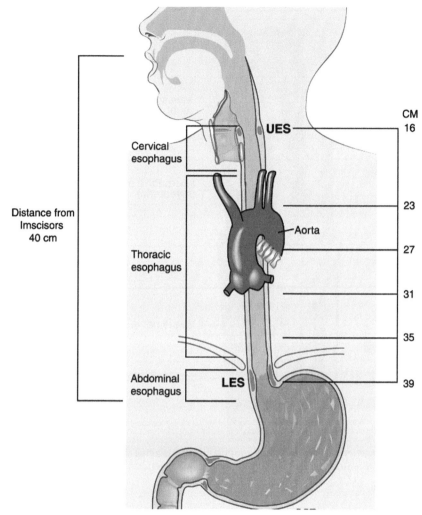

Fig. 1. Schematic view of the esophagus and its relationship to neighboring structures. The esophagus is typically 40 cm long from incisors to end of LES. UES typically is about 16 cm and LES about 38 to 40 cm.

A rapidly progressing pharyngeal contraction then transfers the bolus through the relaxed UES into the esophagus. The UES is opened by relaxation of its muscles, movement of the larynx anteriorly, and pulsation by the bolus. As the UES closes, a progressive circular contraction begins in the upper esophagus and proceeds distally along the esophageal body to propel the bolus through the relaxed LES (**Figs. 3**A and B). Peristaltic pressures normally ranging from 30 to 180 mm Hg are generated.[10,11] The LES subsequently closes with a prolonged contraction preventing movement back into the esophagus. The mechanical effect of peristalsis is a stripping wave that strips the esophagus clean from its proximal to distal end (see **Fig. 3**B).

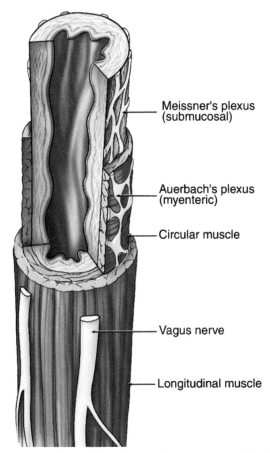

Fig. 2. Cross-sectional anatomy of the esophagus. Vagus nerve supplies the esophageal circular and longitudinal muscles through Meissner and Auerbach plexus.

Secondary peristalsis is a progressive contraction in the esophageal body that is induced by stimulation of sensory receptors, rather than a swallow. This begins approximately at or above the level of the stimulus and resembles primary peristalsis. Its function is to clear the esophagus from food contents poorly cleared by the primary peristalsis and to push refluxed gastric contents back into the stomach.

The UES and LES are tonically contracted at rest. The closed state for the UES is a result of continuous neural excitation, with a small passive component to tone.[3] The UES pressures are asymmetric being higher anteriorly and posteriorly. It is believed that the tonic contraction of the LES is a function of the muscle itself and not dependent on neural innervation. Stimulation of inhibitory fibers results in LES relaxation. LES relaxation occurs not only in response to swallowing, but may occur in response to esophageal distention (secondary peristalsis) or may occur without peristalsis. This is referred to as transient LES relaxation (TLESR), defined as periods lasting 10 to 60 seconds of spontaneous (not preceded by swallow), simultaneous relaxation of the LES and crural diaphragm.[12] TLESR is thought to be a vagally mediated reflex that

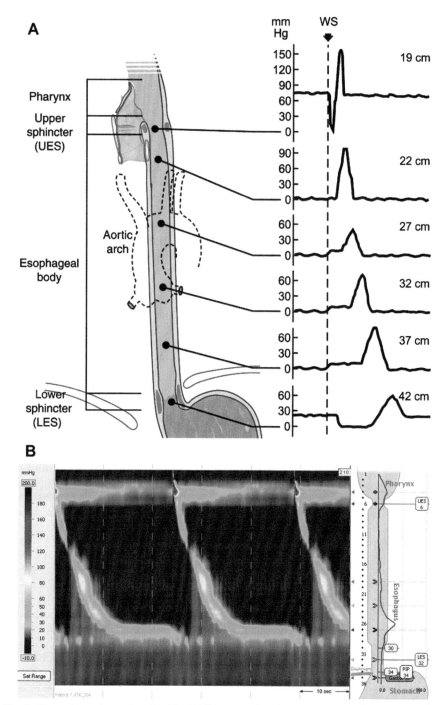

Fig. 3. Normal esophageal peristalsis. (*A*) Water perfused measurement of normal esopha-geal peristalsis showing relaxation of UES with a swallow at 19 cm from the mouth followed by peristaltic contraction of the esophagus along its axis with relaxation of the LES to accommodate the bolus shown at 42 cm from the oral cavity. (*B*) High-resolution manometry showing normal esophageal peristalsis. UES shown in the top and the LES at the bottom of the page with normal peristalsis showing in *yellow* and *orange* colors representing different pressure amplitude as referenced on the *left panel*.

is part of normal digestion and triggered by gastric distention based on observations that it can be diminished with vagal cooling or vagotomy in dogs.[13] TLESR is also absent in patients with achalasia, a condition in which the inhibitory innervation is defective.[8] TLESR represents the primary mechanism for gastroesophageal reflux in normal individuals.[12]

GASTROESOPHAGEAL REFLUX DISEASE

Approximately 25 to 75 million people in the United States are affected by gastroesophageal reflux disease (GERD), and 13% of Americans use medications for GERD at least twice weekly.[14] GERD is a spectrum of disease usually producing symptoms of heartburn and acid regurgitation, which are considered to be part of the esophageal syndromes. Symptoms may also include chest pain or atypically may present as extraesophageal manifestations, such as dental erosion, laryngitis, asthma, chronic obstructive pulmonary disease, cough, hoarseness, postnasal drip disease, sinusitis, otitis media, and recurrent pneumonia, which are among the extraesophageal syndromes (**Fig. 4**).

Extraesophageal reflux (EER) symptoms can occur concurrently with typical GERD symptoms or alone. The diagnosis of GERD is more difficult in those presenting solely with EER symptoms because it is not initially suspected. GERD has become an important public health problem because of the considerable economic burden, lack of productivity, medications, and required consultations. Annual direct cost for GERD management is reported at $971 per patient,[15] with national expenditures ranging from $9.3 billion[16] to $12.1 billion.[17] However, the cost of treating EER is even more impressive. According to recent data,[18] the cost of caring for patients with EER is five times that of GERD at approximately $50 billion (**Fig. 5**).

LARYNGOPHARYNGEAL REFLUX

Laryngopharyngeal reflux (LPR) is an extraesophageal variant of GERD, because the main symptomatic region involves the laryngopharynx.[19,20] Although the hallmark symptoms of GERD include heartburn and regurgitation, symptoms of LPR often include hoarseness, chronic cough, sore throat, globus pharyngeus, and throat-clearing (**Box 1**). Approximately 10% of all otolaryngologic clinic patients overall and 50% of patients with voice complaints have been diagnosed with LPR.[21] However, the prevalence of LPR is difficult to determine because of lack of clear diagnostic gold standard and can certainly be exaggerated because even healthy individuals can have some findings consistent with LPR.[22,23]

Pathophysiology

Laryngeal manifestation of GERD is thought to be related to direct acid-peptic injury to the larynx by esophagopharyngeal reflux (the microaspiration theory)[24] or acidification of the distal esophagus through vagally mediated reflexes (the esophageal-brochial reflex theory) (**Fig. 6**).[25–29] Laryngeal tissue certainly lacks protective mechanisms of the esophagus (production of bicarbonate, physical barriers) and intrinsic acid clearance mechanism (peristalsis) and is highly vulnerable to any acid exposure. In addition to acidic pH levels, substances that can contribute to the noxious quality of the refluxate include pepsin, bile salts, and pancreatic enzymes. Earlier studies suggested that pepsin may be the main cause for LPR symptoms[30,31]; however, later studies suggested the coimportance of acid, pepsin, and bile acids.[32] There is now a resurgence of publications on the role of pepsin in LPR. Some suggest that reflux of pepsin into the larynx with subsequent pepsin

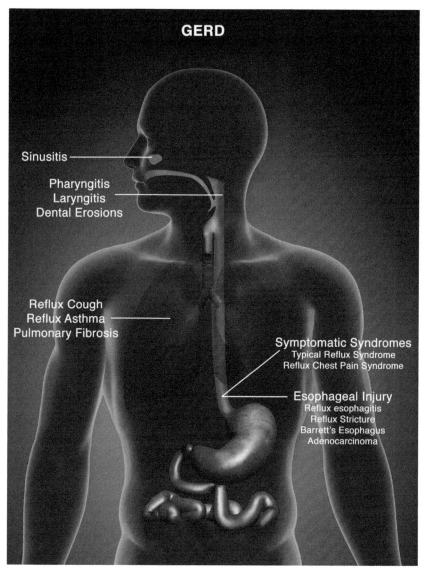

Fig. 4. Esophageal and extraesophageal manifestations of GERD. Esophageal syndromes include typical and chest pain syndromes and reflux esophagitis, stricture, Barrett esophagus, and adenocarcinoma. Extraesophageal syndromes include pharyngitis, laryngitis, dental erosion, cough, asthma, and pulmonary fibrosis.

transfer into the cytoplasm of the laryngeal cells and later activation in the cell organelles with lower pH ranges than the lumen may be an important contributor to LPR.[33] Dilation of intercellular spaces is reported to be an early morphologic marker in GERD; however, recent studies assessing dilation of intercellular spaces in patients suspected of LPR and GERD did not show a difference in epithelial space separation between patients and a group of control subjects.[34]

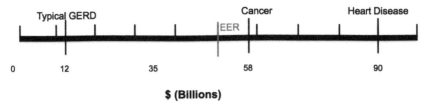

$ (Billions)

Fig. 5. Comparison of estimated economic burden of extraesophageal reflux (EER) initial evaluation with typical GERD, cancer, and heart disease. The annual cost of caring for patients with EER is four to five times that of typical GERD. (*Adapted from* Francis DO, Rymer JA, Slaughter JC, et al. High economic burden of caring for patients with suspected extraesophageal reflux. Am J Gastroenterol 2013;108(6):909.)

Diagnosis and Evaluation

Current diagnostic tests for LPR have many shortcomings and can lead to misdiagnosis of the disease (**Table 1**) and other causes of chronic laryngeal inflammation must be kept in the differential diagnosis (**Fig. 7**). For instance, fever, fatigue, and acute onset is much more indicative of infectious origin, whereas more systemic symptoms with joint involvement or rash might indicate autoimmune causes. Thus, a careful history is critical for diagnosis including factors that may predispose a patient to esophageal reflux, such as tobacco use; diet (soda, spicy foods, fatty foods); alcohol use; and certain drugs (calcium channel blockers, nitrates, steroids).[35]

Some investigators use a self-administered survey consisting of nine questions known as the Reflux Symptom Index to help diagnose patients with LPR.[36–39] However, others are not as optimistic about the predictive potential of the Reflux Symptom Index in LPR.[40–42] Laryngoscopic findings often attributed to LPR (**Box 2**) include erythema, edema, ventricular obliteration, postcricoid hyperplasia, and pseudosulcus.[27] Laryngoscopy as the most frequently used test in those suspected with LPR is highly sensitive to changes within the larynx but is nonspecific for establishing reflux as the cause.

Box 1
Symptoms associated with gastroesophageal reflux laryngitis

- Hoarseness
- Dysphonia
- Sore or burning throat
- Excessive throat clearing
- Chronic cough
- Globus
- Apnea
- Laryngospasm
- Dysphagia
- Postnasal drip
- Neoplasm

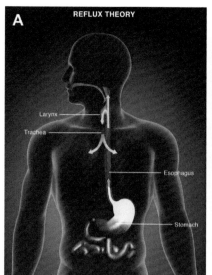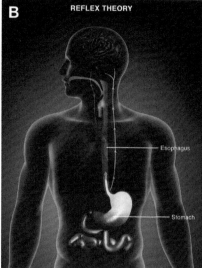

Fig. 6. The two mechanisms, reflux (*A*) and reflex (*B*) theories, underlying the pathophysiology of the extraesophageal manifestations of GERD including LPR.

Table 1
Advantages and disadvantages of methods for detecting esophageal reflux

Method	Advantages	Disadvantages
Endoscopy	Easy visualization of mucosal damage/erosions	Poor sensitivity/specificity/positive predictive value Requires sedation High cost
Laryngoscopy	No sedation required Direct visualization of the larynx and laryngeal pathology	No specific laryngeal signs for reflux Over diagnoses reflux as the cause for patients' symptoms
pH monitoring	Easy to perform Relatively noninvasive Prolonged monitoring Ambulatory	Many are catheter-based May have up to 30% false-negative rate No pH predictors of treatment response for extraesophageal reflux
Impedance monitoring	Easy to perform Relatively noninvasive Prolonged monitoring Ambulatory Measures acidic and nonacidic gas and liquid reflux (combined with pH)	Catheter based False-negative rate unknown but most likely similar to catheter-based pH monitoring Unknown clinical relevance when abnormal on proton pump inhibitor therapy Unknown importance in extraesophageal reflux
ResTech Dx-pH	Faster detection rate and faster time to equilibrium pH than traditional pH catheters	Unknown if clinically useful in patients with LPR Awaiting controlled outcome studies
Lateral flow device for pepsin	Fast and easy detection of salivary pepsin Acceptable sensitivity and specificity	Limited outcome studies Potentially useful but controlled studies needed

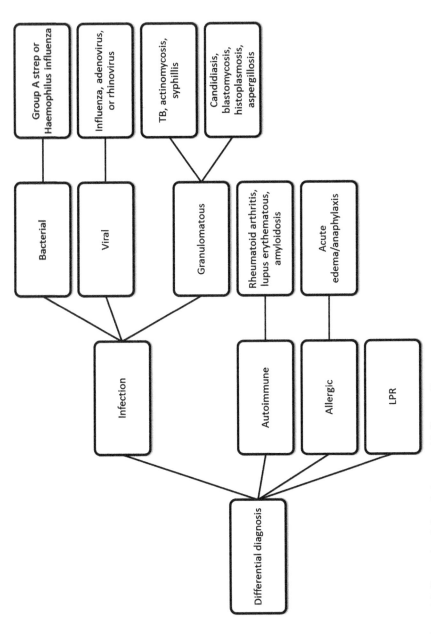

Fig. 7. Differential diagnosis of chronic laryngeal inflammation.

Box 2
Potential laryngopharyngeal signs associated with gastroesophageal reflux laryngitis

- Edema and hyperemia of larynx
- Hyperemia and lymphoid hyperplasia of posterior pharynx (cobblestoning)
- Contact ulcers
- Laryngeal polyps
- Granuloma
- Interarytenoid changes
- Subglottic stenosis
- Posterior glottic stenosis
- Reinke edema
- Tumors

Ambulatory 24-hour pH monitoring was considered the gold standard for diagnosing reflux, but recent studies have shown it to be unreliable in patients with laryngeal symptoms.[27,43] A recent meta-analysis of trials comparing 16 studies involving 793 subjects (264 normal and 529 with LPR) showed that upper probe does give accurate and consistent information in normal subjects and patients with LPR.[23] However, there is lack of consensus on normal pH limits and number of events to diagnose LPR. More importantly, a study by Ulualp and colleagues[44] found that patients with pharyngeal reflux documented by pH monitoring were no more likely to respond to acid-suppressive therapy than patients with no documented reflux.

In patients who remain symptomatic despite aggressive acid-suppressive therapy, recent studies suggest that nonacid reflux may play a role in their symptoms measured by ambulatory intraluminal pH-impedance monitoring.[45] Despite initial enthusiasm,[46] outcome studies with impedance monitoring are lacking and their clinical significance with regards to medically recalcitrant LPR patients still remains unclear.[47] The most recent uncontrolled surgical study in patients suspected of having LPR found that on or off therapy impedance monitoring does not predict LPR symptom response to fundoplication, but presence of hiatal hernia, significant acid reflux at baseline, and presence of regurgitation concomitantly with the LPR symptoms were important predictors of symptom response.[48] Thus, use of impedance monitoring in those refractory to proton pump inhibitor (PPI) therapy continues to be uncertain. We recommend the use of pH monitoring off PPI therapy to provide baseline esophageal reflux parameters. Impedance monitoring may be used on PPI therapy and should be reserved for those who continue to have symptoms despite acid-suppressive therapy. Impedance monitoring findings alone should not be used to determine the need for surgical fundoplication. In the setting of moderate to severe baseline acid reflux off therapy and continued nonacid reflux on PPI therapy, antireflux surgery may be entertained but with caution.

Additional recent tests in LPR include the Restech oropharyngeal pH monitoring and salivary pepsin assay. The Dx-pH measurement system (Respiratory Technology Corp, San Diego, CA) is a sensitive and minimally invasive device for detection of acid reflux in the posterior oropharynx.[49] It uses a nasopharyngeal catheter (the Restech pH catheter) to measure pH in either liquid or aerosolized droplets (**Fig. 8**).[50]

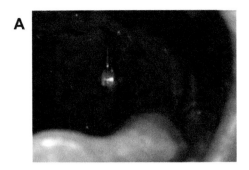

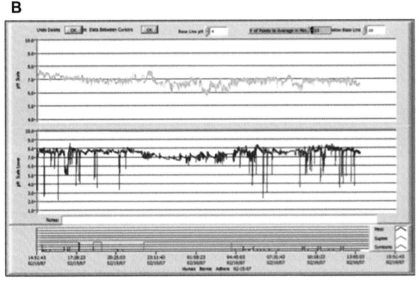

Fig. 8. (*A*) Dx-pH probe and light-emitting diode positioned in the oropharynx. (*B*) Typical tracing of distal esophageal (*lower tracing*) and oropharyngeal (*upper tracing*) pH monitoring in a healthy volunteer.

A comparison of this device with the traditional pH catheters has shown faster detection rate and faster time to equilibrium pH (**Fig. 9**) and a significantly higher number of reflux events detected by Restech pH in patients with LPR than patients with GERD and healthy volunteers.[51] However, controlled outcome-driven studies are needed to assess the future role of this new device in this group of patients. Recently, a novel pepsin rapid test (Peptest-Biomed, RD Biomed Limited, Hull, HU [UK]) was used as a convenient, office-based, noninvasive, quick, and inexpensive technique in LPR diagnosis. This lateral flow device uses two monoclonal antibodies to human pepsin (**Fig. 10**). A prospective, masked study of salivary pepsin assay in 59 patients with objective GERD (esophagitis or abnormal pH testing) compared with 51 control subjects found positive and negative predictive values of 87% and 78%, respectively.[52] The sensitivity and specificity of the assay was 87% by in vitro bench testing. Thus, the study suggests that rapid lateral flow device for salivary pepsin has acceptable test characteristics in GERD. However, the clinical role of this assay in those with LPR is unknown and is the subject of ongoing study.

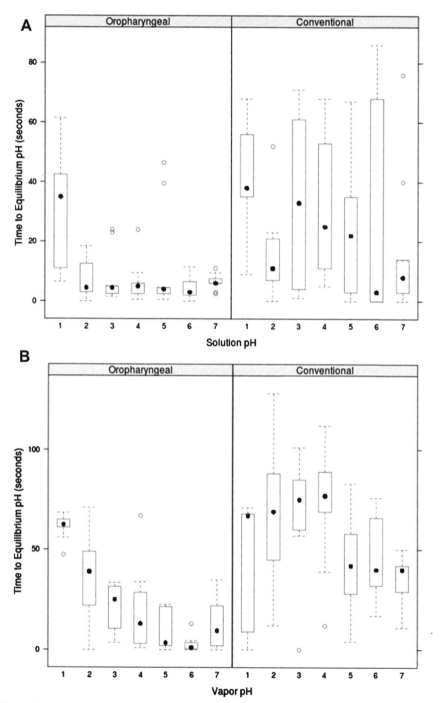

Fig. 9. (*A, B*) Time to reach equilibrium pH (seconds) was significantly (*P*<.001) faster with the oropharyngeal than the conventional pH probe in the liquid and vapor phases.

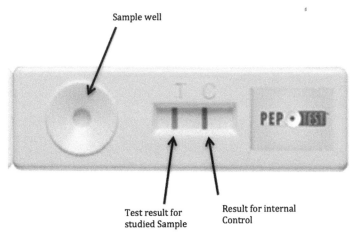

Sample well

Test result for
studied Sample

Result for internal
Control

Fig. 10. Pepsin lateral flow device of a gastric juice sample showing positive pepsin test relative to the control band. C, control band; T, test sample band.

Management

Empiric therapy with a PPI twice daily is considered to be the best diagnostic test in those with LPR. A schematic view of evaluation for patients with LPR based on evidence-based recommendations and risk stratification proposed by our group is shown in **Fig. 11**.[53] Based on this model empiric therapy initially in the low-risk group (no alarm symptoms) followed by diagnostic testing is a reasonable approach in those initially suspected of having LPR. If the patient responds to therapy, then tapering to once-daily PPI initially and then to minimal acid suppression to control symptoms is appropriate. In those with moderate to high risk (weight loss, dysphagia, anemia, odynophagia, hematemesis, or respiratory distress) initial diagnostic test is warranted.[53]

The results from controlled studies with acid-suppressive therapy have been disappointing when PPIs were compared with placebo in clinical trials and recent meta-analysis.[54] The reason for the disappointing results may be because of biases in patient selection. Given lack of knowledge about PPI-responsive LPR symptoms it is most likely that those with non–reflux-related symptoms or signs diluted the enrolled patient groups in these trials resulting in negative outcome. Addition of histamine2 receptor antagonist in those unresponsive to initial empiric PPI therapy is not recommended and has not been showed to have a significant effect on acid suppression.[55] Furthermore, surgical fundoplication is another option, but should not be considered in patients whose symptoms persist despite aggressive PPI therapy unless regurgitation is a dominant concomitant symptom. In a study of 72 patients with LPR who underwent PPI therapy for 4 months, 25 patients had less than a 50% improvement in symptoms and 10 of these patients underwent surgical fundoplication with only one surgical patient (10%) reporting improvement in laryngeal symptoms.[56] Thus, surgery is not recommended for patients whose symptoms do not respond to aggressive PPI therapy.[56,57] The most recent uncontrolled surgical study in patients suspected of having LPR found that presence of hiatal hernia, significant acid reflux at baseline, and presence of regurgitation concomitantly with the LPR symptoms were important predictors of symptom response.[48]

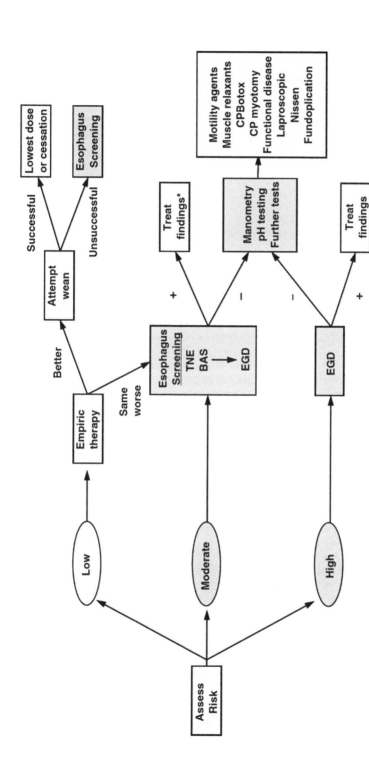

Fig. 11. Clinical protocol for reflux disease based on risk assessment. Low risk includes those without alarm symptoms; moderate risk includes those older than the age of 50 with dysphagia, odynophagia, anemia, or weight loss; high risk includes those with severe odynophagia, hemoptysis or hematemesis, significant weight loss, respiratory distress, and abdominal mass or pain. (*From* Altman KW, Prufer N, Vaezi MF. The challenge of protocols for reflux disease: a review and development of a critical pathway. Otolaryngol Head Neck Surg 2011;145(1):7–14.)

SUMMARY

The diagnosis of LPR is difficult with current understanding of the pathophysiology and available tests. Laryngoscopy has high interrater variability and the results of pH monitoring do not dependably predict who will respond to treatment. A 2-month treatment course of PPI is typically safe in those without accompanying warning symptoms. A trial of twice-daily PPI for evaluation and management in addition to dietary and behavioral changes should be emphasized. All PPI therapy should be tapered to the minimum dose of acid suppression to control patient symptoms. Future studies with oropharyngeal pH monitoring and salivary pepsin assay need to provide controlled outcome data to better understand their role in this difficult-to-diagnose group of patients.

REFERENCES

1. Goyal RK, Martin SB, Shapiro J, et al. The role of cricopharyngeus muscle in pharygoesophageal disorders. Dysphagia 1993;8:252–8.
2. Lang IM, Dantas RO, Cook IJ, et al. Videographic, manometric, and electromyographic assessment of upper esophageal sphincter. Am J Physiol 1991;260: G911–9.
3. Ashoh R, Goyal RK. Manometry and elctromyography of the upper esophageal sphincter in the opossum. Gastroenterology 1978;74:514–20.
4. Elidan J, Gonen B, Shochna M, et al. Electromyography of the inferior constrictor and cricopharyngeal muscles during swallowing. Ann Otol Rhinol Laryngol 1990;99:46–9.
5. Van Overbeek JJ, Wit HP, Paping RH, et al. Simultaneous manometry and electromyography in the pharyngoesophageal segment. Laryngoscope 1985;95:582–4.
6. Mittal RK, Balaban DH. The esophagogastric junction. N Engl J Med 1997;336: 924–32.
7. Cunningham ET, Sawchenko PE. Central neural control of esophageal motility: a review. Dysphagia 1990;5:35–51.
8. Hershcovici T, Mashimo H, Fass R. The lower esophageal sphincter. Neurogastroenterol Motil 2011;23:819–30.
9. Meyer GW, Austin RM, Brady CE, et al. Muscle anatomy of the human esophagus. J Clin Gastroenterol 1986;8:131–4.
10. Crist J, Gidda JS, Goyal RK. Intramural mechanism of esophageal peristalsis: roles of cholinergic and noncholinergic nerves. Proc Natl Acad Sci U S A 1984;81(11):3595–9.
11. Bassotti G, Bacci G, Biangini A, et al. Manometric investigation of the entire esophagus in healthy subjects and patients with high-amplitude peristaltic contractions. Dysphagia 1988;3:93–6.
12. Dodds WJ, Dent J, Hogan WJ, et al. Mechanisms of gastroesophageal reflux in patients with reflux esophagitis. N Engl J Med 1982;307:1547–52.
13. Martin CJ, Patrikios J, Dent J. Abolition of gas reflux and transient lower esophageal sphincter relaxation by vagal blockade in the dog. Gastroenterology 1986;91:890–6.
14. Sontaj SJ. The medical management of reflux esophagitis. Role of antacids and acid inhibition. Gastroenterol Clin North Am 1990;19:683–712.
15. Fenter TC, Naslund MJ, Shah MB, et al. The cost of treating the 10 most prevalent diseases in men 50 years of age or older. Am J Manag Care 2006; 12(Suppl 4):S90–8.
16. Sandler RS, Everhart JE, Donowitz M, et al. The burden of selected digestive diseases in the United States. Gastroenterology 2002;122(5):1500–11.

17. Everhart JE, Ruhl CE. Burden of digestive diseases in the United States part I: over-all and upper gastrointestinal diseases. Gastroenterology 2009;136(2):376–86.
18. Francis DO, Rymer JA, Slaughter JC, et al. High economic burden of caring for patients with suspected extraesophageal reflux. Am J Gastroenterol 2013; 108(6):905–11.
19. Koufman JA, Aviv JE, Casiano RR, et al. Laryngopharyngeal reflux: position state-ment of the committee on speech, voice, and swallowing disorders of the Ameican Academy of Otolaryngology-Head and Neck Surgery. Otolaryngol Head Neck Surg 2002;127:32–5.
20. Koufman JA. Laryngopharyngeal reflux is different from classic gastroesopha-geal reflux disease. Ear Nose Throat J 2002;81(9 Suppl 2):7–9.
21. Koufman JA. The otolaryngologic manifestations of gastroesophageal reflux dis-ease (GERD): a clinical investigation of 225 patients using amblatory 24-hour pH monitoring and an experimental investigation of the role of acid and pepsin in the development of laryngeal injury. Laryngoscope 1991;101:1–78.
22. Hicks DM, Ours TM, Abelson TI, et al. The prevalence of hypopharynx findings associated with gastroesophageal reflux in normal volunteers. J Voice 2002;16: 564–79.
23. Merati AL, Lim HJ, Ulualp SO, et al. Meta-analysis of upper probe measure-ments in normal subjects and patients with laryngopharyngeal reflux. Ann Otol Rhinol Laryngol 2005;114:177–82.
24. Cherry J, Margulies SI. Contact ulcer of the larynx. Laryngoscope 1968;78(11): 1937–40.
25. Tokayer AZ. Gastroesophageal reflux disease and chronic cough. Lung 2008; 186(Suppl 1):S29–34.
26. Wright RA, Miller SA, Corsello BF. Acid-induced esophagobronchial-cardiac re-flexes in humans. Gastroenterology 1990;99(1):71–3.
27. Vaezi MF, Hicks DM, Abelson TI, et al. Laryngeal signs and symptoms and gastroesophageal reflux disease (GERD): a critical assessment of cause and ef-fect association. Clin Gastroenterol Hepatol 2003;1(5):333–44.
28. Irwin RS. Chronic cough due to gastroesophageal reflux disease: ACCP evidence-based clinical practice guidelines. Chest 2006;129(Suppl 1):80S–94S.
29. Chang AB, Lasserson TJ, Gaffney J, et al. Gastro-oesophageal reflux treatment for prolonged non-specific cough in children and adults. Cochrane Database Syst Rev 2005;(2):CD004823.
30. Samuels TL, Johnston N. Pepsin as a causal agent of inflammation during nonacidic reflux. Otolaryngol Head Neck Surg 2009;141(5):559–63.
31. Wood JM, Hussey DJ, Woods C, et al. Biomarkers and laryngopharyngeal re-flux. J Laryngol Otol 2011;125(12):1218–24.
32. Adhami T, Goldblum J, Richter JE, et al. The role of gastric and duodenal agents in laryngeal injury: an experimental canine model. Am J Gastroenterol 2004; 99(11):2098–106.
33. Johnston N, Wells CW, Blumin JH, et al. Receptor-mediated uptake of pepsin by laryngeal epithelial cells. Ann Otol Rhinol Laryngol 2007;116(12):934–8.
34. Vaezi MF, Slaughter JC, Smith BS, et al. Dilated intercellular space in chronic laryngitis and gastro-oesophageal reflux disease: at baseline and post-lansoprazole therapy. Aliment Pharmacol Ther 2010;32(7):916–24.
35. Barry DW, Vaezi MF. Laryngopharyngeal reflux: more questions than answers. Cleve Clin J Med 2010;77:327–34.
36. Belafsky PC, Postma GN, Koufman JA. Validity and reliability of the reflux symp-tom index (RSI). J Voice 2002;16:274–7.

37. Belafsky PC, Postma GN, Koufman JA. Laryngopharyngeal reflux symptoms improve before changes in physical findings. Laryngoscope 2001;111: 979–81.

38. Belafsky PC, Postma GN, Amin MR, et al. Symptoms and findings of laryngo-pharyngeal reflux. Ear Nose Throat J 2002;81:10–3.

39. Belafsky PC, Postma GN, Koufman JA. The association between laryngeal pseu-dosulcus and laryngopharyngeal reflux. Otolaryngol Head Neck Surg 2002;126: 649–52.

40. Milstein CF, Charbel S, Hicks DM, et al. Prevalence of laryngeal irritation signs associated with reflux in asymptomatic volunteers: impact of endoscopic tech-nique (rigid vs flexible scope). Laryngoscope 2005;115:2256–61.

41. Branski RC, Bhattacharya N, Shapiro J. The reliability of the assessment of endoscopic laryngeal findings associated with laryngopharyngeal reflux dis-ease. Laryngoscope 2002;112:1019–24.

42. Belafsky PC, Postma GN, Koufman JA. The validity and reliability of the reflux finding score (RFS). Laryngoscope 2001;111:1313–7.

43. Gupta R, Sataloff RT. Laryngopharyngeal reflux: current concepts and ques-tions. Curr Opin Otolaryngol Head Neck Surg 2009;17:143–8.

44. Ulualp SO, Toohill RJ, Shaker R. Outcomes of acid suppressive therapy in patients with posterior laryngitis. Otolaryngol Head Neck Surg 2001;124: 16–22.

45. Tutuian R, Castell DO. Use of multichannel intraluminal impedance to document proximal esophageal and pharyngeal nonacidic reflux episodes. Am J Med 2003;115(Suppl 3):119S–23S.

46. Mainie I, Tutuian R, Agrawal A, et al. Combined multichannel intraluminal impedance-pH monitoring to select patients with persistent gastro-oesophageal reflux for laparoscopic Nissen fundoplication. Br J Surg 2006;93(12):1483–7.

47. Vaezi MF. Laryngitis and gastro-oesophageal reflux disease (GERD): improve laryngoscopic specificity, don't do pH monitoring. Dig Liver Dis 2004;36(2): 103–4.

48. Francis DO, Goutte M, Slaughter JC, et al. Traditional reflux parameters and not impedance monitoring predict outcome after fundoplication in extraesophageal reflux. Laryngoscope 2011;121(9):1902–29.

49. Wiener GJ, Tsukashima R, Kelly C, et al. Oropharyngeal pH monitoring for the detection of liquid and aerosolized supraesophageal gastric reflux. J Voice 2009;23(4):498–504.

50. Sun G, Muddana S, Slaughter JC, et al. A new pH catheter for laryngopharyng-eal reflux: normal values. Laryngoscope 2009;119(8):1639–43.

51. Yuksel ES, Slaughter JC, Mukhtar N, et al. An oropharyngeal pH monitoring de-vice to evaluate patients with chronic laryngitis. Neurogastroenterol Motil 2013; 25(5):e315–23.

52. Yuksel ES, Strugala V, Slaughter JC, et al. Rapid salivary pepsin test: blinded assessment of test performance in GERD. Laryngoscope 2012;6:1312–6.

53. Altman KW, Prufer N, Vaezi MF. The challenge of protocols for reflux disease: a review and development of a critical pathway. Otolaryngol Head Neck Surg 2011;145(1):7–14.

54. Qadeer MA, Phillips CO, Lopez AR, et al. Proton pump inhibitor therapy for sus-pected GERD-related chronic laryngitis: a meta-analysis of randomized controlled trials. Am J Gastroenterol 2006;101(11):2646–54.

55. Fackler WK, Ours TM, Vaezi MF, et al. Long term effect of H2RA therapy on nocturnal gastric acid breakthrough. Gastroenterology 2002;122:625–32.

56. Swoger J, Ponsky J, Hicks DM, et al. Surgical fundoplication in laryngeal reflux unresponsive to aggressive acid suppression: a controlled study. Clin Gastroenterol Hepatol 2006;4:433–41.
57. So JB, Zeitels SM, Rattner DW. Outcome of atypical symptoms attributed to gastroesophageal reflux treated by laparoscopic fundoplication. Surgery 1998; 124:28–32.

Esophageal Pathology
A Brief Guide and Atlas

Sita Chokhavatia, MD[a], Latifat Alli-Akintade, MD[b],*,
Noam Harpaz, MD, PhD[c], Richard Stern, MD[d]

KEYWORDS

- Esophageal pathology • Dysphagia • Esophageal disorders • Endoscopic evaluation

KEY POINTS

- *Dysphagia* refers to an abnormality with food propulsion.
- Dysphagia may be caused by oropharyngeal or esophageal disorders.
- Radiological modalities, endoscopy, and manometry play an important role in both the diagnosis and management of esophageal disorders.

INTRODUCTION

Dysphagia occurs when there is an abnormality in the propulsion of the ingested bolus during its course from the mouth to the stomach.[1] Difficulties can occur in the oropharyngeal or esophageal phases of swallowing because of functional disorders (dysmotility) or structural lesions (mechanical obstruction) (**Table 1**).

Oropharyngeal (transfer) dysphagia symptoms include difficult initiation of swallows, food sticking in the upper throat or neck, coughing when swallowing, nasal regurgitation, halitosis, or pain on swallowing (odynophagia). Esophageal (transport) dysphagia symptoms include a lower cervical, suprasternal, or retrosternal location of obstruction to food bolus; odynophagia; chest pain; bland regurgitation; nausea; emesis; heartburn; halitosis; or weight loss. In addition to a thorough history directed to elicit dysphagia as well as other symptoms of associated systemic disease, the diagnostic evaluation includes a barium swallow (esophagogram),

The authors have no disclosure.
[a] Division of Gastroenterology, Rutgers-Robert Wood Johnson School of Medicine, One Robert Wood Johnson Place, MEB 478A, New Brunswick, NJ 08903, USA; [b] Division of Gastroenterology, University of California, Davis Medical Center, 2315 Stockton Boulevard South 3, Room 3016, Sacramento, CA 95817, USA; [c] Department of Pathology, The Icahn School of Medicine at Mount Sinai, Annenberg Building, 15th Floor, Room 321468, Madison Avenue, New York, NY 10029, USA; [d] Department of Radiology, The Icahn School of Medicine at Mount Sinai, Radiology Associates, Klingenstein Pavillion 1176 5th Avenue, MC Level, New York, NY 10029, USA
* Corresponding authors.
E-mail address: latifat.alli@gmail.com

0030-6665/13/$ – see front matter © 2013 Elsevier Inc. All rights reserved.

Table 1
Causes of dysphagia

	Oropharyngeal (Transfer) Dysphagia	Esophageal (Transport) Dysphagia
Extrinsic structural obstruction	Cervical osteophytes Goiter Zenker diverticulum Head/neck neoplasm	Vascular compression Mediastinal lesions Cervical osteoarthritis
Intrinsic structural obstruction (mucosal/ submucosal)	Cricopharyngeal bar Webs Esophageal, pharyngeal neoplasms	Rings/webs Strictures: peptic, malignant Diverticula Esophageal tumors
Neuromuscular diseases	Cerebrovascular accident Parkinson disease Multiple sclerosis Amyotrophic lateral sclerosis Myasthenia gravis	Achalasia Abnormal peristalsis (hypercontractility or hypocontractility) Diffuse esophageal spasm Scleroderma
Metabolic diseases	Thyroid disease	Thyroid disease Amyloidosis Wilson disease
Infectious diseases	Viral/bacterial meningitis Diphtheria	Candidiasis Cytomegalovirus Herpes simplex
Rheumatologic diseases	—	Sjögren syndrome Systemic lupus erythematosus Inflammatory myopathies Mixed connective tissue disease Rheumatoid arthritis
Iatrogenic causes	Postsurgical anatomic changes Postradiation strictures Medications	Anastomotic strictures Postradiation strictures Medications
Miscellaneous	—	Eosinophilic esophagitis

Adapted from Gasiorowska A, Fass R. Current Approach to Dysphagia. Gastroenterol Hepatol 2009;5(4):269–79.

Esophagogastroduodenoscopy (EGD), and esophageal manometry. Neck and chest computed tomography (CT) scans and endoscopic ultrasound (EUS) help in the diagnosis of submucosal neoplasms and the staging of malignant tumors.

CERVICAL OSTEOPHYTES

Cervical osteophytes are common in the elderly population. Bridging anterior osteophytes of the cervical spine are usually caused by diffuse idiopathic skeletal hyperostosis (DISH), also referred to as *senile ankylosing hyperostosis, ankylosing vertebral hyperostosis, osteoarthritis,* or *Forestier disease.* The C5-C6 vertebrae levels are the most commonly involved.[2] Cervical osteophytes may cause dysphagia through mechanical obstruction of the esophagus or inflammation causing pharyngitis or periesophagitis. In addition to back or neck stiffness, which is associated with pain, patients report solid food dysphagia and aspiration with swallows. Osteophytes impinging on esophageal lumen can be seen on the barium swallow (**Fig. 1**A). CT and magnetic resonance imaging (MRI) of the neck (see **Fig. 1**B) can be useful to visualize

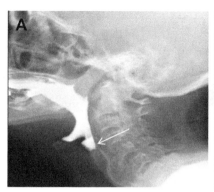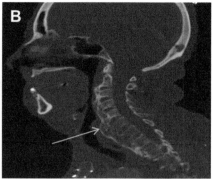

Fig. 1. (A) Esophagram: *Arrow* showing extrinsic compression of the esophagus by cervical osteophytes. (B) MRI: *Arrow* showing bridging osteophytes in the cervical spine.

osteophytes and evaluate infection of the larynx and pharyngeal abscess. The treatment is conservative and directed toward antiinflammatory and antibiotic medications. Surgical intervention for the removal of osteophytes is undertaken in a select few patients for treating severe dysphagia and/or dyspnea.[3]

ZENKER DIVERTICULUM

Zenker diverticulum occurs because of esophageal mucosal and submucosal herniation in the weak area between the transverse fibers of the cricopharyngeus and the oblique fibers of the inferior pharyngeal constrictor (Killian triangle). It is presumed to result from abnormal upper esophageal motility. It is more prevalent in men than women and usually seen in patients aged 60 years and older. The prevalence in the general population is estimated to be 0.01% to 0.11 %.[4] The symptoms include foul breath (halitosis) caused by retained contents in the diverticulum, aspiration, bland regurgitation of food into the mouth, cough, and hoarseness. In some cases, the diverticulum enlarges and encroaches anteriorly into the esophageal lumen causing an extrinsic mechanical obstruction of the upper esophagus. Diagnosis is based on a barium swallow, which shows the contrast retained within the diverticulum (**Fig. 2**A). Care should be taken when endoscopic examination is attempted (see **Fig. 2**B). If the diverticulum is inadvertently intubated instead of the esophageal lumen, further advancing the scope may lead to esophageal perforation.

Symptomatic patients are treated with endoscopic incision or surgical diverticulectomy. The significant surgical morbidity has led to a development of less invasive endoscopic techniques, including the needle-knife technique.[4]

CRICOPHARYNGEAL BAR

Cricopharyngeal bar refers to the posterior barlike indentation caused by the pharyngoesophageal segment of the upper esophageal sphincter. Barium swallow shows this indentation at the C5-C6 vertebrae level. This finding is usually an incidental radiological finding unless there is severe impingement on the esophageal lumen, which can cause dysphagia (**Fig. 3**).

Patients aged 60 years and older may report that multiple swallows are required to propel a food bolus and that choking or aspiration occurs during swallows.

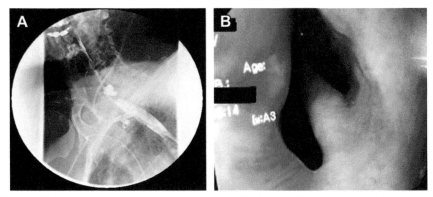

Fig. 2. (*A*) Esophagogram showing Zenker diverticulum with narrowing of the cervical esophagus. (*B*) EGD showing the 2 lumen; true esophageal lumen above the Zenker diverticulum.

Dilation with bougienage or endoscopic injection of botulinum toxin into the cricopharyngeal muscle may relieve dysphagia symptoms. Cricopharyngeal myotomy, an endoscopic or surgical intervention, provides a definitive treatment option for symptomatic patients.[5]

ESOPHAGEAL NEOPLASMS

Mucosal intraluminal tumors and submucosal polypoid lesions compromise the esophageal lumen, leading to the mechanical obstruction of the swallowed food bolus transit. EGD can be used to view and biopsy mucosal lesions. EUS can evaluate submucosal lesions, and fine-needle aspiration biopsies can be obtained. Squamous and adenocarcinoma are the 2 main histologic types of esophageal cancers. EUS and CT/ MRI (**Fig. 4**A) play a key role in the diagnosis and staging of esophageal tumors. Chronic gastroesophageal reflux disease (GRD) can lead to specialized intestinal metaplasia (Barrett esophagus) and is considered a premalignant condition for esophageal adenocarcinoma (see **Fig. 4**B).

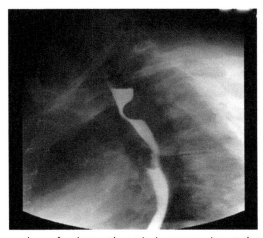

Fig. 3. Esophagogram shows focal smooth extrinsic compression at the posterior aspect of the proximal esophagus.

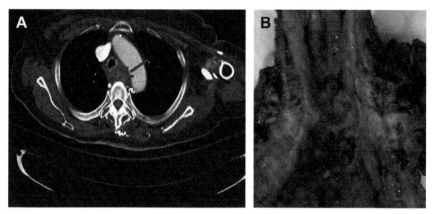

Fig. 4. (*A*) CT scan: *Arrow* showing anterior esophageal compression by mass. (*B*) Barrett esophagus associated adenocarcinoma at the gastroesophageal junction, ulcerated tumor mass with transmural infiltration of the wall.

NEUROLOGIC DISORDERS

Neuromuscular diseases, including muscular dystrophy, inflammatory myopathies, and mitochondrial myopathies, can cause both oropharyngeal and esophageal dysphagia, with the former more common. Cerebrovascular accidents (strokes), multiple sclerosis, Parkinson disease, amyotrophic lateral sclerosis, and cranial neuropathies cause dysphagia by affecting different parts of the central and peripheral nervous system. Neurologic disorders are not reviewed in this article.[6]

SCHATZKI RING

Schatzki ring is a lower esophageal mucosal ring located just above the gastroesophageal junction that can cause intermittent dysphagia to solids. The mechanism of the formation of the Schatzki ring (**Fig. 5**) remains unclear. GERD has been implicated in its pathogenesis because a decreased risk of recurrence is seen after acid suppression treatment. Patients generally become symptomatic only when the internal ring diameter is less than 13 mm.[7] Patients present with intermittent dysphagia to solid food

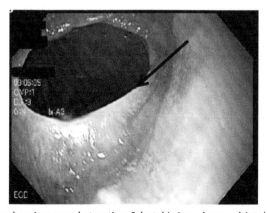

Fig. 5. EGD: *Arrow* showing nonobstructing Schatzki ring above a hiatal hernia.

(steak house syndrome), especially when the ingested bolus is large. Subtle luminal narrowing is best visualized on a barium swallow and may be missed during an endoscopic examination. Endoscopy is less sensitive than the esophagogram for diagnosis but enables therapeutic intervention of balloon dilation of the ring. One study reported 68% of patients were symptom free at 1 year, 35% at 2 years, and only 11% at 5 years following balloon dilation. The rate of recurrent dysphagia was independent of the initial size of the ring and presence or absence of esophagitis.[7] If dysphagia persists despite repeated dilations, other treatment options include biopsy forceps or electrosurgical incision.

ESOPHAGEAL DIVERTICULA

Esophageal diverticula (**Fig. 6**) may be congenital or acquired. The latter occurs because of the herniation of the mucosa and submucosa through the muscle layers of the esophageal as a result of increased intraluminal pressures or external traction from benign or neoplastic mediastinal disease. Only about 37% to 63% of patients with diverticulum are symptomatic.[8] A primary esophageal motility disorder, such as achalasia, is thought to contribute to the development of the diverticulum.

Symptoms may include dysphagia, regurgitation of undigested food, chest pain, and weight loss. Respiratory symptoms caused by aspiration may also occur. Although diagnosed by a barium swallow, an evaluation with endoscopic ultrasound may be useful for ruling out neoplasms. Asymptomatic patients or patients with mild symptoms do require therapeutic interventions. The treatment is directed toward underlying disease, such as a peptic stricture or achalasia. Surgical resection of the diverticulum is recommended for patients with severe dysphagia and weight loss attributed to diverticular disease.

GERD AND ESOPHAGEAL STRICTURE

Gastroesophageal reflux occurs because of the disruption of the gastroesophageal barrier allowing the reflux of gastric contents into the esophageal lumen. A decreased resting lower esophageal sphincter (LES) pressure occurs from a variety of causes, including systemic diseases, such as scleroderma, or medications, such as anticholinergics. Recurrent transient relaxation of the LES, hiatal hernia, and obesity are other causes that can contribute to GERD. Although hiatal hernia is

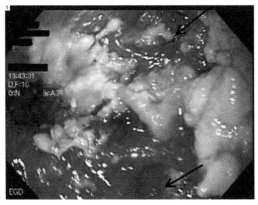

Fig. 6. EGD: *Arrows* showing multiple esophageal diverticula in the distal esophagus (*arrows*).

seen in up to 10% to 80% of US adults,[9] symptoms are usually reported by patients with large herniation. Heartburn, regurgitation, and chest pain are the most common esophageal symptom of GERD. Extraesophageal GERD symptoms include chronic cough, nausea, asthma, hoarseness, laryngitis, pharyngitis, and sinusitis. In one study, 37% of patients with endoscopy-confirmed esophagitis had dysphagia, 43% had severe esophagitis, and 35% had mild esophagitis.[10] Esophagitis and esophageal strictures are GERD complications that predispose to dysphagia. EGD allows mucosal evaluation, biopsy, and therapeutic interventions for the balloon dilation of strictures. The degree of severity of esophagitis, based on endoscopy, is classified by the Los Angeles (LA) grade scale from A to D. Grade A (**Fig. 7**A) refers to one or more mucosal breaks no longer than 5 mm; grade B refers to the presence of one or more mucosal breaks more than 5 mm, not extending between the tops of the

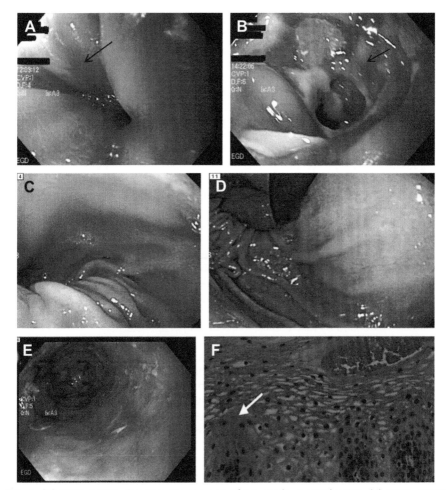

Fig. 7. (*A*) EGD: *Arrow* showing appearance of LA grade A esophagitis. (*B*) EGD: *Arrow* showing appearance of LA grade D esophagitis. (*C, D*) EGD shows hiatal hernia on forward view and on retroflexion. (*E*) Endoscopic appearance of peptic esophagitis. (*F*) H&E stain: *Arrow* showing vascular lakes and patchy squamous cell ballooning which reflects chemically induced intracellular edema and leakage of plasma albumin.

2 mucosal folds; grade C refers to mucosal breaks extending between the top of 2 or more mucosal folds but less than 75% of the esophageal circumference; and grade D (see **Fig. 7**B) has mucosal breaks involving more than 75% of the esophageal circumference. Acid suppressant is the mainstay of treatment.[11] Symptomatic patients with minimal response or no response to medical treatment after 4 to 8 weeks of therapy should be further evaluated, initially with EGD and, if indicated, a pH test. Patients with large hernias (see **Fig. 7**C, D) or complications of GERD despite aggressive medical treatment, such as strictures, ulcers, bleeding, or pulmonary complications, may benefit from antireflux surgery or, more recently, antireflux endoscopic interventions.[12]

Esophageal luminal narrowing may be caused by intrinsic narrowing by fibrosis or tumors or external compression by thoracic tumors. Strictures may be benign or malignant lesions. Peptic, infectious, and autoimmune disease or caustic and radiation injury can cause esophageal strictures. In addition to dysphagia, other symptoms may include chest pain, odynophagia, weight loss, anorexia, and food impaction. A barium study provides information on the location, diameter, and extent of the disease. A chest radiograph and CT scan are useful in evaluating the cause of an extrinsic compression, especially for malignancy and its staging. EGD is also useful to establish the diagnosis, obtain a biopsy and brush cytology, and for therapeutic intervention. EGD is more sensitive than esophagram in the diagnosis of small flat mucosal lesions and has the advantage of allowing biopsies to be taken for histology. Endoscopic ultrasound (EUS) allows for the evaluation of submucosal lesions and staging malignant lesions.

Benign strictures are treated with endoscopic balloon dilatation and aggressive acid suppression using a proton pump inhibitor (PPI). Malignant strictures are managed based on the prognosis. The treatment options include curative surgery or palliative treatment, including esophageal stents for relieving dysphagia.

ACHALASIA

Achalasia is an esophageal motility disorder of an unknown cause. Infectious, autoimmune, and degenerative causes have been implicated. Because the inhibitory neurons of the myenteric (Auerbach) plexus are primarily affected and the excitatory neurons are spared, there is a loss of inhibition leading to high resting lower esophageal spincter (LES) pressures and a failure of relaxation with swallows. The sequential peristaltic contraction preceded by relaxation is lost resulting in aperistalsis.

Chagas disease occurs in Central and South America and is caused by infection with the parasite *Trypanosoma cruzi*. The loss of intramural ganglion cells causes aperistalsis. Malignancy, either by direct invasion into the esophageal nerve bundles (as seen in adenocarcinoma of the gastroesophageal junction) or part of a paraneoplastic syndrome, may have a similar effect and is termed *pseudoachalasia*. The diagnosis is based on symptoms of gradually progressive dysphagia to solids and liquids; bland regurgitation; halitosis; heartburn; nausea; weight loss; emesis; nocturnal coughing; choking; aspiration; maneuvers to force bolus propulsion or transit, such as multiple swallows; and carbonated beverages and positioning to aid bolus passage. In addition to typical symptoms, endoscopy may reveal dilated proximal esophagus (**Fig. 8**A). Barium swallow shows classic bird's beak appearance (**Fig 8**B). Manometry can also support the diagnosis (**Fig. 8**C). Chest and abdomen CT should be obtained if there is clinical suspicion for malignancy. Nitrates and calcium channel blockers have been used with variable success, but therapy is often limited by side effects, including headache and tachyphylaxis. Endoscopic treatment includes

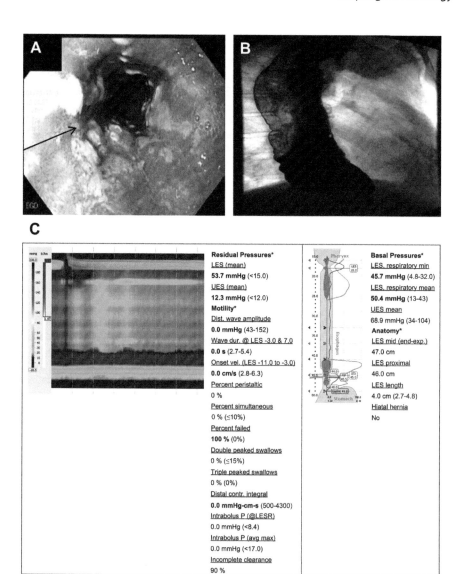

Fig. 8. (*A*) EGD: *Arrow* showing candidiasis and distal narrowing suggesting achalasia. (*B*) Esophagram showing high-grade narrowing in the distal esophagus with dilated corkscrew seen proximally. (*C*) Manometry: Shows aperistalsis, high lower esophageal sphincter pressure as well as abscent relaxation with swallowing.

botulinum toxin injection to decrease LES pressure and pneumatic dilation to disrupt the LES. About 10% to 15% of patients do poorly with pneumatic dilation but do well with surgical myotomy. Surgical myotomy using minimally invasive intervention provides good to excellent relief of symptoms in 70% to 90% of patients.[13] Because up to 11% of patients develop postoperative reflux esophagitis, fundoplication may be done to reduce the incidence of reflux, but this may increase the rate of postoperative dysphagia. Recent reports of successful endoscopic myotomy (POEMS) provide yet another treatment option.[14]

DIFFUSE ESOPHAGEAL SPASM

Diffuse esophageal spasm (DES) is a neuroinhibitory dysfunction characterized by simultaneous high-amplitude contractions of the esophageal smooth muscle with intervening normal peristaltic contractions. The symptoms include dysphagia, odynophagia, or retrosternal chest pain, which may occur after the ingestion of solids or liquids. The symptoms can vary from absent to mild to severe. The diagnosis is based on typical manometric findings of synchronous pressure waves (>8 cm/s), with a minimum amplitude of 30 mm Hg in more than 20% of 10 swallows and some normal peristaltic waves (**Fig. 9**A). A barium swallow may show a corkscrew esophagus or an area of focal spasm (see **Fig. 9**B). Smooth muscle relaxants, such as anticholinergics, calcium channel blockers, and long-acting nitrates, may decrease high-amplitude simultaneous esophageal contractions. Endoscopic injections of botulinum toxin may provide some benefit. In one study, 48% of patients had symptom relief that continued over 7 months.[15] Antidepressants can decrease the discomfort experienced and improve patients' reaction to pain without significantly changing esophageal motility.[16]

INFECTIOUS ESOPHAGITIS

Infectious esophagitis (**Fig. 10**) is an important cause of dysphagia and could be a fungal (*Candida*), viral (herpes simplex virus [HSV], cytomegalovirus [CMV], human immunodeficiency virus [HIV]), or bacterial infection. *Candida*, the most common cause of infectious esophagitis, is seen mostly in immunocompromised patients (HIV, malignancy, or those who have received steroids or chemotherapy). About 25% of patients with Candida esophagitis also have esophageal stasis from diseases, such as scleroderma and achalasia, that allow for growth of the fungus.[17] Presenting symptoms include chest pain, vomiting, dysphagia, odynophagia, and fever. Although oropharyngeal candidiasis is commonly associated with esophageal candidiasis, only 50% to 75% of patients with Candida esophagitis have concurrent oropharyngeal disease. Therefore, the presence of esophageal disease cannot be excluded in the absence of oral thrush.[18] Barium studies show plaquelike lesions separated by segments of normal mucosa. In severe cases, it may appear cobblestonelike, snakeskinlike, or with a pseudo intramural diverticulosis or dumbbell-shaped appearance. Endoscopy-guided biopsy for histopathology and culture remains the best means of diagnosis and guidance of appropriate antifungal therapy. Candida esophagitis is treated with topical or oral antifungal agents, such as nystatin, fluconazole, itraconazole, and intravenous amphotericin (for severe cases). Intravenous ganciclovir is the treatment of choice for CMV in patients with HIV. Foscarnet is used as second-line of treatment. In infectious esophagitis caused by HSV, acyclovir is the preferred treatment.

EOSINOPHILIC ESOPHAGITIS

Eosinophilic esophagitis (EoE) is a chronic disease that occurs because of the immunologic response of the esophagus on exposure to foods or other aeroallergens. The diagnosis is based on the clinical history, endoscopic appearance, and histology. EGD may show mucosal friability, circumferential ringed appearance, longitudinal furrows (**Fig. 11**A, B), altered mucosal vascular pattern, white exudates, mucosal tears, and strictures. A high number of eosinophils (more than 15 per high-power field) have been described in association with dysphagia, hence the term EoE (**Fig. 11**C). There may be an EoE response to acid suppression therapy with PPI suggesting an

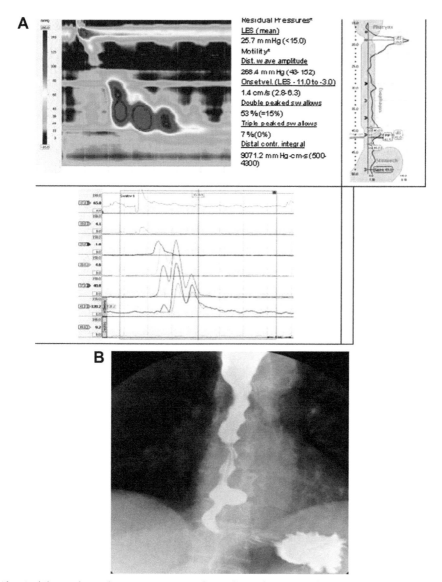

Fig. 9. (*A*) Esophageal manometry: Distal esophageal spasm, which is a variant of jack-hammer esophagus, a cause of dysphagia and chest pain. (*B*) Esophagogram shows appearance of corkscrew esophagus.

association between EoE and GERD. Initially thought to be a pediatric disease, EoE has been increasingly diagnosed in young adults aged between 20 and 40 years. Symptoms include solid food dysphagia, food impaction, heartburn, nausea, and vomiting. Up to 80% of these patients have a history of atopic disease, and only 55% have increased serum immunoglobulin E.[19] Up to 32% of symptomatic patients may have a normal appearance on EGD.[20–24] Radiographic imaging may show a concentric appearance, hence the terms *ring esophagus*, *concentric esophagus*, *feline esophagus*, or *corrugated esophagus*. Treatment is directed toward avoidance

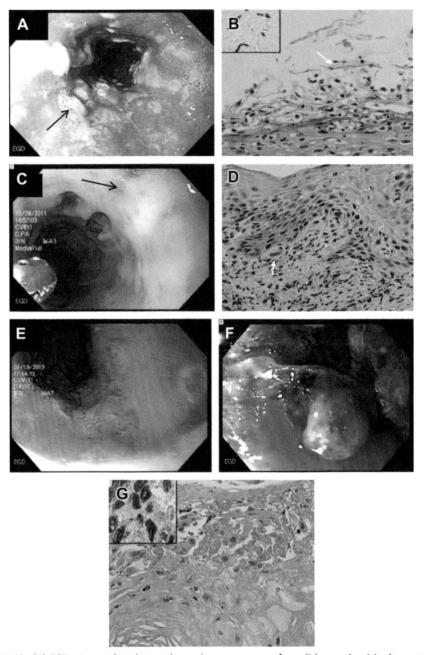

Fig. 10. (*A*) EGD: *Arrow* showing endoscopic appearance of candida esophagitis characterized by multiple grey-white pseudomembranes. (*B*) Candida H&E stain: *Arrow* showing neutrophil infiltration of the squamous mucosa and superficial epithelial sloughing corresponding to the endoscopic pseudomembranes. Arrow designates bluish candida pseudohyphae. Inset: Candida pseudohyphae and spores highlighted with methenamine silver stain. (*C*) EGD: *Arrow* pointing at punched out lesions seen in cytomegalovirus esophagitis. (*D*) H&E stain: *Arrow* showing inflamed squamous esophageal mucosa with enlarged, cytomegalovirus-infected cell featuring intranuclear inclusion and pale cytoplasm. (*E–F*) EGD showing intraluminal ulcerated (*E*) and necrotic mass (*F*) in the esophagus. (*G*) H&E stain showing sharply circumscribed irregular ulcers with erythematous borders. Inset: immunostain positive for herpes.

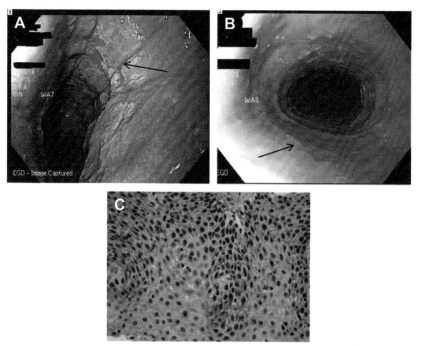

Fig. 11. (*A*) EGD: *Arrow* showing longitudinal furrows and plaques in midesophagus. (*B*) EGD: *Arrow* showing feline appearance with circumferential rings, longitudinal furrows, abscesses. (*C*) Histology: marked increased intraepithelial eosinophils (50 per high-power field) with degranulation (original magnification ×400).

of food allergens by instituting an elimination diet. Topical therapy consists of swallowed steroids, fluticasone, or budesonide in slurry form. There are less adverse events related to topical treatment than with use of systemic steroids. There is an increased risk of perforation associated with endoscopic dilation of EoE strictures.

RHEUMATOLOGIC DISEASES

Dysphagia is a feature of many common rheumatologic diseases. Dysphagia is a well-known complication of scleroderma (component of Calcinosis, Raynauds, Esophageal dysmotility, Sclerodacyl and Telangectasia syndrome [CREST]), with esophageal manifestations in up to 90% of patients. It is seen in up to a third of patients with Sjögren, 13% of patients with systemic lupus erythematosus, 38% of patients with mixed connective tissues disease, and up to 30% of patients with rheumatoid arthritis.[25] The diagnosis is based on the correlation between a history of underlying disease and imaging modalities, showing defective peristalsis and motility. Management is directed toward the treatment of the underlying rheumatologic disease.

REFERENCES

1. Gasiorowska A, Fass R. Current approach to dysphagia. Gastroenterol Hepatol 2009;5(4):269–79.
2. Goh PY, Dobson M, Iseli T, et al. Forestier's disease presenting with dysphagia and dysphonia. J Clin Neurosci 2010;17(10):1336–8. http://dx.doi.org/10.1016/j.jocn.2010.04.002.

3. Maiuri F, Stella L, Sardo L, et al. Dysphagia and dyspnea due to an anterior cervical osteophyte. Arch Orthop Trauma Surg 2002;122:245–7.

4. Ferreira LE, Simmons DT, Baron TH. Zenker's diverticula: pathophysiology, clinical presentation, and flexible endoscopic management. Dis Esophagus 2008; 21:1–8. http://dx.doi.org/10.1111/j.1442-2050.2007.00795.x.

5. Cook IJ. Diagnostic evaluation of dysphagia. Nat Clin Pract Gastroenterol Hepatol 2008;5:393–403. http://dx.doi.org/10.1038/ncpgasthep1153.

6. Pfeiffer RF. Neurogenic dysphagia. Daroff: Bradley's neurology in clinical practice. 6th edition. 2012. p. 153–63.

7. Müller M, Gockel I, Hedwig P, et al. Is the Schatzki ring a unique esophageal entity? World J Gastroenterol 2011;17(23):2838–43. http://dx.doi.org/10.3748/wjg. v17.i23.2838.

8. Soares R, Herbella FA, Prachand VN, et al. Epiphrenic diverticulum of the esophagus. From pathophysiology to treatment. J Gastrointest Surg 2010;14(12): 2009–15. http://dx.doi.org/10.1007/s11605-010-1216-9.

9. Hyun JJ, Bak YT. Clinical significance of hiatal hernia. Gut Liver 2011;5(3): 267–77. http://dx.doi.org/10.5009/gnl.2011.5.3.267.

10. Vakil NB, Traxler B, Levine D. Dysphagia in patients with erosive esophagitis: prevalence, severity, and response to proton pump inhibitor treatment. Clin Gastroenterol Hepatol 2004;2(8):665–8.

11. Katz PO, Gerson LB, Vela MF. Guidelines for the diagnosis and management of gastroesophageal reflux disease. Am J Gastroenterol 2013;108:308–28. http://dx. doi.org/10.1038/ajg.2012.444.

12. Arts J, Tack J, Galmiche JP. Endoscopic antireflux procedures. Gut 2004;53(8): 1207–14. http://dx.doi.org/10.1136/gut.2003.025460.

13. Richter JE. A young man with new diagnosis of Achalasia. Clin Gastroenterol Hepatol 2008;6:859–63.

14. Swanstrom LL, Kurian A, Dunst CM, et al. Long-term outcomes of an endoscopic myotomy for achalasia: the POEM procedure. Ann Surg 2012;256(4):659–67. http://dx.doi.org/10.1097/SLA.0b013e31826b5212.

15. Miller LS, Pullela SV, Parkman HP, et al. Treatment of chest pain in patients with noncardiac, nonreflux, nonachalasia spastic esophageal motor disorders using botulinum toxin injection into the gastroesophageal junction. Am J Gastroenterol 2002;97(7):1640–6.

16. Grübel C, Borovicka J, Schwizer W, et al. Diffuse esophageal spasm. Am J Gastroenterol 2008;103:450–7. http://dx.doi.org/10.1111/j.1572-0241.2007.01632.x.

17. Sam JW, Levine MS, Rubesin SE, et al. The "foamy" esophagus. A radiographic sign of Candida esophagitis. Am J Roentgenol 2000;174:999–1002.

18. Baig MA, Rasheed J, Subkowitz D, et al. Severe esophageal candidiasis in an immunocompetent patient. Int J Infect Dis 2006;5(1). http://dx.doi.org/10.5580/ a1f.

19. Nonevski IT, Downs-Kelly E, Falk GW. Eosinophilic esophagitis: an increasingly recognized cause of dysphagia, food impaction and refractory heartburn. Cleve Clin J Med 2008;75(9):623–33.

20. Liacouras CA, Spergel JM, Ruchelli E, et al. Eosinophilic esophagitis: a 10-year experience in 381 children. Clin Gastroenterol Hepatol 2005;3(12): 1198–206.

21. Dellon ES, Gonsalves N, Hirano I, et al. ACG Clinical guideline: evidence based approach to the diagnosis and management of esophageal eosinophilia and eosinophilic esophagitis (EoE). Am J Gastroenterol 2013;108:679–92. http://dx. doi.org/10.1038/ajg.2013.71.

22. Pregun I, Hritz I, Tulassay Z, et al. Peptic esophageal stricture: medical treatment. Dig Dis 2009;27(1):31–7. http://dx.doi.org/10.1159/000210101.
23. Ali MA, Lam-Himlin D, Voltaggio L. Eosinophilic esophagitis: a clinical, endoscopic, and histopathologic review. Gastrointest Endosc 2012;76(6):1224–37.
24. Smith MS. Esophageal webs and rings. In: Richter JE, Castell DO, editors. The esophagus. 5th edition. Oxford (United Kingdom): Wiley-Blackwell; 2012. http://dx.doi.org/10.1002/9781444346220.ch16.
25. Sheehan NJ. Dysphagia and other manifestations of oesophageal involvement in the musculoskeletal diseases. Rheumatology 2008;47(6):746–52. http://dx.doi.org/10.1093/rheumatology/ken029.

Malnutrition, Dehydration, and Ancillary Feeding Options in Dysphagia Patients

Michael A. Via, MD[a],*, Jeffrey I. Mechanick, MD[b]

KEYWORDS

- Malnutrition • Dehydration • Metabolic support • Dysphagia

KEY POINTS

- All patients with or at risk for dysphagia should be assessed for nutritional status.
- Minor nutritional deficiencies may be addressed by dietary modification or supplementation.
- Judicious use of nutritional support is recommended in both moderately and severely malnourished patients.
- Enteral nutrition support is preferred and generally well tolerated.

INTRODUCTION

Any medical condition that leads to dysphagia can directly reduce dietary intake and increase nutritional risk. The complex process that allows for the safe passage of masticated food boluses through the pharynx to the esophagus for subsequent digestion and absorption can be disrupted by several physical and neurologic pathologic phenomena. Moreover, a vicious cycle emerges as malnutrition can worsen the dysphagia itself, leading to increased morbidity and mortality.

Adequate nutrition entails the regular intake of calories in the form of carbohydrates, protein, and fats in addition to consumption of certain essential nutrients, such as water, vitamins, minerals, trace elements, certain amino acids, and certain fatty acids. Adequate nutrition is crucial for the maintenance of homeostasis and a healthy physiologic state. In contrast, a state of malnutrition may arise if one or more of these essential dietary components are consumed insufficiently, whether subtle micronutrient insufficiency or overt, severe, and symptomatic protein-calorie malnutrition. Therefore, the comprehensive care of patients with dysphagia must include diligent nutritional assessment and management to optimize clinical outcomes.

[a] Division of Endocrinology and Metabolism, Albert Einstein College of Medicine, Beth Israel Medical Center, 55 East 34th Street, New York, NY 10016, USA; [b] Division of Endocrinology, Diabetes and Bone Disease, Icahn School of Medicine at Mount Sinai, 1 Gustave Levy Place, New York, NY 10029, USA
* Corresponding author.
E-mail address: mvia@chpnet.org

Otolaryngol Clin N Am 46 (2013) 1059–1071
http://dx.doi.org/10.1016/j.otc.2013.08.002
0030-6665/13/$ – see front matter Crown Copyright © 2013 Published by Elsevier Inc. All rights reserved.

Abbreviations: Ancillary Feeding in Dysphagia	
SGA	Subjective Global Assessment
NRI	Nutrition Risk Index
NRS2002	Nutritional Risk Screen 2002
ABW	Adjusted body weight
cf	Corrective factor (for adjusted body weight)
PN	Parenteral nutrition
EN	Enteral nutrition
GI	Gastrointestinal
NG	Nasogastric
PEG	Percutaneous endoscopically inserted gastrostomy

PREVALENCE OF DYSPHAGIA

It is estimated that in the United States alone 300,000 to 600,000 people are diagnosed with clinically significant dysphagia annually.[1] Nearly 70% of these patients are greater than 60 years old.[2]

Common causes of dysphagia include neurologic conditions such as stroke, dementia, cerebral palsy, and Parkinson disease, physical obstruction such as cancer of the oropharynx, chemotherapy or radiation treatment, traumatic endotracheal intubation, or rheumatologic disease such as systemic sclerosis.[1] In the case of stroke, 30% to 65% exhibit dysphagia, which is associated with malnutrition and dehydration, leading to worse overall outcome.[3,4] Pneumonia, the leading cause of mortality following stroke, is associated with dysphagia and aspiration.[5]

For institutionalized dementia patients, the prevalence of dysphagia has been observed to be as high as 45%, again associated with a high risk of pneumonia and aspiration in this population.[6] Most patients with head and neck cancer experience significant dysphagia that leads to malnutrition during the course of the disease.[7] This dysphagia that leads to malnutrition is especially true during or after radiation therapy, chemotherapy, or surgery.[8] Up to 25% of deaths from head and neck cancer may be attributed directly to malnutrition.[9]

MALNUTRITION: MACRONUTRIENT DEFICIENCIES

The direct effect of dysphagia on oral food intake places these patients at high risk for malnutrition. In one study of adults with dysphagia, high-calorie oral supplements were given to 30% and placement of a feeding tube was required in an additional 12%.[10] In another group of older adults, protein-calorie malnutrition was present in 19% of those with dysphagia compared with 12% of individuals without dysphagia.[11]

Several methods have been used to assess a patient's nutritional status and classify their degree of malnutrition as mild, moderate, or severe. Of these, the subjective global assessment (SGA) is easily adapted in most clinical practices. The SGA combines the amount of unintentional weight lost with physical signs of malnutrition (eg, lower extremity edema, muscle wasting), an assessment of GI tract function, and overall health and performance of the patient to provide a nutritional status score.[12,13]

The nutrition risk index (NRI) is also a useful tool that combines weight loss and a measure of serum albumin according to the equation: NRI = 0.417 × (current weight − usual weight)/(usual weight) × 100 + serum albumin (mg/dL) × 15.9.[14] A patient with an NRI of less than 83.5 is considered severely malnourished. If their NRI is between 83.5 and 97.5, they are considered moderately malnourished.

Table 1
Nutritional risk screening 2002

Nutritional status	1 Point	2 Points	3 Points
	Weight loss >5% in 3 mo or dietary intake 50%–75% of normal	Weight loss >5% in 2 mo, dietary intake 25%–50% of normal, or BMI of 18.5–20.5	Weight loss >5% in 1 mo, dietary intake 0%–25% of normal, or BMI <18.5
Medical condition	Chronic pulmonary disease, oncologic disease, diabetes, hepatic cirrhosis,	Stroke, hematologic malignancy, severe pneumonia, major abdominal surgery	Head injury, bone marrow transplant, critical illness
Age	>70		

A total score of 3 or higher is considered at risk for malnutrition; a score of 5 or higher is considered severe malnutrition.

A third nutritional evaluation tool that has been validated in clinical trials is the Nutritional Risk Screen 2002 (NRS2002).[15,16] This method incorporates information about unintentional weight loss, severity of illness, and age (**Table 1**) and is especially useful in hospitalized patients.[16–19]

REFEEDING SYNDROME

Patients that are severely malnourished for prolonged periods undergo a physiologic compensation that includes catabolism of lean body mass and reduced energy expenditure. These patients are generally deficient in multiple micronutrients and electrolytes, and they are at risk for the development of refeeding syndrome.[20] If adequate nutrition is rapidly reintroduced, cellular metabolic pathways are activated and consume the available micronutrients while driving potassium, magnesium, and phosphorus electrolytes into cells, leading to a rapid decline in circulating levels. Severe hypokalemia or hypomagnesemia may cause cardiac arrhythmias, while hypophosphatemia may lead to muscle weakness and respiratory failure.

Many patients, including those that are only mildly malnourished, may experience a decline in serum phosphorus levels after the introduction of nutritional support; however, this condition of refeeding hypophosphatemia is mild in comparison to the rapid decline in serum phosphorus in severely malnourished individuals.[21] Consequently, refeeding syndrome is potentially fatal. To prevent this condition, nutrition is slowly reintroduced to severely malnourished patients. Current guidelines recommend starting at a daily calorie intake of 10 kcal/kg and advancing over a 4- to 7-day period to the

Table 2
Estimated daily requirements for macronutrients and water

Calories	25–35 kcal/kg[a]
Protein	1–1.5 g/kg 0.8–1 g/kg Renal insufficiency 1.5–2 g/kg Renal failure on dialysis
Dietary fats	0.8–1 g/kg
Water	30–40 mL/kg

[a] Use ABW for daily calorie goals in obese patients.

goal calorie intake. Adequate supplementation with thiamine, potassium, magnesium, and phosphorus is recommended.[22]

MACRONUTRIENT TARGET INTAKE

An appropriate amount of calories and protein must be consumed to meet daily requirements and expenditures (**Table 2**). There are several methods that have been developed to estimate a patient's protein and calorie requirements that are in clinical use.[23] Care should be taken to avoid overfeeding as this may lead to hyperglycemia, hepatosteatosis, accumulation of adipose tissue, and worsened obesity.

A simple and generally accurate estimation of daily calorie requirements is weight-based and is approximated as 25 to 35 kcal/kg, depending on nutritional risk, objectives, and body composition.[24] This estimate generally provides enough energy for metabolic processes to maintain homeostasis with a low rate of overfeeding.

In obese individuals, an adjusted body weight (ABW) is substituted for actual weight, and 25 to 35 kcal/kg of ABW is used to estimate calorie needs. This adjustment is predicated on the increased lean weight that attends increased adiposity and safe, permissive underfeeding to promote lipolysis without excessive restriction in protein based on a corrective factor (*cf*). ABW may be calculated by the following equation: ABW = Ideal weight + ([current weight − ideal weight] × *cf*), where published values of *cf* range from 0.25 to 0.5.[25] In common practice, a conservative value for *cf* is 0.25.[26]

Because there are no protein stores, patients require dietary protein every day. In general, daily protein intake should be approximately 1 g/kg/d in the nonstressed state, with increased amounts to 1.2 to 1.5 g/kg/d in the stressed state. One exception is for patients with renal insufficiency, who require 0.8 to 1 g/kg of protein daily, and for renal failure patients on dialysis that require 1.5 to 2 g/kg to make up for protein loss in dialysis. Obese stressed patients that are permissively underfed should be given close to 1.5 g/kg of protein to optimize nitrogen balance, nearly always necessitating the use of protein supplements.[24]

MALNUTRITION: MICRONUTRIENT DEFICIENCY

Patients with dysphagia that reduce their overall dietary intake or selectively choose foods that are easier to swallow are at risk of micronutrient deficiencies. Commonly observed deficiencies include iron, folate, cobalamin (B12), and vitamin D.[27,28] Other micronutrients, such as thiamin (B1) and zinc, may also be deficient, especially in severely malnourished patients.[29] Even with nutritional support, micronutrient deficiencies may develop that contribute to a decline in the overall health of the patient.[30] Trace metal deficiencies, including iron, zinc, copper, and manganese, have been reported in patients with long-term use of enteral tube feeds.[31]

Empiric supplementation with multivitamins and vitamin D can help to reduce this risk. Periodic testing for serum levels of iron, folate, B12, and vitamin D at 4- to 6-month intervals can ensure adequate micronutrient intake over the course of the disease.[27–29]

In some individuals, micronutrient deficiencies may contribute to the dysphagia itself. A case of dysphagia that was associated with severe B12 deficiency and resolved with the administration of B12 has been reported.[32] This same phenomenon of reversible dysphagia has also been noted in severe B1 deficiency.[33] Adequate supplementation and empiric treatment of these micronutrients can reduce these effects.

DEHYDRATION

Water is an essential component of the diet that is necessary to replace fecal, urinary, and other insensible fluid losses. Daily water requirements are approximately 30 to 40 mL/kg, depending on age, body composition, and energy expenditure. Some of this is ingested as water contained within foods, which generally provide 15% to 25% of the daily requirements of water, while most is consumed separately as a liquid.[34]

Dysphagia patients are at high risk for dehydration, which represents a common cause of morbidity and rehospitalization in this group.[35,36] The actual prevalence of dehydration is difficult to quantify because there is no agreement for the standard clinical definition. Some authors argue that an elevated blood urea nitrogen to creatinine ratio (>15) is sufficient for the diagnosis of dehydration,[37] while a more traditional approach involves a complete assessment of electrolytes for hypernatremia, hyponatremia, and renal function, urine studies for highly concentrated urine, and physical examination findings, such as poor skin turgor and dry mucous membranes.[38]

Patients with dysphagia should be evaluated frequently for signs of dehydration, and if present, further evaluation of other nutritional deficiencies may be warranted.[8,39]

DIETARY MODIFICATION

Components of the diet may be adjusted or modified to facilitate the swallowing process. In general, solid foods are softened and liquids are thickened. Although clinical evidence for this practice is limited, its widespread use is largely based on experience and anecdotal evidence.[40] In one study comparing use of dietary liquids of varying thickness in dysphagia patients, no difference in rates of pneumonia were observed among the different study groups.[41] Some authors speculate that the decreased palatability of these thickened foods and other dietary modifications may contribute to diminished intake and may worsen nutritional status.[1] In one study, the intake of dietary liquids is reduced when thickening agents, such as honey, are added, increasing the risk of dehydration in these patients.[42]

NUTRITIONAL SUPPLEMENTS

Oral supplements in the form of high-calorie, protein, and micronutrient-containing beverages or puddings are available. These products may be added for regular consumption to the diet of dysphagia patients to augment their nutritional intake.

In patients with head and neck cancer, the addition of oral dietary supplements can reduce weight loss and improve tolerability of radiation therapy and surgery.[43] In patients with dementia, oral supplements reduced cognitive decline and weight loss.[44] The inclusion of oral supplements alongside food during mealtime or with snacks increases their consumption and overall caloric intake.[45]

Dysphagia patients treated with oral supplements that continue to lose weight or that show signs of dehydration or other nutritional deficiencies should be assessed for more aggressive nutritional support.

NUTRITIONAL SUPPORT: ENTERAL FEEDING

The enteral feeding route is generally preferred for nutrition support.[24,46] The use of enteral nutrition (EN) in patients with dysphagia can significantly improve nutritional status. A review of feeding practices following stroke that included 33 randomized controlled trials demonstrates the use of enteral feeding through either nasogastric (NG) tube or percutaneous endoscopically inserted gastrostomy (PEG) tube led to increased protein and calorie intake.[39] Although there were no demonstrable differences in mortality, or in functional dependence following stroke, a reduction in decubitus ulcers was noted. Patients with PEG tube feeding also had lower incidence of gastrointestinal (GI) bleeding, higher amount of food delivery, and higher serum albumin levels compared with patients fed with NG tubes.[39]

Patients with long-term and progressive neurologic disorders may also be considered for PEG tube insertion and provision of enteral tube feeds.[47–49] In advanced neurologic disease, patients are unable to meet daily caloric requirements because of dysphagia coupled with diminished appetite due to effects of the underlying disorders on the appetite centers of the hypothalamus and elsewhere in the central nervous system.

The practice of providing EN to patients with advanced dementia is controversial and is currently not recommended.[50,51] The use of EN has been advocated in Parkinson disease patients with dysphagia; however, these patients may require higher calorie intake because of a higher resting energy expenditure associated with muscle rigidity or dyskinesias.[47,52]

Patients with head and neck cancer are at significant risk of dysphagia because of the erosive direct effects of the cancer and the indirect effects of the treatment (surgical, external radiation, and/or and chemotherapy). The prophylactic insertion of a PEG feeding tube before treatment in head and neck cancer remains controversial.[8,53] In some uncontrolled studies, early PEG tube insertion has been associated with lower than expected weight loss in this population.[54,55] Two small randomized trials that compare the use prophylactic PEG tube insertion versus no insertion in patients with head and neck cancer have been published.[56,57] Results of these small trials demonstrate improved quality of life at 6 months of follow-up and slightly lower rates of malnutrition at 6 months and 1 year of follow-up, suggesting the prophylactic management of nutrition may be beneficial in these patients.

The use of NG tubes for enteral feeding has also been advocated in patients with head and neck cancer.[58] The cost of NG tube insertion is approximately 10-fold less than that of PEG tube insertion[59]; however, because patients tend to require several months of tube feed administration, NG tubes need to be replaced every 14 to 20 days to avoid epithelial erosion.[60]

To date, only one small randomized controlled trial (n = 33) has been published comparing PEG versus NG tube feeding in patients with head and neck cancer.[59] In this study, the group of patients in the PEG tube group lost only 1.25 kg at 6 weeks of follow-up, compared with a loss of 3 kg in the NG tube group. By 6 months, no differences were noted.

Current guidelines recommend that patients with head and neck cancer be given EN, especially during radiation treatment. The decision for mode of delivery, either NG or PEG tube, should be made on an individual basis. If a prolonged duration of EN administration is expected, then PEG placement is reasonable.[8,24,46]

JEJUNOSTOMY TUBES

Direct enteral access via the small intestine may also be obtained for provision of EN. Feeding tubes are placed directly into the proximal jejunum either endoscopically, during a laparotomy, or as a gastrostomy or NG tube that extends through the pylorus into the duodenum or jejunum. It is argued that the delivery of tube feeds more distally in the GI tract can reduce reflux and potentially reduce the risk of aspiration; however, no differences in these complications have been observed in patients fed through either prepyloric tube or postpyloric tubes.[61,62]

In patients that have undergone esophagectomy, placement of a jejunostomy allows the administration of tube feeds distal to the anastomosis created during the procedure for improved healing.[63]

Gastric feeding is generally preferred over jejunal feeding because it is considered more physiologic.[24,64] The ability of the stomach to expand to accommodate food boluses allows flexibility in feeding schedule; feeds may be given continuously or as boluses. Jejunal expansion is comparatively limited and jejunal feeds are typically given as a continuous infusion[65] but may limit the patient's mobility and lifestyle. Some patients can tolerate 12-hour or 18-hour jejunal tube feed infusion cycles, which allow for extended periods of time in between cycles and greater flexibility of daily activities; however, feeding rates greater than 120 mL/h are associated with increased rates of diarrhea.[24]

FORMULA SELECTION

A wide range of tube feed formula choices are available for clinical use. These formulas are highly processed foods made from water, corn syrup, starches, oils, soy protein, caseins, and other components. Standard tube feeds are generally the least expensive and adequate in many patients. They contain 1 to 2 kcal/mL. Approximately 50% to 55% of the calories are derived from carbohydrates, 30% to 35% from lipids, and 15% to 20% from protein. Tube feed formulas also contain vitamins and trace elements and generally provide 100% of the recommended daily allowance of these essential micronutrients when greater than 1400 calories are given as tube feeds.

Modified and specialized tube feed formulas are available and may be appropriate in specific clinical conditions.[24] Semi-elemental tube feeds are enzymatically processed to hydrolyzed peptides of varying lengths for easier digestion and absorption. They also typically contain higher amounts of medium-chain triglycerides as their fat source compared with standard intact protein formulas, which are also more easily absorbed.

Semi-elemental tube feeds may be beneficial to patients with intestinal malabsorption because of intestinal ischemia, prior intestinal surgeries, or pancreatic insufficiency.[66] Patients receiving jejunal feeds may also have increased absorption with semi-elemental formulas to prevent diarrhea. If diarrhea develops while on standard tube feeds, switching to a semi-elemental formula may improve absorption and reduce symptoms.[24]

Diabetes-specific tube feed formulas contain a relatively low carbohydrate content. Approximately 35% to 40% of calories are in the form of sugars and starches, compared to 50% to 55% of standard formulas. Minor reductions in blood glucose levels have been observed in randomized trials.[67,68] These formulas can be considered for use in patients with diabetes that exhibit elevated blood glucose levels while receiving tube feeds.[69] There are also several tube feed formulas that contain a relatively low carbohydrate content and may be beneficial in patients with diabetes, even though they are not specifically marketed for use in diabetes.

For patients with renal insufficiency, several concentrated tube feed formulas are available that limit fluid intake and contain low levels of potassium, magnesium, and phosphorus that can reduce the risk of electrolyte abnormalities.[70]

Several other specialized tube feeds exist that are marketed for conditions such as hepatic or pulmonary disease. The use for many of these formulas is limited and generally discouraged as studies have shown minimal clinical benefits.[24,71]

Some specialized formulas are fortified with nutritional substances thought to modulate the immune system, such as glutamine, arginine, ω-3 fatty acids, among others.[72] In randomized trials, the use of these immune-modulating formulas has been shown to reduce time on ventilators and improve mortality in critically ill patients with acute lung injury, acute respiratory distress syndrome, and severe sepsis.[73] The use of immune-modulating tube feeds is reserved for these specific patient populations.

FEED SCHEDULE

Tube feeds are generally initiated at a low rate and slowly titrated to monitor for nausea, vomiting, diarrhea, or other signs of intolerance. An initial continuous infusion allows slow feeding rates to be gradually increased over a 24-hour to 48-hour period. As a patient is shown to tolerate the feeds, conversion to a bolus schedule is possible for those with gastric tubes (NG or PEG tubes).[74] Tube feeds are generally given in 250 to 500 mL boluses several times per day. Each bolus is followed by the administration of 50 to 100 mL of tap water that helps to clear the tube of any residual formula and prevent feeding tube obstruction. The tap water may be substituted with one-half normal saline or normal saline if renal or GI sodium losses are suspected. Greater amounts of water may be given as boluses or between tube feeds in dehydrated patients.[24]

As mentioned, patients receiving jejunal tube feeds are generally kept on continuous feeds. For convenience, the infusion rates can be increased to a 12-hour to 18-hour feeding cycle. As with gastrostomy tubes, jejunostomy tubes must also be flushed after each cycle. Jejunostomy tube flushes should consist of one-half normal saline or normal saline rather than tap water to reduce osmotic injury to intestinal epithelial cells[24] (if the patient has hypernatremia and free water is required, 5% dextrose in water can be used as flushes).

NUTRITION SUPPORT: PARENTERAL NUTRITION

Parenteral nutrition (PN) allows the delivery of essential dietary components and calories intravenously, bypassing the GI tract. Patients may fully meet their nutritional needs with the administration of PN and in some cases have relied on this form of nutrition for greater than 20 to 25 years (Jeffrey I. Mechanick, MD, personal experience).[75] Often the need for PN is temporary and it is typically given acutely or subacutely.

PN is generally associated with higher infection rates and hepatic injury when compared with EN in well-nourished or only mildly malnourished individuals.[17,76,77] However, in these studies, the subgroup of severely malnourished patients demonstrated a benefit from the addition of PN. Thus PN is generally reserved for patients with either severe malnutrition or for those patients that either have loss of GI function or are expected to be unable to tolerate use of the GI tract for at least 7 days.[24] PN is also indicated as a preoperative preparation in severely malnourished patients that are scheduled for surgery.[19,76] All other patients that cannot meet their nutritional requirements should be considered for EN.

Each PN formula is carefully designed to deliver appropriate amounts of dextrose, amino acids, lipids, electrolytes, multivitamins, and trace elements. As with enteral feeding, the daily PN formula should contain 25 to 30 kcal/kg, with 1 to 1.5 g amino acids per kilogram. A physician nutrition specialist should be consulted for the development of each individualized formula to assure compatibility and adequacy of each component.[26]

There are several important risks associated with use of PN, including infection, thrombus formation, hyperglycemia, and hepatic injury. The rate of thrombosis in patients receiving PN is approximately 1% per year.[75]

The high osmolarity of the infused solution requires use of a central venous catheter, which may become infected or occluded from a thrombus. Rates of infection are approximately 5% to 10% per year for patients on home total PN and 3% to 5% per hospitalization.[26] Line infections associated with PN may be due to gram-positive or gram-negative bacteria, or *Candida sp*, and should be treated with broad spectrum coverage, or appropriate antifungals, until the source of infection has been isolated and identified.[78]

Rates of both hyperglycemia and hepatic injury can be reduced through careful adjustment of the dextrose and insulin content in the PN formula. An infusion rate of dextrose less than 2 to 3 mg/kg/min is recommended to manage hyperglycemia.[26] The addition of carnitine to the PN formula may also reduce the risk of hepatosteatosis in at-risk patients.

PN is reserved for patients with inaccessible and dysfunctional GI tracts, or those with severe malnutrition expected to undergo surgery.[26] Most patients with dysphagia do not meet these requirements and generally benefit from EN alone.

SUMMARY

The high prevalence of malnutrition in patients with dysphagia contributes significantly to the morbidity and mortality that is associated with their underlying medical condition. Current clinical practice includes continual assessment of nutritional status in dysphagia patients with care that addresses their nutritional needs. In mild cases, oral nutritional supplements are sufficient. Continued weight loss and poor oral intake may necessitate a more aggressive form of nutritional support that generally involves the administration of EN through a feeding tube. PN is an appropriate alternative to EN when there is dysfunction of the GI tract or in patients with severe malnutrition that plan to undergo surgery.[26] The application of nutritional support improves the functional status, quality of life, and overall disease outcome.

REFERENCES

1. Sura L, Madhavan A, Carnaby G, et al. Dysphagia in the elderly: management and nutritional considerations. Clin Interv Aging 2012;7:287–98.
2. Leder SB, Suiter DM. An epidemiologic study on aging and dysphagia in the acute care hospitalized population: 2000-2007. Gerontology 2009;55:714–8.
3. Smithard DG, O'Neill PA, Parks C, et al. Complications and outcome after acute stroke. Does dysphagia matter? Stroke 1996;27:1200–4.
4. Altman KW, Yu GP, Schaefer SD. Consequence of dysphagia in the hospitalized patient: impact on prognosis and hospital resources. Arch Otolaryngol Head Neck Surg 2010;136:784–9.
5. Pikus L, Levine MS, Yang YX, et al. Videofluoroscopic studies of swallowing dysfunction and the relative risk of pneumonia. AJR Am J Roentgenol 2003; 180:1613–6.
6. Horner J, Alberts MJ, Dawson DV, et al. Swallowing in Alzheimer's disease. Alzheimer Dis Assoc Disord 1994;8:177–89.
7. Righini CA, Timi N, Junet P, et al. Assessment of nutritional status at the time of diagnosis in patients treated for head and neck cancer. Eur Ann Otorhinolaryngol Head Neck Dis 2013;130:8–14.
8. Nugent B, Lewis S, O'Sullivan JM. Enteral feeding methods for nutritional management in patients with head and neck cancers being treated with radiotherapy and/or chemotherapy. Cochrane Database Syst Rev 2013;(1):CD007904.

9. Senesse P, Assenat E, Schneider S, et al. Nutritional support during oncologic treatment of patients with gastrointestinal cancer: who could benefit? Cancer Treat Rev 2008;34:568–75.

10. Roy N, Stemple J, Merrill RM, et al. Dysphagia in the elderly: preliminary evidence of prevalence, risk factors, and socioemotional effects. Ann Otol Rhinol Laryngol 2007;116:858–65.

11. Serra-Prat M, Palomera M, Gomez C, et al. Oropharyngeal dysphagia as a risk factor for malnutrition and lower respiratory tract infection in independently living older persons: a population-based prospective study. Age Ageing 2012;41: 376–81.

12. Baker JP, Detsky AS, Wesson DE, et al. Nutritional assessment: a comparison of clinical judgement and objective measurements. N Engl J Med 1982;306: 969–72.

13. Gabrielson DK, Scaffidi D, Leung E, et al. Use of an abridged scored patient-generated subjective global assessment (abPG-SGA) as a nutritional screening tool for cancer patients in an outpatient setting. Nutr Cancer 2013;65:234–9.

14. Buzby GP, Knox LS, Crosby LO, et al. Study protocol: a randomized clinical trial of total parenteral nutrition in malnourished surgical patients. Am J Clin Nutr 1988;47:366–81.

15. Kondrup J, Allison SP, Elia M, et al. ESPEN guidelines for nutrition screening 2002. Clin Nutr 2003;22:415–21.

16. Kondrup J, Rasmussen HH, Hamberg O, et al. Nutritional risk screening (NRS 2002): a new method based on an analysis of controlled clinical trials. Clin Nutr 2003;22:321–36.

17. Casaer MP, Mesotten D, Hermans G, et al. Early versus late parenteral nutrition in critically ill adults. N Engl J Med 2011;365:506–17.

18. Kuppinger D, Hartl WH, Bertok M, et al. Nutritional screening for risk prediction in patients scheduled for abdominal operations. Br J Surg 2012;99:728–37.

19. Jie B, Jiang ZM, Nolan MT, et al. Impact of preoperative nutritional support on clinical outcome in abdominal surgical patients at nutritional risk. Nutrition 2012;28:1022–7.

20. Ahmed S, Travis J, Mehanna H. Re-feeding syndrome in head and neck–prevention and management. Oral Oncol 2011;47:792–6.

21. Viana Lde A, Burgos MG, Silva Rde A. Refeeding syndrome: clinical and nutritional relevance. Arq Bras Cir Dig 2012;25:56–9.

22. Stanga Z, Brunner A, Leuenberger M, et al. Nutrition in clinical practice-the refeeding syndrome: illustrative cases and guidelines for prevention and treatment. Eur J Clin Nutr 2008;62:687–94.

23. de Oliveira FC, Alves RD, Zuconi CP, et al. Agreement between different methods and predictive equations for resting energy expenditure in overweight and obese Brazilian men. J Acad Nutr Diet 2012;112:1415–20.

24. Bankhead R, Boullata J, Brantley S, et al. Enteral nutrition practice recommendations. JPEN J Parenter Enteral Nutr 2009;33:122–67.

25. Krenitsky J. Adjusted body weight, pro: evidence to support the use of adjusted body weight in calculating calorie requirements. Nutr Clin Pract 2005;20: 468–73.

26. McClave SA, Martindale RG, Vanek VW, et al. Guidelines for the provision and assessment of nutrition support therapy in the adult critically ill patient: Society of Critical Care Medicine (SCCM) and American Society for Parenteral and Enteral Nutrition (A.S.P.E.N.). JPEN J Parenter Enteral Nutr 2009;33:277–316.

27. Orell-Kotikangas H, Schwab U, Osterlund P, et al. High prevalence of vitamin D insufficiency in patients with head and neck cancer at diagnosis. Head Neck 2012;34:1450–5.

28. Gorgulu O, Selcuk T, Ozdemir S, et al. Evaluation of the roles of serum vitamin B(12), folate and homocysteine levels in laryngeal squamous cell carcinoma. J Int Med Res 2010;38:2047–52.

29. Berger MM, Shenkin A. Vitamins and trace elements: practical aspects of supplementation. Nutrition 2006;22:952–5.

30. Obara H, Tomite Y, Doi M. Serum trace elements in tube-fed neurological dysphagia patients correlate with nutritional indices but do not correlate with trace element intakes: case of patients receiving enough trace elements intake. Clin Nutr 2008;27:587–93.

31. Kajiyama H, Murase K, Miyazaki T, et al. Micronutrient status and glutathione peroxidase in bedridden patients on tube feeding. J Int Med Res 2001;29:181–8.

32. Kayhan B, Olmez S, Ozaslan E, et al. Dysphagia resolved with vitamin B12 therapy: a case of esophageal parakeratosis. Endoscopy 2011;43(Suppl 2 UCTN): E231.

33. Karaiskos I, Katsarolis I, Stefanis L. Severe dysphagia as the presenting symptom of Wernicke-Korsakoff syndrome in a non-alcoholic man. Neurol Sci 2008; 29:45–6.

34. Campbell SM. Hydration needs throughout the lifespan. J Am Coll Nutr 2007;26: 585S–7S.

35. Crary MA, Groher ME. Reinstituting oral feeding in tube-fed adult patients with dysphagia. Nutr Clin Pract 2006;21:576–86.

36. Payne C, Wiffen PJ, Martin S. Interventions for fatigue and weight loss in adults with advanced progressive illness. Cochrane Database Syst Rev 2012;(1):CD008427.

37. Lin LC, Yang JT, Weng HH, et al. Predictors of early clinical deterioration after acute ischemic stroke. Am J Emerg Med 2011;29:577–81.

38. Chassagne P, Druesne L, Capet C, et al. Clinical presentation of hypernatremia in elderly patients: a case control study. J Am Geriatr Soc 2006;54:1225–30.

39. Geeganage C, Beavan J, Ellender S, et al. Interventions for dysphagia and nutritional support in acute and subacute stroke. Cochrane Database Syst Rev 2012;(10):CD000323.

40. Logemann JA, Gensler G, Robbins J, et al. A randomized study of three interventions for aspiration of thin liquids in patients with dementia or Parkinson's disease. J Speech Lang Hear Res 2008;51:173–83.

41. Robbins J, Gensler G, Hind J, et al. Comparison of 2 interventions for liquid aspiration on pneumonia incidence: a randomized trial. Ann Intern Med 2008; 148:509–18.

42. Whelan K. Inadequate fluid intakes in dysphagic acute stroke. Clin Nutr 2001; 20:423–8.

43. Zemanova M, Novak F, Vitek P, et al. Outcomes of patients with oesophageal cancer treated with preoperative chemoradiotherapy, followed by tumor resection: influence of nutritional factors. J BUON 2011;17:310–6.

44. Allen VJ, Methven L, Gosney MA. Use of nutritional complete supplements in older adults with dementia: systematic review and meta-analysis of clinical outcomes. Clin Nutr 2013 (In press).

45. Simmons SF, Zhuo X, Keeler E. Cost-effectiveness of nutrition interventions in nursing home residents: a pilot intervention. J Nutr Health Aging 2010;14: 367–72.

46. Arends J, Bodoky G, Bozzetti F, et al. ESPEN guidelines on enteral nutrition: non-surgical oncology. Clin Nutr 2006;25:245–59.
47. Barichella M, Cereda E, Pezzoli G. Major nutritional issues in the management of Parkinson's disease. Mov Disord 2009;24:1881–92.
48. Loser C, Aschl G, Hebuterne X, et al. ESPEN guidelines on artificial enteral nutrition–percutaneous endoscopic gastrostomy (PEG). Clin Nutr 2005;24: 848–61.
49. Miller RG, Jackson CE, Kasarskis EJ, et al. Practice parameter update: the care of the patient with amyotrophic lateral sclerosis: drug, nutritional, and respiratory therapies (an evidence-based review): report of the Quality Standards Subcommittee of the American Academy of Neurology. Neurology 2009;73:1218–26.
50. Candy B, Sampson EL, Jones L. Enteral tube feeding in older people with advanced dementia: findings from a Cochrane systematic review. Int J Palliat Nurs 2009;15:396–404.
51. Chung AM. Percutaneous gastrostomy feeding tubes in end stage dementia: don't "just do it". Can Assoc Radiol J 2012;63:S5–6.
52. Yamazaki Y, Kobatake K, Hara M, et al. Nutritional support by "conventional" percutaneous endoscopic gastrostomy feeding may not result in weight gain in Parkinson's disease. J Neurol 2011;258:1561–3.
53. Locher JL, Bonner JA, Carroll WR, et al. Prophylactic percutaneous endoscopic gastrostomy tube placement in treatment of head and neck cancer: a comprehensive review and call for evidence-based medicine. JPEN J Parenter Enteral Nutr 2011;35:365–74.
54. Wiggenraad RG, Flierman L, Goossens A, et al. Prophylactic gastrostomy placement and early tube feeding may limit loss of weight during chemoradiotherapy for advanced head and neck cancer, a preliminary study. Clin Otolaryngol 2007;32:384–90.
55. Assenat E, Thezenas S, Flori N, et al. Prophylactic percutaneous endoscopic gastrostomy in patients with advanced head and neck tumors treated by combined chemoradiotherapy. J Pain Symptom Manage 2011;42:548–56.
56. Salas S, Baumstarck-Barrau K, Alfonsi M, et al. Impact of the prophylactic gastrostomy for unresectable squamous cell head and neck carcinomas treated with radio-chemotherapy on quality of life: prospective randomized trial. Radiother Oncol 2009;93:503–9.
57. Silander E, Nyman J, Bove M, et al. Impact of prophylactic percutaneous endoscopic gastrostomy on malnutrition and quality of life in patients with head and neck cancer: a randomized study. Head Neck 2012;34:1–9.
58. Lees J. Nasogastric and percutaneous endoscopic gastrostomy feeding in head and neck cancer patients receiving radiotherapy treatment at a regional oncology unit: a two year study. Eur J Cancer Care (Engl) 1997;6:45–9.
59. Corry J, Poon W, McPhee N, et al. Randomized study of percutaneous endoscopic gastrostomy versus nasogastric tubes for enteral feeding in head and neck cancer patients treated with (chemo)radiation. J Med Imaging Radiat Oncol 2008;52:503–10.
60. Sheth CH, Sharp S, Walters ER. Enteral feeding in head and neck cancer patients at a UK cancer centre. J Hum Nutr Diet 2013;26(5):421–8.
61. Heyland DK, Dhaliwal R, Drover JW, et al. Canadian clinical practice guidelines for nutrition support in mechanically ventilated, critically ill adult patients. JPEN J Parenter Enteral Nutr 2003;27:355–73.
62. Montejo JC, Grau T, Acosta J, et al. Multicenter, prospective, randomized, single-blind study comparing the efficacy and gastrointestinal complications

of early jejunal feeding with early gastric feeding in critically ill patients. Crit Care Med 2002;30:796–800.

63. Fenton JR, Bergeron EJ, Coello M, et al. Feeding jejunostomy tubes placed during esophagectomy: are they necessary? Ann Thorac Surg 2011;92:504–11 [discussion: 11–2].

64. Jabbar A, McClave SA. Pre-pyloric versus post-pyloric feeding. Clin Nutr 2005; 24:719–26.

65. Meeroff JC, Go VL, Phillips SF. Control of gastric emptying by osmolality of duodenal contents in man. Gastroenterology 1975;68:1144–51.

66. Pereira-da-Silva L, Pitta-Gros Dias M, Virella D, et al. Osmolality of elemental and semi-elemental formulas supplemented with nonprotein energy supplements. J Hum Nutr Diet 2008;21:584–90.

67. Craig LD, Nicholson S, SilVerstone FA, et al. Use of a reduced-carbohydrate, modified-fat enteral formula for improving metabolic control and clinical outcomes in long-term care residents with type 2 diabetes: results of a pilot trial. Nutrition 1998;14:529–34.

68. Pohl M, Mayr P, Mertl-Roetzer M, et al. Glycaemic control in type II diabetic tube-fed patients with a new enteral formula low in carbohydrates and high in mono-unsaturated fatty acids: a randomised controlled trial. Eur J Clin Nutr 2005;59: 1221–32.

69. Elia M, Ceriello A, Laube H, et al. Enteral nutritional support and use of diabetes-specific formulas for patients with diabetes: a systematic review and meta-analysis. Diabetes Care 2005;28:2267–79.

70. Stratton RJ, Bircher G, Fouque D, et al. Multinutrient oral supplements and tube feeding in maintenance dialysis: a systematic review and meta-analysis. Am J Kidney Dis 2005;46:387–405.

71. Als-Nielsen B, Koretz RL, Kjaergard LL, et al. Branched-chain amino acids for hepatic encephalopathy. Cochrane Database Syst Rev 2003;(2):CD001939.

72. Marik PE, Zaloga GP. Immunonutrition in critically ill patients: a systematic review and analysis of the literature. Intensive Care Med 2008;34:1980–90.

73. Pontes-Arruda A, Aragao AM, Albuquerque JD. Effects of enteral feeding with eicosapentaenoic acid, gamma-linolenic acid, and antioxidants in mechanically ventilated patients with severe sepsis and septic shock. Crit Care Med 2006;34: 2325–33.

74. Rhoney DH, Parker D Jr, Formea CM, et al. Tolerability of bolus versus continuous gastric feeding in brain-injured patients. Neurol Res 2002;24:613–20.

75. Cotogni P, Pittiruti M, Barbero C, et al. Catheter-related complications in cancer patients on home parenteral nutrition: a prospective study of over 51,000 catheter days. JPEN J Parenter Enteral Nutr 2013;37(3):375–83.

76. Perioperative total parenteral nutrition in surgical patients. The Veterans Affairs Total Parenteral Nutrition Cooperative Study Group. N Engl J Med 1991;325: 525–32.

77. Woodcock NP, Zeigler D, Palmer MD, et al. Enteral versus parenteral nutrition: a pragmatic study. Nutrition 2001;17:1–12.

78. Advani S, Reich NG, Sengupta A, et al. Central line-associated bloodstream infection in hospitalized children with peripherally inserted central venous catheters: extending risk analyses outside the intensive care unit. Clin Infect Dis 2011;52:1108–15.

Surgical and Other Interventions

Nonsurgical Treatment
Swallowing Rehabilitation

Karen W. Hegland, PhD, CCC-SLP[a],*, Thomas Murry, PhD[b]

KEYWORDS

- Dysphagia • Rehabilitation • Behavioral treatment • Non-surgical treatment
- Direct exercise • Indirect exercise • Compensatory techniques

KEY POINTS

- The speech-language pathologist is the primary member of the swallowing team who will provide ongoing nonsurgical and nonpharmacological rehabilitation for the patient with dysphagia.
- Aside from ameliorating aspiration risk, the focus of the speech-language pathologist is to improve or restore swallowing function.
- To this end, there are many direct and indirect therapeutic options whose application will depend on the pathophysiology of the disorder, and other patient variables related to the motivation and ability to participate in therapy.

INTRODUCTION

The speech-language pathologist (SLP) is the primary member of the swallowing team who will provide ongoing nonsurgical rehabilitation for the patient with dysphagia. The nonsurgical, nonpharmacologic approach to dysphagia treatment focuses on ameliorating aspiration risk and on improving or restoring voice, speech, and swallow functions. The treatment schedule should include a plan to monitor treatment effectiveness or ineffectiveness, as well as qualitative and quantitative measures of improvement or decline in function. The SLP must also maintain an awareness regarding the feasibility of treatment based on patient travel, access to the treatment center, reimbursement allotments, and need for a caregiver to monitor swallowing activities away from the treatment center.

Funding Sources: Dr K.W. Hegland, American Heart Association.
Conflict of Interest: Dr T. Murry, Royalties and Board of Directors: Plural Publishing INC.
[a] Department of Speech, Language and Hearing Sciences, College of Public Health and Health Professions, University of Florida, Box 117420, Gainesville, FL 32611, USA; [b] Department of Otolaryngology-Head and Neck Surgery, Weill Cornell Medical College, 1305 York Avenue, New York, NY 10021, USA
* Corresponding author.
E-mail address: Kwheeler@ufl.edu

Otolaryngol Clin N Am 46 (2013) 1073–1085
http://dx.doi.org/10.1016/j.otc.2013.08.003
0030-6665/13/$ – see front matter © 2013 Elsevier Inc. All rights reserved.

oto.theclinics.com

Abbreviations: Management of Dysphagia	
EMST	Expiratory muscle strength training
HLE	Head lift exercise
MEG	Magnetoencephalography
NMES	Neuromuscular electrical stimulation
sEMG	Surface electromyography
SLP	Speech-language pathologist
TES	Transcutaneous electrical stimulation
TTOS	Thermal tactile oral stimulation
UES	Upper esophageal sphincter

Treatment protocols typically include a multimodal approach, including diet or postural modification to address immediate airway protection concerns, as well as rehabilitative therapy targeting the pathophysiologic underpinnings of the disorder. Development of a treatment protocol will depend on the results of screenings and evaluation tests that are discussed in articles in this publication by Speyer: "Oropharyngeal Dysphagia: Screening and Assessment" and by Brady and Donzelli: "The Modified Barium Swallow and the Functional Endoscopic Evaluation of Swallowing." Changes in patients' swallowing resulting from treatment and/or the passage of time may be noted through weight changes, speed of eating, types of foods being consumed, or special scales to assess changes in quality of life brought about through changes to swallowing function. In addition, the clinician must identify those points whereby physiologic reassessment is necessary to document properly whether swallowing function is improving, whether the patient is reaching short and long-term goals, and ultimately to decide whether treatment should continue.

PRINCIPLES OF CARE
Introduction

Based on results of the swallowing evaluation, the treating clinician should have a firm sense of the patient's current swallowing ability, associated risks to airway protection, and the best rehabilitative approaches to apply in treatment. **Box 1** summarizes the primary factors in treatment planning that the rehabilitation team must be cognizant of for all patients with dysphagia. Additional factors that must be considered in treatment planning are the associated medical diagnoses, general health and nutritional

Box 1
Factors in dysphagia treatment planning
1. All medical diagnoses
2. Patients general health
3. Current swallowing ability
4. Known risks of airway protection
5. Previously tried treatments and their outcomes
6. Current nutritional status
7. Cognitive status
8. Available care giver support

status, cognitive and communication status, and whether the patient has family and/or caregivers support.

Assess Aspiration Risk and Deficit Focus

A wide range of deficits may lead to reduced ability to protect the airway, from profound structural and sensory changes due to treatment of head and neck cancer, to sensorimotor changes associated with stroke, or other neurologic disease. Airway protection should always be a consideration of swallowing treatment; however, whether specific instances of aspiration are noted on instrumental swallowing examination should not be the only factor determining the presence or absence of dysphagia, or whether to implement treatment. Focusing on the physiologic deficits found during evaluation allows the clinician to assess both the real (observed) and the assumed risk of aspiration.

If aspiration of material to the airway has been directly observed, did it occur before, during, or after the pharyngeal phase of swallowing is completed? This observation will yield information as to whether there is a problem initiating the swallow (where penetration/aspiration is noted before the pharyngeal swallow is triggered) with the structural movements during the pharyngeal phase of swallowing (where penetration/aspiration is noted during the swallow), or with residual material within the pharynx that enters the airway (where penetration/aspiration is noted after the swallow). If no direct observation of aspiration occurred during the instrumental testing, does material penetrate the airway (enter the laryngeal vestibule, but remain above the level of the vocal cords)? What physiologic findings (whether aspiration is observed) may put the patient *at risk* of aspiration during swallowing? These physiologic findings may include premature spilling into the pharynx, reduced hyolaryngeal excursion, incomplete closure of the laryngeal vestibule, reduced extent or duration or upper esophageal sphincter (UES) opening, or postswallow pharyngeal residue.

During the instrumental examination, it is highly desirable to test candidate interventions to determine if there is a positive effect on swallowing function. This testing will allow the clinician to determine the immediate effect, if any, of a particular consistency or postural change, or of a swallow-specific exercise. This piece of information can then be used to prepare the therapy plan better. For example, if instructing the patient to use a chin tuck while swallowing thin liquids ameliorates observed airway compromise, then it should be part of the treatment plan. However, if continued aspiration is noted with the chin tuck, or the patient cannot coordinate the chin tuck with other swallow events, then it may not be a good therapeutic choice.

Establishing a Treatment Schedule

Once the case history and examination have been completed, the clinician must recommend an appropriate treatment protocol and schedule for treatment. How many days per week will the patient attend treatment sessions? How long will each treatment session last? How many weeks (or months) will treatment continue? Will a maintenance program be possible, whereby the patient continues certain aspects of treatment on his/her own after formal treatment sessions end? The answers will vary by patient, with consideration given not only to severity of the deficit but also to the proximity of the patient to a treatment source, insurance coverage, other treatments/therapies in which the patient participates, and caregiver availability and support.

The treatment schedule should be structured to include short-term and long-term goals, and the timeframe in which meeting those goals should be met. It is imperative to document progress clearly, or lack thereof, toward goals. This documentation is a concrete way for clinicians to monitor progress or decline in function, and whether changes to the treatment and/or treatment schedule are warranted.

When to Reassess

Multiple considerations contribute to the question of when to reassess a patient's swallowing function. **Box 2** outlines the major considerations for reassessment of the patient.

The establishment of long-term goals and incremental short-term goals at treatment initiation should give a clear progression with an associated timeline. In the absence of other factors that may warrant reassessment, this timeline should guide the clinician to a point where he/she must reassess to document treatment progress/lack of progress and any further recommendations. Acute changes to function, whether observed during therapy or reported by the patient, may warrant reassessment.

Oral Care

The most common location of bacteria is in the mouth. Therefore, patients with swallowing disorders should brush their teeth, or someone should do it for them, 3 times per day. Mouth rinse is also suggested provided it does not lead to aspiration if swallowed accidently.

MOTOR AND SENSORY STIMULATION
Electrical Stimulation

Neuromuscular electrical stimulation (NMES) is a technique that has been used for many years by physical therapists and works by applying electrical stimulation, causing muscle fibers to contract when the correct amount of stimulator intensity is applied. NMES can be either percutaneous (intramuscular) or transcutaneous (surface).[1] Percutaneous NMES delivers stimulation via hook-wire electrodes that are inserted directly into the muscle of interest.[2] Transcutaneous electrical stimulation (TES) is a noninvasive form of NMES that applies stimulation to the skin overlaying the target muscles. Thus, TES activates sensory fibers in the skin as well as underlying muscles, when the right amount of intensity is applied.[3]

The primary hypothesis governing the use of TES for dysphagia is that by stimulating the muscles in the neck via surface stimulation, the swallowing musculature will be strengthened and/or the sensory pathways important for swallowing will have heightened awareness. To date, there is a small body of literature supporting the use of TES as a dysphagia treatment. A 2009 review by Clark and colleagues[1] concluded limited evidence suggests positive treatment effect of NMES for

---

Box 2
Conditions that suggest reassessment of the patient

1. After short-term goals are met

2. After a decline in swallow function either noticed or reported

3. After a reported pneumonia

4. After further surgery to the head and neck areas

5. After a change in cognition

6. After a noted change in eating strategies by the patient

7. After failure of current treatments to improve swallowing

swallowing therapy, and an ongoing need for examination of dosage, timing, and applications to specific populations. Moreover, the level of evidence for NMES was limited due to the lack of controlled studies, control groups, and sufficient outcome measures over a long period of time. A more recent review by Humbert and colleagues[3] concludes similarly and discusses data that suggest certain electrode configurations may negatively impact swallowing. In a 2010 report, Ludlow[2] suggests that electrical stimulation is most effective when the electrical stimulus is applied directly to the muscle via intramuscular electrodes. In contrast to surface stimulation, intramuscular stimulation uses a hooked wire electrode inserted into the muscle of interest to direct the current to a specific muscle. However, because of the invasive nature of intramuscular electrode placement, it is not commonly used by most speech-language clinicians at this time.

Thermal-tactile Stimulation

Thermal tactile oral stimulation (TTOS) is the stroking or rubbing of one or more of the structures (typically the anterior faucial pillars) involved with swallowing with an ice stick or cold probe. As well, it can include presentation of boluses with varying temperature, carbonation, and gustatory properties. These methods are used when dysphagia is caused, at least in part, by sensory deficits. The underlying hypothesis is that manipulation of touch, cold, and taste stimulation provide heightened oral awareness and an alerting stimulus to the brainstem and brain, causing the pharyngeal swallow to trigger faster than it would without the stimulation.[4–6] Support for this hypothesis is provided by Teismann and colleagues,[7] whose study of cortical activation during TTOS using whole head magnetoencephalography (MEG) showed functional cortical changes the authors suggest reflect short-term cortical plasticity of sensory swallowing areas.

To date, there is little empiric research to support the extensive use of cold stimulation to the oral-pharyngeal mucosa to improve general swallow function, outside of a short-term acute affect. That is, although results of multiple studies have shown various physiologic changes to oral and pharyngeal swallow function following cold stimulation, that effect is generally limited to the first swallow immediately following the stimulation.[5,6,8] A few studies have combined cold and gustatory stimulation and shown significant results also in terms of swallowing timing. Bove and colleagues[9] found no significant differences in healthy individuals in swallowing durational measures following stimulation with a cold laryngeal mirror, but they did find that swallow times were shorter when swallowing cold water compared with swallowing water warmed to body temperature. A study of stimulation with a sour bolus by Logemann and colleagues[10] found that there was an earlier onset of lingual activity to propel a bolus into the pharynx, triggering the pharyngeal motor response, and a shorter pharyngeal component of the swallow in patients following stroke or mixed neurologic disorders. Other studies of temperature and/or carbonation have been equivocal in showing acute changes in swallow function. It remains to be studied if these acute changes would induce permanent cortical adaptation and consequently enduring functional improvement over time.

EXERCISE-BASED REHABILITATIVE THERAPY
Introduction

Exercise-based therapies apply either direct or indirect maneuvers to facilitate swallowing and swallow rehabilitation. Direct maneuvers include a swallow as part of the therapeutic protocol. Indirect exercises will target muscles and movements important for swallowing, but will not include an actual swallow. Before initiating either a direct or an indirect program, the clinician should assess the following:

A. Does the patient have adequate cognitive skills to follow instruction?
B. Is the patient motivated to improve?
C. Is the patient willing to practice independently?

If the answer to any of these is not yes, these may not be appropriate therapeutic options.

Direct Swallow Maneuvers

Direct swallow maneuvers place various aspects of the pharyngeal swallow under the voluntary control by instructing the patient to modulate specific aspects of their swallow. The major direct maneuvers include the following:

1. Supraglottic swallow
2. Effortful swallow
3. Mendelsohn maneuver

The theories supporting the use of direct swallow maneuvers are 2-fold: first, these maneuvers target physiologic deficits based on results of the evaluation, providing immediate amelioration of aspiration risk. Second, they may act as task-specific exercises that improve coordination and strength of the muscles primarily involved in swallowing, leading to improvement in general swallowing function.[11,12]

These maneuvers should be explained to the patients slowly, tried first without foods or liquids, and then ideally be examined during instrumental studies of swallow function before continuous therapy. Oftentimes, biofeedback (for example, surface electromyography [sEMG]) with video is useful in teaching these maneuvers to patients and during treatment sessions.[13]

The supraglottic swallow is a 4-step maneuver:

1. Inhale and hold breath
2. Place bolus in swallow position
3. Swallow while holding breath
4. Cough after swallow before inhaling.

This technique is often used with patients who have vocal fold paresis, paralysis, or laryngeal sensory deficits. This maneuver is considered a voluntary airway closure technique and, when done properly, closes the vocal folds before the swallow and keeps them closed during the swallow, thus preventing aspiration.[14,15] **Table 1** summarizes the known physiologic effects of these maneuvers.

Table 1	
Summary of direct swallow maneuvers	
Maneuver	**Immediate Physiologic Effect**
Supraglottic swallow	Close the vocal folds (breathhold) during the swallow and then clear any residue that may have entered the laryngeal vestibule (cough) before breathing again
Effortful swallow	Increased retraction of the base of the tongue and pharyngeal pressure to improve bolus clearance from the valleculae
Mendelsohn maneuver	By keeping the larynx tilted and elevated, the UES relaxes to allow food to pass, leaving less residual material in the pharynx.

The effortful swallow is simply a squeeze. The patient is told or shown to "squeeze hard with all of your muscles." This maneuver may be the easiest for patients who have trouble with multiple-stage commands or for those patients with significant sensory loss. The squeeze may help in propelling the bolus into the oropharynx because of weakness in the tongue. Lazarus and colleagues[11] reported that this maneuver produces high pharyngeal pressure and results in reduction or elimination of pharyngeal residue. A more recent study by Hoffmann and colleagues[16] using high-resolution manometry found increased velopharyngeal pressure, and prolonged nadir UES pressure during effortful swallows. Of note, the effortful swallow maneuver should be used with caution if instrumental examination reveals oropharyngeal weakness or lack of vocal fold closure.

The Mendelsohn maneuver is a technique to open the UES by extending the duration of laryngeal elevation. In this maneuver, the patient initiates several dry swallows while trying to feel the thyroid prominence lift.[17] Once the patient is able to identify the lift, he/she is instructed to hold the thyroid up for several seconds. The Mendelsohn maneuver is useful for treating patients who, for reasons of neurologic injury or surgical treatment, cannot obtain adequate laryngeal excursion or elevation or who cannot co-ordinate the elevation motion with bolus passage.[11]

Indirect Swallow Exercises

As the name implies, indirect swallow exercises target the swallowing mechanism indirectly by focusing on structures and movements important for swallowing, but without including actual swallows in their protocol. Indirect exercises that are discussed include

1. Tongue strengthening
2. Shaker head raise
3. Expiratory muscle strength training (EMST)

Each of these exercises has a specific training regimen that is based on principles of training and overload (**Table 2**). Burkhead and colleagues[18] provide a review of these principles as they apply to the muscles of swallowing. It should be remembered that these exercises are not specific to swallowing and there is a need to assess transference to improved swallowing to continue these treatments. Instrumental reassessment (as suggested in **Box 2**) may be necessary to assess the effects of these exercises.

Table 2		
Summary of indirect swallow exercises		
Exercise	**Known Physiologic Effects**	**Training Protocol**
Shaker HLE	Strengthen geniohyoid, thyrohyoid, and digastric muscles. Decrease the hypopharyngeal bolus pressure as it enters the UES	Three 1-min sustained head lifts 30 s of repetitive head lifts 6 wk
Tongue strengthening	Increase isometric anterior and posterior lingual strength Decrease oral transit duration Increase swallowing pressures	60% or 80% maximum tongue pressure 3 sets of 10 repetitions, 3 d/wk 4 or 8 wk
EMST	Increase expiratory muscle strength Increase anterior suprahyoid activation Increase hyolaryngeal movement	75% maximum expiratory pressure 5 sets of 5 repetitions, 5 d/wk 4 wk

Lingual Strengthening

Tongue control provides transmission of the bolus to the pharynx, and as such, lingual strength has received much attention. Decreases in tongue strength occur because of normal aging and as a result of other disorders and pathologic abnormalities.[19–21] Lingual strength exercises may constitute a fundamental aspect of swallowing treatment because of the crucial role that the tongue plays in the oral preparatory, oral, and pharyngeal phases of swallowing. Tongue strength exercises also aim to improve tongue elevation and lateralization. One of the earliest studies to show the value of tongue strengthening exercises was reported by Lazarus and colleagues,[22] using young normal subjects, who were divided into 3 groups. Two groups of subjects were asked to press a rubber bulb or a tongue blade against their hard palate. After a month, both the rubber bulb and the tongue blade groups showed improved tongue strength compared with the third group that performed no exercises. Robbins and colleagues[23] showed similar results with 8 healthy elderly volunteers and found lingual exercises to improve lingual strength using Iowa Oral Performance Instrument (Blaise Inc) with both anterior and posterior lingual pressure bulbs. In 2007, Robbins replicated the study in patients after stroke and found increased isometric lingual strength, and improvement in swallowing outcome measures, including incidence of aspiration, in 10 research participants.[24] Steele and colleagues[25] studied lingual exercises that emphasized strength and accuracy, using a biofeedback technique, to improve tongue strength and swallow function in 6 adults with dysphagia following traumatic brain injury. The study reported improvement in measures of tongue strength and penetration-aspiration, with no differences reported in the amount of pharyngeal residue.

Shaker Head Lift Exercise

An important aspect of swallowing is the ability to open the UES to allow the passage of the bolus. Shaker and colleagues[26] developed a head lift exercise (HLE) that focuses on strengthening the suyprahyoid muscles, which are important for UES opening. The HLE consists of lying in a supine position and doing a series of head lifts while the shoulders remain on the floor or bed. The goals of the Shaker exercise are to

1. Strengthen the muscles that contribute to the opening of the UES, specifically, the geniohyoid, thyrohyoid, and digastric muscles.
2. Decrease the hypopharyngeal bolus pressure as it enters the UES, thus permitting bolus passage with less resistance.

In their 1997 study, Shaker and colleagues[26] studied healthy elderly subjects using manometry and videofluoroscopy to measure intrabolus pressure before and following a program of HLEs, finding increased extent and duration UES opening. Based on results of this and subsequent study, the researchers hypothesized that HLE likely ameliorates aspiration risk by decreasing the amount of residue in the pharynx after a swallow.[26,27] In 2009, Logemann and colleagues[28] compared the HLE to traditional swallowing maneuvers, including the supraglottic swallow and Mendelsohn maneuver, and found decreased instances of aspiration and increased UES opening in the HLE group compared with traditional swallowing maneuver groups (n = 8 in HLE group, n = 11 in traditional swallowing group). Both groups showed significant physiologic changes, including increased superior hyolaryngeal excursion and increased anterior laryngeal movement.[28]

There are several considerations before initiating the Shaker HLE with a patient. Typically, it requires repeated instruction, cueing, and encouragement to perform the exercise accurately, and some research participants did report neck muscle soreness and dizziness during the early weeks of the exercise program.[29] Fatigue may also be a limiting factor for some patients. A study by White and colleagues[27] found that after a 6-week training program, the Shaker HLE fatigues the sternocleidomastoid, which may preclude the continuation of the exercise in some situations, especially with elderly subjects. This fatigue suggests that the Shaker exercise may not be appropriate for individuals with any condition that predisposes them to fatigue quickly (ie, those with amyotrophic lateral sclerosis or other neuromuscular diseases). It is also important to note that the Shaker HLE cannot be used with individuals who have cervical spine deficits or reduced neck movement ability.

Expiratory Muscle Strength Training

In a 2005 study by Baker and colleagues[30] demonstrated EMST improves both ventilatory and nonventilatory (speech) functions in healthy young adults. EMST uses a small, hand-held device that requires the user to blow into the mouthpiece. Once enough expiratory pressure is generated, a spring-loaded valve pops open allowing air to flow through the device. The pressure threshold is set at a percentage of the users maximum expiratory pressure, usually at 75%. Training is then completed at home, 5 days per week.

Multiple studies focusing specifically on swallow function have shown EMST to be a valuable adjunctive rehabilitative technique to use with patients who show muscular weakness resulting from typical aging, neurologic, or neuromuscular diseases.[31–34] Wheeler and colleagues[35] showed increased duration and amplitude of anterior suprahyoid muscle activation during use of EMST compared with saliva and water swallows. In 2009, Wheeler-Hegland and colleagues[12] studied hyoid movement and muscle activation during EMST. They found increased hyoid movement associated with increased muscle activation versus normal swallowing and suggested that the EMST training has the potential to induce strength gains in the anterior suprahyoid musculature. It was subsequently hypothesized that these strength gains would equate to improved hyolaryngeal elevation.[12] Since then, a randomized controlled trial using EMST to improve swallowing function in patients with Parkinson disease has shown improved penetration-aspiration score following training with the device.[31] Beyond swallowing, EMST is associated with improved cough and speech function in Parkinson patients,[36] sedentary elderly,[32] and patients with multiple sclerosis.[33]

PROSTHETIC MANAGEMENT

Prosthodontics is the science of providing suitable substitutes for missing, lost, or removed structures in the oral cavity (**Box 3**). Prostheses are used for 2 main etiologic

---

Box 3
Goals of prosthetic management for dysphagia

1. To normalize the size of the oral cavity to assist with adequate oral-pharyngeal bolus transit

2. To develop appropriate contacts and subsequent pressures between adjacent structures during swallowing

3. To protect the underlying mucosa

4. To improve appearance and psychosocial adjustment

5. To develop appropriate subglottal pressures for swallowing

Table 3	
Primary considerations when planning or modifying dysphagia diets	
Domain	**Consideration**
Physical	Dentition
	Lingual function
	Aspiration risks
Social	Living situation
	Available support (caregivers, living situation)
	Mealtime social interaction (lives alone, lives with others)
Personal	Diet compliance
	Ethnic/religious food preferences
	Taste preferences

factors: (1) congenital defects and (2) acquired defects. Congenital oral defects include cleft lip, cleft palate, cleft mandible, and bifid uvula. Acquired oral defects are those primarily related to surgical treatment of diseases, traumas, pathologies, or burns. Oral prosthodontics takes into account direct swallowing management, including prosthetic management with dental, palatal, or tongue prostheses, medical therapy, and environmental adjustments, such as proper types of utensils to improve and control feeding when a prosthesis is required. Prosthetic appliances such as dental implants, palate lowering, soft palate and lingual prostheses offer an additional supplement to managing the bolus in the oral cavity. The role of the SLP is to assess function during and following the fitting of these devices.

Speaking valves fitted over the tracheotomy are also considered prosthetic devices. They have been in existence for over 25 years and provide adjunctive subglottic pressure to help transfer the bolus to the esophageal inlet.[37–39]

DIET CONSIDERATIONS

Trials of multiple consistencies during the videofluoroscopic examination will help determine what consistencies for liquids and solids will be the safest and minimize the risk of aspiration. Diet modification as a means of mitigating aspiration risk is an option for those patients who demonstrate safe and effective swallowing on certain consistencies but not others. This diet modification offers a way to continue oral intake. Modification of the diet should take the physical, social, and personal considerations of the patient into account when planning a healthy nutritional program. **Table 3** lists the primary nutritional considerations when planning or modifying dysphagia diets.

An important consideration to diet modification is patient and/or caregiver adherence to the recommendation. A recently published study by Kaizer and colleagues[40] suggests that including both patients and caregivers in the decision-making process leading up the recommendation to alter aspects of the diet may lead to increased acceptance and adherence to these recommendations. This process depends heavily on patient and caregiver education about risks, benefits, and overall consequences of the decision.[40]

SUMMARY

Swallowing therapy is now commonly provided for acute and chronic swallowing disorders resulting from surgical excisions of tumors in the head and neck regions, neuromuscular disorders, neurologic disorders, and debilitation associated with a cohort of aging conditions that affect the nerves and muscles involved in swallowing. SLPs are specifically trained in the nonsurgical techniques of treatment. It is to be expected that patients recovering from swallowing disorders will experience occasional aspiration. Using the compensatory swallow maneuvers and the postural techniques reviewed in this article can be efficacious in reducing aspiration events and preventing aspiration pneumonia and may be a patient-by-patient experience, given that patients rarely present with a uniform case history and medical status.

Compensatory therapies continue to evolve and be tested in both normal subjects and in patients who can tolerate the various testing formats. Procedures such as EMST, a treatment that was developed for nonswallowing disorder, are now being explored as treatments for patients with swallowing disorders. The application of neuroplastic principles such as "use it or lose it," transference, repetition, and stimulus intensity in the treatment process offer an improved rationale for the nonsurgical treatment of swallowing. New treatments may provide additional evidence for continued use of nonsurgical treatments for patients with swallowing disorders.

REFERENCES

1. Clark H, Lazarus C, Arvedson J, et al. Evidence-based systematic review: effects of neuromuscular electrical stimulation on swallowing and neural activation. Am J Speech Lang Pathol 2009;18(4):361–75. http://dx.doi.org/10.1044/1058-0360(2009/08-0088).
2. Ludlow CL. Electrical neuromuscular stimulation in dysphagia: current status. Curr Opin Otolaryngol Head Neck Surg 2010;18(3):159–64. http://dx.doi.org/10.1097/MOO.0b013e3283395dec.
3. Humbert IA, Michou E, MacRae PR, et al. Electrical stimulation and swallowing: how much do we know? Semin Speech Lang 2012;33(3):203–16. http://dx.doi.org/10.1055/s-0032-1320040.
4. Rosenbek JC, Robbins J, Willford WO, et al. Comparing treatment intensities of tactile-thermal application. Dysphagia 1998;13(1):1–9.
5. Regan J, Walshe M, Tobin WO. Immediate effects of thermal-tactile stimulation on timing of swallow in idiopathic Parkinson's disease. Dysphagia 2010;25(3):207–15. http://dx.doi.org/10.1007/s00455-009-9244-x.
6. Sciortino K, Liss JM, Case JL, et al. Effects of mechanical, cold, gustatory, and combined stimulation to the human anterior faucial pillars. Dysphagia 2003;18(1):16–26.
7. Teismann IK, Steinstrater O, Warnecke T, et al. Tactile thermal oral stimulation increases the cortical representation of swallowing. BMC Neurosci 2009;10:71. http://dx.doi.org/10.1186/1471-2202-10-71.
8. Kaatzke-McDonald MN, Post E, Davis PJ. The effects of cold, touch, and chemical stimulation of the anterior faucial pillar on human swallowing. Dysphagia 1996;11(3):198–206.
9. Bove M, Mansson I, Eliasson I. Thermal oral-pharyngeal stimulation and elicitation of swallowing. Acta Otolaryngol 1998;118(5):728–31.
10. Logemann JA, Pauloski BR, Colangelo L, et al. Effects of a sour bolus on oropharyngeal swallowing measures in patients with neurogenic dysphagia. J Speech Hear Res 1995;38(3):556–63.
11. Lazarus C, Logemann JA, Song CW, et al. Effects of voluntary maneuvers on tongue base function for swallowing. Folia Phoniatr Logop 2002;54(4):171–6.

12. Wheeler-Hegland KM, Rosenbek JC, Sapienza CM. Submental sEMG and hyoid movement during Mendelsohn maneuver, effortful swallow, and expiratory muscle strength training. J Speech Lang Hear Res 2008;51(5):1072–87.

13. Crary MA, Carnaby Mann GD, Groher ME, et al. Functional benefits of dysphagia therapy using adjunctive sEMG biofeedback. Dysphagia 2004;19(3):160–4. http://dx.doi.org/10.1007/s00455-004-0003-8.

14. Lazarus C, Logemann JA, Gibbons P. Effects of maneuvers on swallowing function in a dysphagic oral cancer patient. Head Neck 1993;15(5):419–24.

15. Ohmae Y, Logemann JA, Kaiser P, et al. Effects of two breath-holding maneuvers on oropharyngeal swallow. Ann Otol Rhinol Laryngol 1996;105(2):123–31.

16. Hoffman MR, Mielens JD, Ciucci MR, et al. High-resolution manometry of pharyngeal swallow pressure events associated with effortful swallow and the Mendelsohn maneuver. Dysphagia 2012;27(3):418–26. http://dx.doi.org/10.1007/s00455-011-9385-6.

17. Ding R, Larson CR, Logemann JA, et al. Surface electromyographic and electroglottographic studies in normal subjects under two swallow conditions: normal and during the Mendelsohn manuever. Dysphagia 2002;17(1):1–12.

18. Burkhead LM, Sapienza CM, Rosenbek JC. Strength-training exercise in dysphagia rehabilitation: principles, procedures, and directions for future research. Dysphagia 2007;22(3):251–65. http://dx.doi.org/10.1007/s00455-006-9074-z.

19. Nicosia MA, Hind JA, Roecker EB, et al. Age effects on the temporal evolution of isometric and swallowing pressure. J Gerontol A Biol Sci Med Sci 2000;55(11): M634–40.

20. Clark HM. Neuromuscular treatments for speech and swallowing: a tutorial. Am J Speech Lang Pathol 2003;12(4):400–15. http://dx.doi.org/10.1044/1058-0360(2003/086).

21. Lazarus C, Logemann JA, Pauloski BR, et al. Effects of radiotherapy with or without chemotherapy on tongue strength and swallowing in patients with oral cancer. Head Neck 2007;29(7):632–7. http://dx.doi.org/10.1002/hed.20577.

22. Lazarus C, Logemann JA, Huang CF, et al. Effects of two types of tongue strengthening exercises in young normals. Folia Phoniatr Logop 2003;55(4): 199–205.

23. Robbins J, Gangnon RE, Theis SM, et al. The effects of lingual exercise on swallowing in older adults. J Am Geriatr Soc 2005;53(9):1483–9. http://dx.doi.org/10.1111/j.1532-5415.2005.53467.x.

24. Robbins JA, Kays SA, Gangnon RE, et al. The effects of lingual exercise in stroke patients with dysphagia. Arch Phys Med Rehabil 2007;88(2):150–8.

25. Steele CM, Bailey GL, Polacco RE, et al. Outcomes of tongue-pressure strength and accuracy training for dysphagia following acquired brain injury. Int J Speech Lang Pathol 2013. http://dx.doi.org/10.3109/17549507.2012.752864.

26. Shaker R, Kern M, Bardan E, et al. Augmentation of deglutitive upper esophageal sphincter opening in the elderly by exercise. Am J Physiol 1997;272(6 Pt 1):G1518–22.

27. White KT, Easterling C, Roberts N, et al. Fatigue analysis before and after Shaker exercise: physiologic tool for exercise design. Dysphagia 2008;23(4):385–91. http://dx.doi.org/10.1007/s00455-008-9155-2.

28. Logemann JA, Rademaker A, Pauloski BR, et al. A randomized study comparing the Shaker exercise with traditional therapy: a preliminary study. Dysphagia 2009; 24(4):403–11. http://dx.doi.org/10.1007/s00455-009-9217-0.

29. Easterling C, Grande B, Kern M, et al. Attaining and maintaining isometric and isokinetic goals of the shaker exercise. Dysphagia 2005;20(2):133–8. http://dx.doi.org/10.1007/s00455-005-0004-2.

30. Baker S, Davenport P, Sapienza C. Examination of strength training and detraining effects in expiratory muscles. J Speech Lang Hear Res 2005;48(6):1325.
31. Troche MS, Okun MS, Rosenbek JC, et al. Aspiration and swallowing in parkinson disease and rehabilitation with EMST: a randomized trial. Neurology 2010;75(21): 1912–9. http://dx.doi.org/10.1212/WNL.0b013e3181fef115.
32. Kim J, Davenport P, Sapienza C. Effect of expiratory muscle strength training on elderly cough function. Arch Gerontol Geriatr 2009;48(3):361–6.
33. Chiara T, Martin D, Sapienza C. Expiratory muscle strength training: speech production outcomes in patients with multiple sclerosis. Neurorehabil Neural Repair 2007;21(3):239–49. http://dx.doi.org/10.1177/1545968306294737.
34. Saleem AF, Sapienza CM, Okun MS. Respiratory muscle strength training: treatment and response duration in a patient with early idiopathic Parkinson's disease. NeuroRehabilitation 2005;20(4):323–33.
35. Wheeler KM, Chiara T, Sapienza CM. Surface electromyographic activity of the submental muscles during swallow and expiratory pressure threshold training tasks. Dysphagia 2007;22(2):108–16.
36. Pitts T, Bolser D, Rosenbek J, et al. Impact of expiratory muscle strength training on voluntary cough and swallow function in Parkinson disease. Chest 2009; 135(5):1301–8. http://dx.doi.org/10.1378/chest.08-1389.
37. Prigent H, Lejaille M, Terzi N, et al. Effect of a tracheostomy speaking valve on breathing-swallowing interaction. Intensive Care Med 2012;38(1):85–90. http://dx.doi.org/10.1007/s00134-011-2417-8.
38. Suiter DM, McCullough GH, Powell PW. Effects of cuff deflation and one-way tracheostomy speaking valve placement on swallow physiology. Dysphagia 2003; 18(4):284–92. http://dx.doi.org/10.1007/s00455-003-0022-x.
39. Dettelbach MA, Gross RD, Mahlmann J, et al. Effect of the Passy-Muir Valve on aspiration in patients with tracheostomy. Head Neck 1995;17(4):297–302.
40. Kaizer F, Spiridigliozzi AM, Hunt MR. Promoting shared decision-making in rehabilitation: development of a framework for situations when patients with dysphagia refuse diet modification recommended by the treating team. Dysphagia 2012;27(1):81–7. http://dx.doi.org/10.1007/s00455-011-9341-5.

Management of Cricopharyngeus Muscle Dysfunction

Maggie A. Kuhn, MD, Peter C. Belafsky, MD, MPH, PhD*

KEYWORDS

- Dysphagia • Cricopharyngeal muscle • Cricopharyngeus muscle
- Pharyngoesophageal segment • Upper esophageal sphincter
- Cricopharyngeal muscle dysfunction • Cricopharyngeus muscle dysfunction

KEY POINTS

- The cricopharyngeus muscle (CPM) is one component of the upper esophageal sphincter, and the failure of its coordinated relaxation or expansion is termed *cricopharyngeus muscle dysfunction* (CPD).
- Many conditions cause CPD; the clinical manifestations vary from asymptomatic to profound dysphagia.
- The diagnosis of CPD may be accomplished with a combination of clinical and instrumental swallowing evaluations, including flexible endoscopic evaluation of swallowing, video-fluoroscopic swallow study, and high-resolution manometry.
- The success of intervention at the CPM relies heavily on the accuracy of diagnosis, which is often challenging.
- Patients with dysphagia with CPD who retain sufficient pharyngeal strength and hyolaryngeal elevation will fair best with interventions targeting the CPM.
- Interventions include nonsurgical, pharyngoesophageal segment dilation, botulinum toxin injection, and cricopharyngeus myotomy.

INTRODUCTION

The upper esophageal sphincter (UES) is a 2.5- to 4.5-cm high-pressure zone extending from the distal pharynx to the proximal esophagus. This anatomic region is also referred to as the *pharyngoesophageal segment* (PES). The cricopharyngeus muscle (CPM) is positioned in the transition zone between the inferior pharyngeal constrictor and cervical esophageal musculature, which compose the PES. The CPM is 1 to 2 cm wide and C shaped, attaching to the lateral portions of the cricoid cartilage without a median raphe. It is composed of a horizontal portion termed the *pars fundiformis* and an oblique portion known as the *pars oblique*. Uniquely composed of skeletal muscle and abundant connective tissue, the CPM small fibers originate and insert within the

Department of Otolaryngology/Head and Neck Surgery, Center for Voice and Swallowing, University of California, Davis, 2521 Stockton Boulevard, Suite 7200, Sacramento, CA 95817, USA
* Corresponding author.
E-mail address: peter.belafsky@ucdmc.ucdavis.edu

Otolaryngol Clin N Am 46 (2013) 1087–1099
http://dx.doi.org/10.1016/j.otc.2013.08.006
0030-6665/13/$ – see front matter © 2013 Elsevier Inc. All rights reserved.

Abbreviations: Cricopharyngeus Muscle Dysfunction	
BTx	Botulinum toxin
CPB	Cricopharyngeus muscle bar
CPD	Cricopharyngeus muscle dysfunction
CPM	Cricopharyngeus muscle
FEES	Flexible endoscopic evaluation of swallowing
FOSS	Functional outcome swallowing scores
HRM	High-resolution impedance manometry
PCR	Pharyngeal constriction ratio
PES	Pharyngoesophageal segment
PSM	Pharyngeal squeeze maneuver
RLN	Recurrent laryngeal nerve
UES	Upper esophageal sphincter
VFSS	Video-fluoroscopic swallow study

fibroelastic connective tissue.[1] The CPM contains mostly slow type 1 muscle fibers but also fast type 2 fibers enabling baseline tonicity as well as rapid reflexive relaxation or tightening. Anatomic studies have demonstrated that the CPM receives dual innervation from the ipsilateral pharyngeal plexus and the recurrent laryngeal nerve (RLN). Sensory information is carried along the glossopharyngeal nerve and cervical sympathetics.

At rest, the tonically contracted UES protects against aspiration of refluxed gastric contents as well as aerophagia during respiration. Reflexive tightening of the UES is induced by esophageal distention or acid exposure, pharyngeal stimuli and emotional stress.[2–5] During deglutition, eructation and vomiting, the UES reflexively opens. During swallowing, opening of the PES relies on CPM relaxation, anterosuperior movement of the hyolaryngeal complex, pharyngeal contraction, and distension by the passing bolus.[6] Although the CPM is only one component of effective PES function, it is the only portion that actively participates in all reflexive relaxation and tightening activities. Consequently, the CPM is an important target for therapy in several disease processes affecting the UES. Cricopharyngeus muscle dysfunction (CPD) describes impaired or uncoordinated PES relaxation or expansion and results from a variety of causes as listed in **Table 1**.

EVALUATION OF CPD

Accurately diagnosing CPD is challenging but essential for therapeutic decision making. Individuals with poor CPM relaxation but intact laryngeal elevation and pharyngeal contraction generally respond well to surgical CPM intervention. However, those demonstrating intact CPM behavior with impaired pharyngeal strength or hyolaryngeal elevation are more appropriate candidates for therapy than surgery. Dysphagia clinicians rely on several diagnostic tools to identify and differentiate pharyngeal weakness, poor hyolaryngeal elevation, loss of PES elasticity, and impaired CPM relaxation. Available tools include the clinical swallow evaluation, flexible endoscopic evaluation of swallowing (FEES), video-fluoroscopic swallow study (VFSS) and manometry of the pharynx, and UES.

Clinical Swallow Evaluation

Information gathered during the clinical swallow evaluation is useful for generating a hypothesis for the cause or site of dysphagia and for choosing a potential instrumental tool

Table 1 Conditions responsible for PES dysfunction	
Neoplastic	Oropharyngeal carcinoma Esophageal carcinoma Benign esophageal neoplasm Brainstem neoplasm
Neurologic/Neuromuscular	Cerebrovascular accident Traumatic brain injury Parkinson disease Amyotrophic lateral sclerosis Huntington chorea Inflammatory myopathy Spinocerebellar degeneration Syringobulbia Muscular dystrophy
Inflammatory/Autoimmune	Laryngopharyngeal reflux Pharyngitis Dermatomyositis Inclusion body myositis Polymyositis Scleroderma
Infectious/Toxic	Poliomyelitis Diphtheria Rabies Botulism Lead poisoning
Metabolic	Hyperthyroidism Myxedema Diabetes
Trauma/Iatrogenic	Foreign body Postsurgical changes Radiation therapy Aerodigestive injury
Other	Zenker diverticulum Idiopathic

for further swallowing assessment. A history of solid food or combined solid food and liquid dysphagia suggests impaired pharyngeal strength, PES dysfunction, or an esophageal cause, whereas isolated dysphagia to thin liquids indicates laryngopharyngeal sensory impairment or oropharyngeal dysphagia. Furthermore, patients identifying their dysphagia as cervical may have a pharyngeal or UES abnormality, whereas those localizing complaints to the chest assuredly have an esophageal cause for their dysphagia.

The physical examination is helpful in assessing hyolaryngeal mobility. Poor palpable elevation of the hyoid bone or thyroid notch during a dry swallow reveals a probable cause for poor PES distension. During bolus trials, repeated swallows or throat clearing after swallowing suggests hypopharyngeal residue, which is frequently encountered with PES dysfunction or pharyngeal weakness.

Although the clinical swallow evaluation is important for the initial evaluation of patients complaining of dysphagia, it is inadequate to fully characterize all phases of swallowing and definitively identify the sites of abnormality. Furthermore, previous studies have shown that a bedside swallow evaluation may fail to detect aspiration in up to 40% of individuals.[7]

FEES

A potentially useful component of the office-based dysphagia evaluation is FEES. It is particularly important for assessing laryngopharyngeal anatomy as well as sensory and motor integrity. Although FEES does not directly evaluate PES function, the presence of pooled hypopharyngeal secretions with intact pharyngeal strength assessed by the pharyngeal squeeze maneuver (PSM) (**Fig. 1**) indicates obstruction at the PES. However, observing an impaired PSM suggests pharyngeal weakness as a potential cause for dysphagia but reveals little regarding PES function.

Video-fluoroscopy

Improved evaluation of PES opening is afforded during the VFSS. Impaired CPM function may manifest radiographically as a cricopharyngeus muscle bar (CPB) with varying degrees of obstruction or complete PES obstruction (**Fig. 2**). To improve interpretation and comparison of sequential studies, Leonard and colleagues[8,9] reported validated displacement and timing measures that allow extraction of objective data from VFSS. Particularly important for assessing CPM function are the PES opening size and duration; laryngohyoid approximation; oropharyngeal and hypopharyngeal transit times; and pharyngeal constriction ratio (PCR), which is a surrogate measure for pharyngeal strength. The PES opening enlarges with increasing bolus size and is, on average, smaller in adults older than 65 years. CPBs are frequently encountered during VFSS and were identified in nearly one-third of a cohort of nondysphagic elderly (>65 years of age) individuals.[10] Such incidental findings lend support to measuring the PES opening because it remains adequate in many individuals with radiographic evidence of CPBs. Furthermore, measurement of the PES opening preoperatively and postoperatively in patients with obstructing CPM dysfunction helps to quantify the effect of the intervention.

A decreased PES opening in the presence of poor laryngohyoid approximation suggests that dysphagia is a consequence of more than CPD; more importantly, it may not respond favorably to CPM surgery. Additionally, pharyngeal weakness, indicated by an elevated PCR, may account for impaired bolus transport through the PES. The PCR is also a useful measure to monitor the treatment effect after intervention

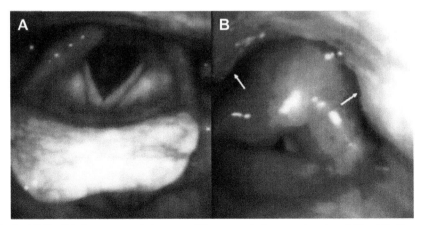

Fig. 1. (*A*) Flexible laryngoscopic images of the normal pharynx at rest and (*B*) while the patient says a forceful /eee/ demonstrating an intact PSM. Note that the lateral hypopharyngeal walls contract and obliterate the pyriform sinuses (*yellow arrows*).

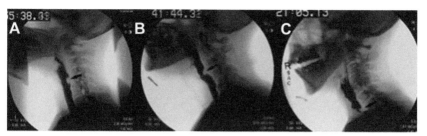

Fig. 2. Images captured during VFSS performed on 3 unique patients. (*A*) A nonobstructing cricopharyngeal (CP) bar (*arrow*) does not impede bolus flow. (*B*) A moderately obstructing CP bar (*arrow*) occupies nearly half of the UES lumen. (*C*) A severely obstructing CP bar (*arrow*) causes near complete UES narrowing.

downstream at the CPM. The ability of video-fluoroscopy to demonstrate the interrelationship of the PES opening, laryngohyoid elevation, and pharyngeal contraction is uniquely valuable and particularly important for therapeutic decision making in patients with suspected CPD.

Pharyngeal and UES Manometry

High-resolution impedance manometry (HRM) can be a useful adjunctive diagnostic tool in the evaluation of CPD (**Fig. 3**). It enables the assessment of pharyngeal strength, UES relaxation, and the coordination of pharyngeal and UES activity as well as abnormally elevated intrabolus pressure. The authors perform HRM using a 36-channel, 2.75-mm diameter ManoScan esophageal catheter (Given Imaging Ltd, Los Angeles, CA) and ManoViewZ software (Given Imaging Ltd, Los Angeles, CA). Elevated UES resting pressure may not clinically manifest as CPD but rather may indicate CPM spasm, which has been associated with gastroesophageal reflux and globus pharyngeus.[11,12] During deglutition, in the presence of normal pharyngeal contraction, elevated UES residual pressure suggests CPD (**Fig. 4A**). Furthermore, during failed UES relaxation, elevated hypopharyngeal bolus pressure may be observed, which further supports the diagnosis of CPD (see **Fig. 4B**).

One shortcoming of pharyngeal and UES HRM is the expected motion of the manometry catheter during swallowing, which decreases the accuracy of identifying

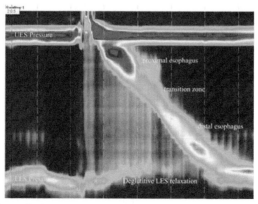

Fig. 3. Normal high-resolution manometry pressure topography plot with appropriate UES relaxation (*asterisk*). LES, lower esophageal sphincter.

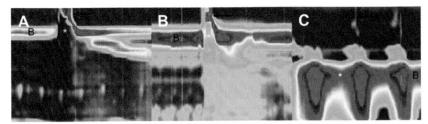

Fig. 4. Pharyngeal and UES HRM. (A) Complete relaxation of the UES (*asterisk*) and normal hypopharyngeal pressure wave (*black arrow*). (B) Incomplete UES relaxation (*asterisk*) with a preserved, normal hypopharyngeal pressure wave (*black arrow*). (C) Hypertensive and absent UES relaxation (*asterisk*) with absent pharyngeal contraction (*black arrow*). B, baseline UES pressure.

where pressures are generated. To address this, pairing manometry with fluoroscopy has allowed the intraluminal pressure with exact anatomic locations depicted on a lateral fluoroscopic view (**Fig. 5**).

MANAGEMENT OF CPD

Individuals with dysphagia caused by CPD may benefit from interventions targeted at the CPM. Choosing the appropriate candidate and correct intervention can be challenging and requires thoughtful consideration of patients' overall well-being and the results of the instrumental evaluations described earlier. Those most likely to benefit from intervention report solid food or combined liquid and solid food dysphagia and demonstrate radiographic evidence of PES narrowing or manometric evidence of elevated UES residual and intrabolus pressure with preserved pharyngeal strength and hyolaryngeal elevation.

Nonsurgical

Although not intended for cure, nonsurgical interventions may play an important role in the comprehensive management of CPD. Patients who struggle with viscous or

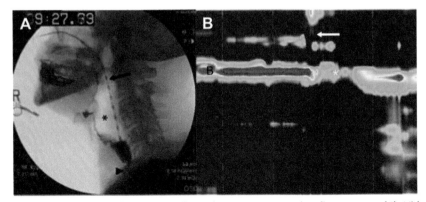

Fig. 5. High-resolution pharyngoesophageal manometry under fluoroscopy. (A) Videofluoroscopic image demonstrates the transnasal small-diameter catheter in place (*black arrow*) and (B) the output of pressures transduced. A large, dilated pharynx (*black asterisk*) corresponds to poor pharyngeal contractility (*white arrow*). There is relative obstruction at the UES (*arrowhead*) and incomplete UES relaxation (*white asterisk*) on manometry. B, baseline UES pressure.

solid food may improve ease of swallowing or intake by diet modification to thin or slippery consistencies. Additionally, gastroesophageal reflux has been implicated in CPM hypertrophy and dysfunction.[13,14] Antireflux therapy, usually proton pump inhibitor, is warranted in patients with symptomatic or objectively confirmed gastroesophageal reflux. Given its implication in the development of CPD, empiric reflux therapy may be indicated in all individuals with dysphagia caused by CPD. Although volitional expansion of the UES with the Mendelsohn maneuver has been shown,[15] traditional dysphagia therapy and exercises are unlikely to benefit patients with CPD.

Dilation

Esophageal dilation has been performed for centuries beginning primitively with a dilator fashioned from whalebone in the seventeenth century. The first bougienage dilators were introduced in the nineteenth century.[16] For the past several decades, dilation has targeted the UES in the setting of stenosis or fibrosis. Published reports confirm both the efficacy and safety of such dilations.[17,18] PES dilation may also be indicated in individuals with CPD. In the largest published series, Clary and colleagues[19] reviewed their experience with 46 patients undergoing bougie PES dilation for CPD. They found an overall improvement in two-thirds of patients reflected by functional outcome swallowing scores (FOSS), with a median duration of efficacy of more than 2 years. However, there was significant variability in the time to benefit as well as the duration of improvement. Of note, there were no major complications in a total of 59 CPM dilation procedures.

Esophageal dilation has traditionally been performed with fixed-diameter dilators (Maloney bougies [Teleflex Medical, Research Triangle Park, NC] or Savory dilators [Cook Medical, Bloomington, IN]) and usually under general anesthesia. Gaining popularity is balloon dilation with single-use, variably sized, saline-inflated balloons. These dilators offer the advantage of incremental enlargement under direct visualization, the use of 2 balloon dilators, and performance on lightly sedated patients (**Fig. 6**). However, unlike fixed-size dilators, balloons are single use and carry added expense.

Botulinum Toxin Injection

Botulinum toxin (BTx) is a purified neurotoxin that irreversibly binds to presynaptic nerve terminals and consequently inhibits the release of acetylcholine into

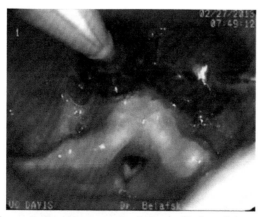

Fig. 6. Flexible endoscopic view demonstrating balloon dilation of the UES for a moderately obstructing cricopharyngeal bar. Two balloons are used to better approximate the oblong shape of the UES.

neuromuscular junctions. The result is chemical denervation and temporary muscle paralysis. Seven BTx serotypes have been isolated, with serotypes A and B commercially available for clinical use, most commonly by neurologists, ophthalmologists, otolaryngologists, and plastic surgeons, among others for a variety of conditions. The CPM has long been a popular target for BTx in laryngectomies with dysphagia or voicing difficulties. In 1989, Schneider and colleagues[20] first described the injection of BTx into the CPM for CPD.

Different techniques for instilling BTx into the CPM have been described. Awake, in-office CPM BTx injection with electromyogram and/or fluoroscopic guidance is performed transcervically (**Fig. 7**) or via flexible endoscopy.[21,22] Operative CPM BTx injection involves rigid laryngoscopy and esophagoscopy with direct visualization of the CPM (**Fig. 8**), allowing for a more controlled BTx injection and concurrent UES dilation. Often patients who may derive benefit from CPM BTx injection have comorbidities that preclude procedures requiring general anesthesia and are, thus, better suited for in-office procedures. Dosing is variable depending on the clinician but usually ranges from 20 to 100 units, with higher quantities used in feeding tube–dependent patients who are unlikely to get worse if too much toxin is injected. BTx is prepared in low-volume, high-concentration dilutions to minimize the potential for undesired diffusion of the toxin. The effects of BTx are appreciated within weeks of injection and typically last up to 5 or 6 months, although some individuals have experienced long-term effects.[23]

The reported results of CPM BTx are favorable, although mainly consist of case reports or series without standardized indications, dosage, or outcome measures. In 2006, Moerman[24] reviewed 16 publications and found reported improvement in 74% of patients, with nearly half of the publications reporting improvement in 100% of patients. The largest published series of patients undergoing CPM BTx injection for CPD suggests modest results. Zaninotto and colleagues[25] reported improved symptoms in only 9 of 21 patients (43%). The 12 patients who failed to improve with

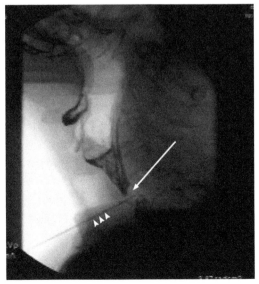

Fig. 7. Video-fluoroscopic image of BTx injection into the cricopharyngeus muscle (*white arrow*) using an electromyography needle (*white arrowheads*).

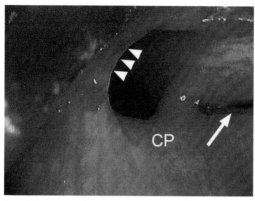

Fig. 8. Endoscopic view during microdirect laryngoscopy showing injection of BTx (*white arrow*) into CPM. Also visible is a cricopharyngeal web (*white arrowheads*).

BTx underwent surgical myotomy, with 73% experiencing improved swallowing, suggesting that the response to CPM BTx injection may not accurately predict the effect of future definitive surgical management as had previously been proposed.[26] In a recent retrospective review of 49 patients with CPD from various causes, Kelly and colleagues[27] reported 65% had improved EAT-10 scores following CPM BTx injection without a major complication.

Excluding the negative effects of anesthesia or rigid endoscopy, most complications of CPM BTx result from diffusion into neighboring structures causing dyspnea or dysphonia if the intrinsic laryngeal musculature are affected or worsening dysphagia from pharyngeal weakness.[24]

Myotomy

The first report of a surgical CPM myotomy was by Kaplan[28] in 1951 for a patient with dysphagia related to poliomyelitis. Surgical CPM myotomy remains the gold standard treatment of CPD. As with other interventions at the CPM, patients with adequate hyolaryngeal elevation and pharyngeal strength are favored. A trial of PES dilation or CPM BTx injection may predict the efficacy of surgical CPM myotomy.[26] However, surgical myotomy should still be considered in patients with severe CPD and a marginal response to CPM dilation or BTx if they are sound surgical candidates and meet the criteria for intervention.

Manometric studies have demonstrated a 50% reduction in UES pressure with CPM myotomy, and the effect is enhanced when the myotomy is extending into the inferior constrictors and, to a lesser extent, into the muscular fibers of the cervical esophagus.[29] These findings are the rationale for performing a 5- to 6-cm myotomy during an open surgical procedure. The pharynx and esophagus are distended with a bougie, and the incision is carried through all visible muscle fibers leaving the pharyngeal and esophageal mucosa intact. Luminal injuries must be identified immediately, repaired, and monitored closely to prevent serious consequences. Open CPM myotomy caries the risk of potentially life-threatening complications that may be poorly tolerated by decompensated patients with multiple comorbidities. A review of 253 traditional CPM myotomies performed by a single surgeon reported 5 patients developing wound infection or hematoma, 3 developing fistulae, and 8 experiencing pulmonary complications, with 4 progressing to fatal respiratory distress.[30] Additional risks include injury to the RLN and aspiration. Awareness of these risks should guide patient counseling and perioperative care. Oral intake is generally delayed several days or longer in the absence of luminal injury, and some advocate video-fluoroscopy or chest radiography before initiating oral feeding.

Reports on the outcomes of CP myotomy are largely limited to retrospective case series. Efficacy is related to dysphagia severity and the underlying cause of CPD as well as its effects on other swallowing physiology. Therefore, individuals with focal neurologic deficits or idiopathic, isolated CPD are more likely to perform better after CPM myotomy than those with central neurologic processes, such as amyotrophic lateral sclerosis and Parkinson disease or systemic myopathy.[31,32]

Surgical approaches to CPM myotomy include the traditional transcervical procedure and the endoscopic, laser-assisted technique. The latter was introduced in 1994 and uses a laryngoscope or diverticuloscope to isolate the CPM, which is divided with its overlying mucosa using a laser.[33] Care is taken to avoid disrupting the underlying fascia to minimize the risk of pneumomediastinum or mediastinitis (**Fig. 9**). Treatment of the incised overlying mucosa following myotomy varies among surgeons and includes primary suture closure, application of fibrin glue, and, most commonly, healing by secondary intention.[33–35]

The endoscopic laser-assisted approach to CPM myotomy has gained popularity because early results suggest its effectiveness with earlier reintroduction of oral diet and less morbidity than the traditional open approach.[35–37] However, comparison of the 2 techniques has not yet been prospectively performed. Bachy and colleagues[37] recently reported their long-term outcomes of more than 30 patients who underwent endoscopic CPM myotomy. At least three-quarters reported improved swallowing symptoms measured by the deglutition handicap index at up to 99 months following intervention. No cases of mediastinitis or death were reported, but 3 minor complications of pulmonary infection, contained fistula, and subcutaneous emphysema were encountered. Additional risks of endoscopic CPM myotomy include bleeding, pain, oral or dental injury, and laryngeal edema.

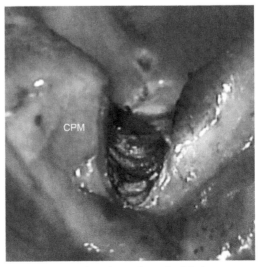

Fig. 9. Endoscopic CPM myotomy using the carbon dioxide laser.

SUMMARY

CPD may result from a variety of causes, including neurologic, autoimmune, neuromuscular, neoplastic, and traumatic. Clinically, it manifests as solid food or combined liquid and solid food dysphagia, with symptoms ranging from mild to severe. Identifying CPD may be challenging, but it is imperative for selecting appropriate interventions that target the CPM. Clinicians rely on the clinical swallow evaluation, FEES, VFSS, and HRM to assist in the diagnosis of CPD. These tools also assist in the identification of patients with dysphagia who have adequate pharyngeal strength and laryngohyoid elevation, which are important positive prognosticators for treatments targeting the CPM. Interventions for CPD include PES dilation, CPM BTx injection, and CPM myotomy.

REFERENCES

1. Brownlow H, Whitmore I, Willan PL. A quantitative study of the histochemical and morphometric characteristics of the human cricopharyngeus muscle. J Anat 1989;166:67–75.
2. Andreollo NA, Thompson DG, Kendall GP, et al. Functional relationships between cricopharyngeal sphincter and oesophageal body in response to graded intraluminal distension. Gut 1988;29:161–6.
3. Kahrilas PJ, Dodds WJ, Dent J, et al. Effect of sleep, spontaneous gastroesophageal reflux, and a meal on upper esophageal sphincter pressure in normal human volunteers. Gastroenterology 1987;92:466–71.
4. Shaker R, Ren J, Xie P, et al. Characterization of the pharyngo-UES contractile reflex in humans. Am J Physiol 1997;273:G854–8.
5. Cook IJ, Dent J, Shannon S, et al. Measurement of upper esophageal sphincter pressure. Effect of acute emotional stress. Gastroenterology 1987;93:526–32.
6. Cook IJ, Dodds WJ, Dantas RO, et al. Opening mechanisms of the human upper esophageal sphincter. Am J Physiol 1989;257:G748–59.
7. Linden P, Kuhlemeier KV, Patterson C. The probability of correctly predicting subglottic penetration from clinical observations. Dysphagia 1993;8:170–9.
8. Leonard RJ, Kendall KA, McKenzie S, et al. Structural displacements in normal swallowing: a videofluoroscopic study. Dysphagia 2000;15:146–52.
9. Kendall KA, McKenzie S, Leonard RJ, et al. Timing of events in normal swallowing: a videofluoroscopic study. Dysphagia 2000;15:74–83.
10. Leonard R, Kendall K, McKenzie S. UES opening and cricopharyngeal bar in nondysphagic elderly and nonelderly adults. Dysphagia 2004;19:182–91.
11. Stanciu C, Bennett JR. Upper oesophageal sphincter yield pressure in normal subjects and in patients with gastro-oesophageal reflux. Thorax 1974;29:459–62.
12. Corso MJ, Pursnani KG, Mohiuddin MA, et al. Globus sensation is associated with hypertensive upper esophageal sphincter but not with gastroesophageal reflux. Dig Dis Sci 1998;43:1513–7.
13. Gerhardt DC, Shuck TJ, Bordeaux RA, et al. Human upper esophageal sphincter. Response to volume, osmotic, and acid stimuli. Gastroenterology 1978;75:268–74.
14. Freiman JM, El-Sharkawy TY, Diamant NE. Effect of bilateral vagosympathetic nerve blockade on response of the dog upper esophageal sphincter (UES) to intraesophageal distention and acid. Gastroenterology 1981;81:78–84.
15. Kahrilas PJ, Logemann JA, Krugler C, et al. Volitional augmentation of upper esophageal sphincter opening during swallowing. Am J Physiol 1991;260:G450–6.

16. Hildreth CT. Stricture of the esophagus. N Engl J Med Surg 1821;10:235.
17. Wang YG, Tio TL, Soehendra N. Endoscopic dilation of esophageal stricture without fluoroscopy is safe and effective. World J Gastroenterol 2002;8: 766–8.
18. Ahlawat SK, Al-Kawas FH. Endoscopic management of upper esophageal strictures after treatment of head and neck malignancy. Gastrointest Endosc 2008;68: 19–24.
19. Clary MS, Daniero JJ, Keith SW, et al. Efficacy of large-diameter dilatation in cricopharyngeal dysfunction. Laryngoscope 2011;121:2521–5.
20. Schneider I, Thumfart WF, Pototschnig C, et al. Treatment of dysfunction of the cricopharyngeal muscle with botulinum A toxin: introduction of a new, noninvasive method. Ann Otol Rhinol Laryngol 1994;103:31–5.
21. Murry T, Wasserman T, Carrau RL, et al. Injection of botulinum toxin A for the treatment of dysfunction of the upper esophageal sphincter. Am J Otolaryngol 2005; 26:157–62.
22. Parameswaran MS, Soliman AM. Endoscopic botulinum toxin injection for cricopharyngeal dysphagia. Ann Otol Rhinol Laryngol 2002;111:871–4.
23. Chiu MJ, Chang YC, Hsiao TY. Prolonged effect of botulinum toxin injection in the treatment of cricopharyngeal dysphagia: case report and literature review. Dysphagia 2004;19:52–7.
24. Moerman MB. Cricopharyngeal Botox injection: indications and technique. Curr Opin Otolaryngol Head Neck Surg 2006;14:431–6.
25. Zaninotto G, Marchese Ragona R, Briani C, et al. The role of botulinum toxin injection and upper esophageal sphincter myotomy in treating oropharyngeal dysphagia. J Gastrointest Surg 2004;8:997–1006.
26. Blitzer A, Brin MF. Use of botulinum toxin for diagnosis and management of cricopharyngeal achalasia. Otolaryngol Head Neck Surg 1997;116:328–30.
27. Kelly EA, Koszewski IJ, Jaradeh SS, et al. Botulinum toxin injection for the treatment of upper esophageal sphincter dysfunction. Ann Otol Rhinol Laryngol 2013; 122:100–8.
28. Kaplan S. Paralysis of deglutition, a post-poliomyelitis complication treated by section of the cricopharyngeus muscle. Ann Surg 1951;133:572–3.
29. Pera M, Yamada A, Hiebert CA, et al. Sleeve recording of upper esophageal sphincter resting pressures during cricopharyngeal myotomy. Ann Surg 1997; 225:229–34.
30. Brigand C, Ferraro P, Martin J, et al. Risk factors in patients undergoing cricopharyngeal myotomy. Br J Surg 2007;94:978–83.
31. Orringer MB. Extended cervical esophagomyotomy for cricopharyngeal dysfunction. J Thorac Cardiovasc Surg 1986;80:669.
32. Poirier NC, Bonavina L, Taillefer R, et al. Cricopharyngeal myotomy for neurogenic oropharyngeal dysphagia. J Thorac Cardiovasc Surg 1997;113:233–40 [discussion: 240–1].
33. Halvorson DJ, Kuhn FA. Transmucosal cricopharyngeal myotomy with the potassium-titanyl-phosphate laser in the treatment of cricopharyngeal dysmotility. Ann Otol Rhinol Laryngol 1994;103:173–7.
34. Ho AS, Morzaria S, Damrose EJ. Carbon dioxide laser-assisted endoscopic cricopharyngeal myotomy with primary mucosal closure. Ann Otol Rhinol Laryngol 2011;120:33–9.
35. Lawson G, Remacle M. Endoscopic cricopharyngeal myotomy: indications and technique. Curr Opin Otolaryngol Head Neck Surg 2006;14:437–41.

36. Takes RP, van den Hoogen FJ, Marres HA. Endoscopic myotomy of the cricopharyngeal muscle with CO2 laser surgery. Head Neck 2005;27:703–9.
37. Bachy V, Matar N, Remacle M, et al. Long-term functional results after endoscopic cricopharyngeal myotomy with CO2 laser: a retrospective study of 32 cases. Eur Arch Otorhinolaryngol 2013;270:965–8.

Zenker Diverticulum

Eitan Prisman, MD, FRCSC[a],*, Eric M. Genden, MD, FACS[b]

KEYWORDS

- Zenker diverticulum • Myotomy • Killian triangle • Diverticulum • Diverticulectomy
- CO_2 laser • Endoscopic stapling

KEY POINTS

- Zenker diverticulum is a pseudodiverticulum through Killian triangle between the oblique and fundiform parts of the cricopharyngeus.
- It is thought to be caused by repeated incoordination between upper esophageal sphincter relaxation and pharyngeal contraction resulting in increased intraesophageal pressure and subsequent pseudoherniation through Killian triangle.
- It is most commonly presents in males in their seventh and eighth decades.
- The most common symptoms are dysphagia, regurgitation of food, and halitosis.
- It is seen on esophagram as a cricopharyngeal bar and associated diverticulum that can vary in size.
- Most diverticula, both small and large, can be successfully treated endoscopically with minimal morbidity and a 95% success rate.
- Open surgery is reserved for failed endoscopic treatment or inability to obtain adequate endoscopic exposure.

INTRODUCTION

Zenker diverticulum (ZD) is an outpouching of mucosa without muscle through a dehiscence in a triangular area of weakness within the cricopharyngeus (CP) muscle, on the dorsal wall of the hypopharynx, and is therefore more correctly classified as a pseudodiverticulum. Originally described in Great Britain by Ludlow as an autopsy finding in 1769, a more detailed description was put forth by the German Pathologists

Both Eitan Prisman and Eric Genden have no conflicts of interests to disclose.

[a] Division of Otolaryngology Head and Neck Surgery, Gordon and Leslie Diamond Health Care Centre, Vancouver General Hospital, University of British Columbia, 4th Floor-2775 Laurel Street, Vancouver, British Columbia V5Z 1M9, Canada; [b] Otolaryngology- Head and Neck Surgery, Department of Otolaryngology, The Head Neck, and Thyroid Center, The Mount Sinai Medical Center, The Icahn School of Medicine at Mount Sinai, One Gustave Levy Place, Box 1189, New York, NY 10029-6574, USA
* Corresponding author.
E-mail address: eitan.prisman@gmail.com

Zenker and von Ziemssen in 1877. They proposed the generally accepted pathophysiology of "forces within the lumen acting against restriction". Later, in 1907, Killian observed this pharyngeal pseudodiverticulum as emanating posteriorly in the midline between the thyropharyngeus above and the CP below (**Fig. 1**).

ANATOMY

The inferior pharyngeal constrictor consists of 2 muscles, the *thyropharyngeus* and the *cricopharyngeus*. The latter muscle has 2 components, the oblique, or superior part of the CP and the fundiform, or inferior part of the CP. Both the superior and inferior portions arise bilaterally from the posterolateral border the thyroid lamina. Although the *superior fibers* meet at a median raphe on the posterior border of the hypopharynx, the *inferior fibers* circle the esophageal lumen without attaching to a median raphe. The triangular area between these components is defined as Killian triangle[1] and is the triangle through which ZD herniates. This should be differentiated from the Killian-Jamieson diverticulum, located more inferolaterally, in close proximity to the recurrent laryngeal nerve, between the inferior CP muscle above and the superior border of the longitudinal muscle fibers of the proximal esophageal muscle below.

PATHOPHYSIOLOGY

The upper esophageal sphincter (UES) is approximately 1 cm in craniocaudal dimension and is principally formed by the CP. The CP, which is contracted at rest, generates the zone of maximal UES pressure with a resting pressure of 60 mm Hg and 30 mm Hg in the sagittal and transverse dimensions, respectively.[2] As originally proposed by Zenker, it is generally accepted that the repeated dyscoordination between UES relaxation and pharyngeal contraction during deglutition, known as circopharyngeal dysfunction (CPD), causes increased intra-esophageal pressure and contributes to the anatomic weakness of the posterior pharyngeal musculature, thereby predisposing to the development of a pseudodiverticulum.[3] Various age-related changes in deglutition contribute to cricopharyngeal dysfunction and support the presentation of ZD in a relatively older population. These include dyssynchronous oral and pharyngeal phases of swallow, degenerated Auerbach plexus and delayed anterior displacement of the hyoid as well as on overall decreased elevation of the hyolaryngeal complex. Similarly, cricopharyngeal achalasia, incomplete or delayed CP relaxation, premature UES closure, and neuropathic injuries leading to uncoordinated deglutition

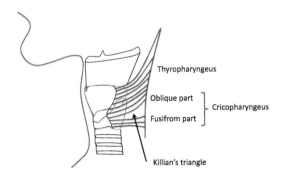

Fig. 1. Anatomy of the cricopharyngeus.

may also contribute to an elevated UES pressure and predispose to the development of a ZD.[4] Although gastroesophageal reflux (GERD) has been implicated in the development of ZD by some, it is difficult to differentiate GERD as a cause or effect of CPD or ZD.[5] Certainly, histologic studies of the cricopharyngeus of ZD demonstrate fibrosis, increased collagen deposition, and fat replacement, which confirm the hypothesis of a poorly compliant cricopharyngeal system.[6]

SYMPTOMS

ZD is a relatively rare entity with a reported prevalence of 0.11%, presenting most commonly in men in their seventh or eighth decades. Symptoms relate to the size of the pharyngeal diverticulum and most commonly manifest as dysphagia. Other symptoms include regurgitation of undigested food, halitosis, aspiration, gurgling in the throat, neck mass, dysphonia, and malnutrition.

SIGNS

Most patients do not have pertinent clinical signs on physical examination. However, a minority of patients with very large diverticulum may present with malnutrition, dysphonia, a soft swelling on the left side of the neck known as Boyce sign, cervical borborygmi, or crepitus. Although the diagnosis is suspected based on history, it is confirmed by esophageal studies (**Fig. 2**).

OPEN SURGICAL TREATMENT

Surgical treatment of ZD can be categorized as either external or endoscopic. Traditionally, an open transcervical resection of ZD was the treatment of choice.[7] However, as the underlying contribution of the cricopharyngeus to the pathophysiology of ZD was appreciated, a CP myotomy, with or without diverticulopexy or diverticulectomy, gained favor as a significant component of the surgical therapy. Once the diverticulum is exposed through an external approach, there remain several options to manage the diverticulum including diverticulectomy followed by hand sewn closure or applying a staple-assisted device to complete both the resection and closure of the esophagotomy. These open techniques must be accompanied by a myotomy to address the underlying pathophysiology and prevent recurrence. Earlier on in the evolution of managing ZD, to avoid the concern of post-diverticulectomy dehiscence and leaking, the techniques of diverticulopexy and diverticular imbrication were designed to negate an esophagotomy. Diverticulopexy involves suturing the base of the diverticulum to the prevertebral fascia or pharyngeal constrictors, whereas diverticular imbrication involves tying a purse string around the diverticulum followed by inversion into the lumen.[8,9] However, diverticulopexy is associated with a higher recurrence rate, and inversion is likely only beneficial for a small diverticulum. Furthermore, with careful attention to sewing techniques, particularly the canal stitch, as well as the reliability of the gastrointestinal anastomotic stapler, leaking post-diverticulectomy has become much less of a concern. Although the risks of diverticulectomy are low, they must be considered and discussed with the patients. These include mediastinitis, recurrent laryngeal nerve injury, pneumonia, hematoma, and infection.

Open Myotomy or Diverticulectomy Technique

The patient is placed in the supine position under general anesthesia. A horizontal 4-cm incision is performed on the left side just inferolateral to the cricoid cartilage. The fascia

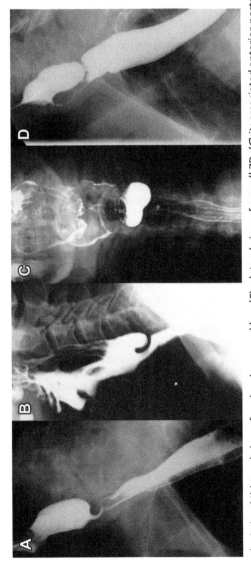

Fig. 2. Esophagram depicting (*A*) lateral view of a cricopharyngeal bar, (*B*) a lateral view of a small ZD, (*C*) its associated anterior-posterior view, and (*D*) a lateral view of a large ZD.

separating the sternocleidomastoid muscle and the strap muscles is incised and the carotid sheath is gently retracted laterally. Blunt dissection is carried down onto the esophagus and posterolaterally to the prevertebral fascia exposing the diverticulum. The diverticulum is grasped with a Babcock and suspended superolaterally to allow for the diverticulectomy to be performed. When available, an endostapler is used to simultaneously perform the diverticulectomy and pharyngeal repair. Alternatively a diverticulectomy can be performed with a scissor or scalpel, and a 3–0 Vicryl on a tapered needle is used to perform vertical canal stitches in an interrupted fashion (**Fig. 3**). Inferior to the diverticulum the dysfunctional cricopharyngeus is exposed and a myotomy is performed using a fresh scalpel. A nasogastric tube is inserted and the patient is kept NPO for 48 hours, after which a barium swallow study is performed before resumption of an oral diet. When only a small diverticulum is present, or in the case of a symptomatic cricopharyngeal bar, a myotomy alone is performed (**Fig. 4**). The cricopharyngeus is exposed as described earlier. These patients can resume an oral liquid diet following a barium swallow study on the first post-operative day.

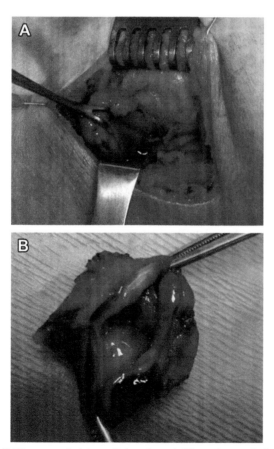

Fig. 3. (*A*) A small ZD suspended by a Babcock and (*B*) an internal view of the excised diverticulum.

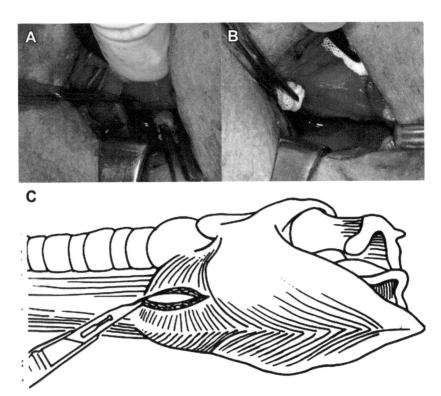

Fig. 4. Intraoperative exposure of (*A*) the cricopharyngeus and (*B*) the resulting myotomy and (*C*) a schematic of the cricopharyngeal myotomy.

ENDOSCOPIC TREATMENT

Although Mosher and colleagues reported the first endoscopic management of ZD in 1917, it was not until the 1960s that Dohlman and Mattson reported a large series of successful endoscopic management with a specially designed laryngoscope (Dohlman diverticuloscope) to isolate the partying wall separating the diverticulum from the esophagus.[10] Although they reported the use of electrocautery, more recent series have reported on the success of using the CO_2, KTP, or Argon laser.[11] The next significant development was the introduction of the endoscopic stapling device, which has since become the method most commonly used.[12] The critical step in this technique is adequate exposure of the partying septum; this may be difficult in patients with prominent teeth, cervical kyphosis, retrognathia, or temporomandibular joint disease. These factors contribute to an overall 5% conversion rate to open surgery. When exposure is not hindered, this minimally invasive technique is quick and associated with much less morbidity compared with open surgery. This technique has a reported leak rate that is negligible and is associated with an overall 5% recurrence rate. However, the endoscopic stapling technique cannot effectively address small diverticula (<2 cm). In these situations, a traction stitch may be placed through the partying wall to suspend the cricopharyngeus and aid in dividing the diverticulum. Additional techniques have been developed to treat small diverticula including using a CO_2 laser or a harmonic scalpel to perform a cricopharyngeal myotomy through mucosa and the cricopharyngeus.[13] Others have described performing a flexible endoscopic myotomy

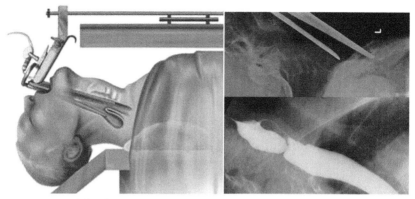

Fig. 5. Exposure of the diverticula using a diverticuloscope.

using electrocautery, argon plasma coagulation, or CO_2 laser on a select group of elderly patients not amenable to rigid endoscopic treatment.[14,15]

Endoscopic Diverticulectomy Technique

The patient is placed in the supine position under general anesthesia and is fully relaxed. The bivalve diverticuloscope (Karl Storz, CA, USA; Tutlingen, Germany) is gently

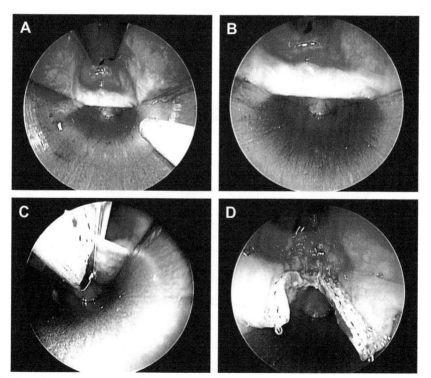

Fig. 6. Endoscopic exposure of the diverticula under (A) low and (B) high power, (C) inserting the endostapler and (D) post-diverticulectomy.

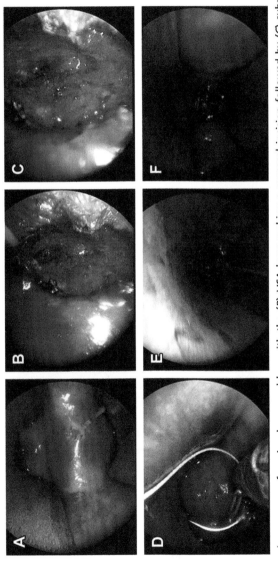

Fig. 7. (A) Endoscopic exposure of a cricopharyngeal bar with the (B) LISA laser making a mucosal incision followed by (C) submucosal dissection through the cricopharyngeus. The (D) endostitch is then used to repair the mucosal incision and suspended followed by (E) applying an endoscopic clip applier to the stitch just superior to the mucosal edges and (F) the repaired endoscopic view.

inserted such that the upper blade is inserted into the esophagus, and the lower blade into the diverticulum, providing exposure of the partying wall of the cricopharyngeus (**Fig. 5**). The diverticuloscope is then suspended. Under direct vision, a disposable endostapler (Ethicon Endo-Surgery, OH, USA) is inserted through the diverticuloscope to straddle the partying septum wall, with the cartridge in the esophagus and the anvil in the diverticulum. A 5-mm 0° telescope is inserted to confirm placement before discharging the endostapler. For diverticula greater than 2 cm, one cartridge will usually suffice; however for diverticula greater than 6 cm, a subsequent endostapler may be required. A traction stitch can be placed through the partying wall with an endostitch device (US Surgical, Normwalk, CT, USA) to aid in exposing the partying septum wall before placement of the endostapler (**Fig. 6**). These patients can resume an oral liquid diet on the first post-operative day following a normal barium swallow study.

Endoscopic CO$_2$ Myotomy

For small diverticula (<2 cm) and associated cricopharyngeal bars, an endoscopic laser technique can be implored. The general anesthesia and positioning are performed as described earlier. If there is no diverticulum, the distal end of the lower blade is inserted 1 cm proximal from the upper end of the cricopharyngeus. A flexible Holmium-YAG LISA laser (LISA laser USA) is inserted under indirect visualization via a 5-mm 0° endoscope. A small incision is performed on the posterior esophageal mucosal wall overlying the cricopharyngeus. The LISA laser is inserted through this incision and then carefully used to submucosally perform a cricopharyngeal myotomy under indirect visualization using the 0° telescope. The flexible LISA laser is not limited by the line of sight, as may be the case when imploring the more traditional microscope and CO$_2$ laser. The mucosal incision can then be repaired either with an endostitch device, which may be challenging to tie, or alternatively, the stitch can be inserted to approximate the mucosal edges and an endoclip device can be used to fasten the 2 suture ends (**Fig. 7**). These patients can resume an oral liquid diet on the first post-operative day following a normal barium swallow study.

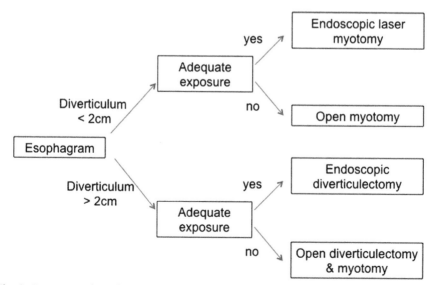

Fig. 8. Treatment algorithm.

TREATMENT ALGORITHM

Endoscopic techniques provide a high success rate with minimal morbidity and therefore every effort should be made to complete the management of a ZD through a minimally invasive endoscopic technique. The choice of endoscopic technique will depend on the size of the diverticulum and the comfort of the surgeon. An open surgical intervention is preferred in the presence of inadequate endoscopic exposure or in the setting of multiple recurrences from endoscopic techniques (**Fig. 8**).

SUMMARY

ZD is a pseudodiverticulum through Killian triangle between the oblique and fundiform parts of the cricopharyngeus muscle, which develops as a consequence of repeated incoordinated UES relaxation and pharyngeal contraction resulting in increased intraesophageal pressure and subsequent pseudoherniation. The treatment of choice, for both small and large diverticula, remains rigid endoscopic management; this is associated with a 95% success rate and minimal morbidity. With the lack of randomized controls trials comparing the different endoscopic techniques, surgeon comfort and training remain the most important factor for successful endoscopic management. Open surgery is reserved for failed endoscopic therapy or inability to provide adequate endoscopic exposure and is associated with excellent results albeit with an increased morbidity compared with endoscopic techniques.

REFERENCES

1. Anagiotos A, Preuss SF, Koebke J. Morphometric and anthropometric analysis of Killian's triangle. Laryngoscope 2010;120(6):1082–8.
2. Broniatowski M, Sonies BC, Rubin JS, et al. Current evaluation and treatment of patients with swallowing disorders. Otolaryngol Head Neck Surg 1999;120(4):464–73.
3. Westrin KM, Ergun S, Carlsoo B. Zenker's diverticulum–a historical review and trends in therapy. Acta Otolaryngol 1996;116(3):351–60.
4. Dzeletovic I, Ekbom DC, Baron TH. Flexible endoscopic and surgical management of Zenker's diverticulum. Expert Rev Gastroenterol Hepatol 2012;6(4):449–65 [quiz: 466].
5. Ekberg O, Lindgren S. Gastroesophageal reflux and pharyngeal function. Acta Radiol Diagn (Stockh) 1986;27(4):421–3.
6. Zaninotto G, Costantini M, Boccù C, et al. Functional and morphological study of the cricopharyngeal muscle in patients with Zenker's diverticulum. Br J Surg 1996;83(9):1263–7.
7. Butcher RB 2nd, Larrabee WF Jr. Surgical treatment of hypopharyngeal (Aenker's) diverticulum. Arch Otolaryngol 1979;105(5):254–7.
8. Holinger PH, Schild JA. The Zenker's (hypopharyngeal) diverticulum. Ann Otol Rhinol Laryngol 1969;78(4):679–88.
9. Johnson JT, Weissman J. Diverticular imbrication and myotomy for Zenker's. Laryngoscope 1992;102(12 Pt 1):1377–8.
10. Dohlman G, Mattsson O. The endoscopic operation for hypopharyngeal diverticula: a roentgencinematographic study. AMA Arch Otolaryngol 1960;71:744–52.
11. Wouters B, van Overbeek JJ. Pathogenesis and endoscopic treatment of the hypopharyngeal (Zenker's) diverticulum. Acta Gastroenterol Belg 1990;53(3):323–9.
12. Collard JM, Otte JB, Kestens PJ. Endoscopic stapling technique of esophagodiverticulostomy for Zenker's diverticulum. Ann Thorac Surg 1993;56(3):573–6.

13. Fama AF, Moore EJ, Kasperbauer JL. Harmonic scalpel in the treatment of Zenker's diverticulum. Laryngoscope 2009;119(7):1265-9.
14. Mulder CJ, den Hartog G, Robijn RJ, et al. Flexible endoscopic treatment of Zenker's diverticulum: a new approach. Endoscopy 1995;27(6):438-42.
15. Rabenstein T, May A, Michel J, et al. Argon plasma coagulation for flexible endoscopic Zenker's diverticulotomy. Endoscopy 2007;39(2):141-5.

Glottal Insufficiency with Aspiration Risk in Dysphagia

Laureano A. Giraldez-Rodriguez, MD*, Michael Johns, III, MD

KEYWORDS

- Dysphagia • Unilateral vocal fold immobility • Vocal fold atrophy
- Postintubation phonatory insufficiency • High vagal paralysis • Glottal insufficiency
- Glottal incompetence

KEY POINTS

- Glottal closure is an important part of the mechanism that protects the airway during the normal swallow.
- Glottal insufficiency disrupts glottal closure and therefore puts patients at risk of aspiration.
- Treatment of glottal insufficiency can be classified as surgical or nonsurgical.
- The objective of treating glottal insufficiency is to avoid aspiration or penetration of secretions or food into the airway.
- Nonsurgical treatment consists of swallowing maneuvers and other measures.
- Surgical treatment of glottal insufficiency includes injection laryngoplasty, medialization thyroplasty with or without arytenoid adduction or with arytenopexy and cricothyroid subluxation, hypopharyngoplasty, cricopharynx muscle dilation, and cricopharynx myotomy.

OVERVIEW

Glottal closure occurs during the normal swallow as part of the mechanism that prevents aspiration of the bolus of foods.[1–8] It also protects the airway from aspiration of respiratory secretions produced by the salivary glands of the upper aerodigestive tract.

Glottal competence is aided by a series of events that begin in the oral cavity and end with closure of the glottis and opening of the upper esophageal sphincter (UES). The oral cavity and oropharynx are responsible for oral propulsion forces that advance the bolus into the pharynx, whereas the esophagus acts as a "suction pump" that propels the bolus further into the UES. Oral competence and velopharyngeal closure are crucial to maintain oronasal separation and thus necessary for bolus propulsion by a series of pressure gradients created.

Disclosure: The authors have no disclosures.
Department of Otolaryngology–Head and Neck Surgery, Emory Voice Center, 550 Peachtree Street Northeast, 9th Floor, Atlanta, GA 30308, USA
* Corresponding author.
E-mail address: laugiraldez@icloud.com

Otolaryngol Clin N Am 46 (2013) 1113–1121
http://dx.doi.org/10.1016/j.otc.2013.09.004   oto.theclinics.com
0030-6665/13/$ – see front matter © 2013 Elsevier Inc. All rights reserved.

Abbreviations	
CP	Cricopharynx
PIPI	Postintubation phonatory insufficiency
UES	Upper esophageal sphincter
UVFI	Unilateral vocal fold immobility

The pharyngeal phase of the swallowing begins as the bolus of food touches the anterior tonsillar pillars. A series of sensory-mediated events that are triggered in the pharynx and the supraglottic larynx occurs that translate into airway protection: the false and true vocal folds close, the pharyngeal constrictors contract, the larynx and the hyoid elevate anteriorly, the epiglottis tilts posteriorly covering the glottic inlet, and the cricopharyngeus muscle relaxes. The fine-tuned interplay of all of these involuntary mechanisms prevents aspiration/penetration of food into the larynx. The risk of dysphagia in the presence of glottal insufficiency is thus heightened by inability of the bolus to have the adequate speed or consistency, by loss of the pressure gradient from oral incompetence or velopharyngeal insufficiency, or because of an inability to pass the bolus into the esophagus.

The primary mechanisms by which glottal incompetence occurs are unilateral vocal fold immobility (UVFI), bilateral vocal fold atrophy, and postintubation phonatory insufficiency (PIPI) (**Box 1**).

CAUSE AND DIAGNOSIS

Vocal fold immobility is most commonly caused by iatrogenic injury to the recurrent laryngeal nerve, idiopathic neural injury (usually related to viral illness), or tumors affecting the vagus nerve (**Box 2**). The term is generally used to describe vocal fold paresis or paralysis.

Vocal atrophy occurs with age because there is loss of vocal fold mass. PIPI occurs with prolonged intubation that leads to medial arytenoid cartilage erosion and vocal fold scarring with subsequent glottic insufficiency.

Glottal insufficiency caused by UVFI, vocal atrophy, or PIPI can be confirmed with laryngeal video stroboscopy. Aspiration, penetration, and reduced laryngeal clearance during the swallow are diagnosed with the aid of different testing tools. The role of each of these testing modalities in dysphagia is further discussed in other articles in this publication (**Box 3**) (see articles Dysphagia Screening and Assessment Instruments by Speyer and The Modified Barium Swallow and Functional Endoscopic Evaluation of Swallowing by Brady).

PATHOPHYSIOLOGY

Inability to achieve glottal closure leads to valvular incompetence that causes a constant pressure leak into the airway that can make the production of voice and

Box 1
Causes of glottal insufficiency
Bilateral vocal fold atrophy
Unilateral vocal fold immobility
Postintubation phonatory insufficiency
High vagal paralysis

Box 2
Causes of UVFI

Iatrogenic (thyroidectomy, mediastinal surgery)

Idiopathic (viral illness)

Neoplasia (skull-base tumors, vagal schwannomas)

Trauma (arytenoid subluxation, neck trauma)

Neural (amyotrophic lateral sclerosis, neuronitis)

Autoimmune (systemic lupus erythematosus)

---

swallowing more difficult. Glottal insufficiency can lead to voice, respiratory, and swallowing symptoms. Cough and choking with liquids or saliva are the most common manifestations of dysphagia in glottal insufficiency. Choking with solids is less frequent, but may also occur in some patients, especially those with high vagal paralysis.

Patients with high vagal paralysis exhibit decreased velopharyngeal closure, decreased and discordant pharyngeal constriction, UVFI, decreased laryngeal sensation, and cricopharyngeal dysfunction. These patients usually present with more severe symptoms of aspiration as these result in decreased bolus propulsion, impaired glottal sensory protection, and decreased esophageal opening. Many of these patients are at risk of becoming tracheostomy- or gastrostomy-dependent to manage secretions and avoid aspiration of food, and some may even require laryngectomy.

The goal of surgical treatment of patients with glottal insufficiency is to restore valve closure to re-establish airway protection during the swallow. The role of injection laryngoplasty and medialization thyroplasty with or without arytenoid repositioning is to re-establish glottal closure. In high vagal paralysis patients, Cricopharynx (CP) myotomy and pharyngoplasty can also be used in the management of glottal insufficiency to decrease the risk of aspiration by increasing the transit time of the pharyngeal bolus.

MANAGEMENT OF DYSPHAGIA IN GLOTTAL INSUFFICIENCY

Treatment of dysphagia in patients with UVFI, bilateral vocal fold atrophy, and PIPI is tailored toward the severity of the patient's symptoms. Patients with mild symptoms who refer occasional choking with thin liquids and who have no history of hospitalizations due to aspiration pneumonia can be managed conservatively with swallowing maneuvers. In-depth discussion can be found in article Swallowing Rehabilitation by Hegland.

Box 3
Diagnostic testing in dysphagia associated with UVFI

Indirect flexible laryngoscopy

Video stroboscopy

Modified barium swallow

Flexible endoscopic evaluation of swallowing

Flexible endoscopic evaluation of swallowing with sensory testing

---

Surgical correction of glottal insufficiency is also indicated in patients with mild symptoms, but is particularly helpful in patients with moderate to severe symptoms of dysphagia or patients who have had multiple hospitalizations from aspiration pneumonia.

CP myotomy is indicated in patients with dysphagia in the setting of glottal insufficiency when there is hypertrophy of the CP muscle or delayed opening of the UES. This hypertrophy causes worsening of aspiration or penetration during the swallow due to decreased hypopharyngeal clearance.

Pharyngoplasty may benefit patients with high vagal paralysis by obliterating a dilated pyriform sinus so that the bolus is preferably transferred to the dominant side of the hypopharynx during the swallow so that it can be propelled with ease into the esophagus (**Box 4**).

INJECTION LARYNGLOPLASTY

Injection laryngoplasty of the vocal folds increases the bulk of an immobile or paretic vocal fold. Hence, the surface area of contact with the contralateral fold is restored at the midline. It restores glottal closure at the time of the pharyngeal phase of the swallow, preventing material to penetrate through the glottis. There are a wide variety of readily available commercial materials that can be used for temporary vocal fold injections: Cymetra (Micronized Alloderm Tissue), Radiesse Voice Gel (carboxymethylcellulose), Radiesse Voice (Calcium Hydroxyapatite), and Restylane (hyaluronic acid) (**Table 1**). Autologous fat injections have also been used to augment the vocal fold temporarily. Teflon has also been used in the past but has fallen into disfavor because of its tendency toward inflammatory reaction and granuloma formation.

Injection laryngoplasty is performed under general anesthesia or awake. The advantage of injecting the vocal fold under general anesthesia with direct laryngoscopy is that it provides the most direct access to the vocal fold. It is also the favored approach in patients who do not tolerate an awake procedure or are unwilling to undergo awake injection. The major disadvantage of this approach is that one cannot have immediate feedback on vocal fold position or quality of the voice. Awake injection laryngoplasty has the advantage of avoiding general anesthesia and immediate feedback can be obtained on vocal fold position as the procedure is performed with continuous visualization using indirect flexible laryngoscopy. It is also performed in the office with minimal complications.

Conscious sedation without intubation as well as general anesthesia with endotracheal intubation can both be considered when undertaking injection laryngoplasty in the operating room setting. The patient is placed in the flexion-extension position and direct laryngoscopy is used to gain direct access to the vocal fold. The vocal

---

Box 4
Management of glottal insufficiency in dysphagia

Swallow maneuvers

Injection laryngoplasty

Medialization thyroplasty ± arytenoid adduction or arytenoidpexy/cricothyroid subluxation

Pharyngoplasty (pyriform sinus imbrication)

Cricopharyngeal muscle myotomy

Tracheostomy

Table 1
Vocal fold injectable materials

Injectable Material	Duration of Action	Advantages	Disadvantages
Cymetra (micronized alloderm tissue)	2–4 mo	Injected through small needle	Theoretic risk of infection transmission, contraindicated in erythromycin allergy
Radiesse voice gel (carboxymethylcellulose)	4–6 mo	Trial before medialization thyroplasty	—
Radiesse voice (CaHa)	1.5–2 y	Long-lasting option	Poor viscoelastic properties, placement has to be exact
Gelfoam	6 wk	Shortest acting, can be used for trial	Large-bore needle leads to extrusion from vocal fold
Teflon	Permanent	None	Granuloma formation
Fat	Variable	Excellent viscoelastic properties	Requires donor site, large-bore needle for harvest

fold is injected using a 23-g or 24-g laryngeal injection needle directly into the superior arcuate line of the vocal fold. The material is injected until the vocal fold is overmedialized.

Injection laryngoplasty in the awake setting can be performed through different approaches: transthyrohyoid membrane, transthyroid cartilage, cricothyroid membrane approach, and transoral approach (**Fig. 1**). The procedure is performed with

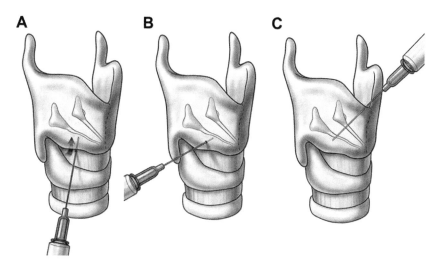

A   **B**   **C**

Fig. 1. (*A*) Transcricothyroid approach. (*B*) Transthyroid approach. (*C*) Transthyrohyoid approach. (*From* Rosen CA, Simpson CB. Percutaneous vocal fold augmentation in the clinic setting. In: Rosen CA, Simpson CB, editors. Operative techniques in laryngology. Heidelberg (Germany): Springer; 2008. p. 215–20; with permission.)

the aid of flexible indirect laryngoscopy and a video camera. Proper topical anesthesia of the larynx should be performed either with a trans-tracheal injection of 3 mL 4% lidocaine or by dripping 10 mL 2% lidocaine into the glottis while the patient holds a sustained 'e' via a flexible laryngoscope with a port.

In the transoral approach an Abraham cannula is used to anesthetize the vallecula and the base of the tongue. Then, a curved laryngeal injection needle is used to augment the vocal fold while under direct visualization with a flexible laryngoscope or a rigid 90° or 70° endoscope.

In the transthyrohyoid approach, after anesthesia of the larynx is performed, the skin immediately external to the thyroid notch is anesthetized with 1% lidocaine with 1:100,000 epinephrine. The flexible laryngoscope is advanced through the nose and the larynx is brought in view. A 23-g needle is bent at the base to 70°. Palpation is critical to identifying the thyrohyoid space. The needle is then inserted through the skin and directed caudal immediately after entering the anatomic space behind the thyroid cartilage. This maneuver directs the needle toward the infrahyoid petiole and then the needle is redirected toward the vocal fold to be augmented.

The transthyroid cartilage approach is performed after anesthesia of the skin of the neck with 1% lidocaine. A 23-g needle is passed 3 mm above the inferior border of the thyroid cartilage 0.5 cm lateral to the midline on the side to be augmented. The needle tip is moved medially to confirm that it is not in a subepithelial position and augmentation of the vocal fold is performed. This approach is well suited to patients with a nonossified laryngeal cartilage.

In the cricothyroid approach the vocal folds are accessed through a submucosal route. Local anesthesia of the skin of the neck is performed at the level of the cricothyroid space. A needle is bent to a 45° angle and passed through the skin, then upward from the inferior border of the cricoid cartilage 0.5 cm lateral to the midline. Medial movement of the tip confirms the position of the needle, and the vocal fold is augmented when positioning is adequate.

Injection laryngoplasty is an immediate but temporary and reversible solution to restore glottal insufficiency. It can be used in the outpatient as well as the hospital setting in patients who have symptoms of dysphagia due to glottal insufficiency. The risk of aspiration pneumonia is potentially decreased. In particular patient populations, especially the elderly or deconditioned hospitalized patients, this may signify prevention of a life-threatening complication.

MEDIALIZATION THYROPLASTY WITH OR WITHOUT ARYTENOID REPOSITIONING

Medialization thyroplasty is the preferred surgical treatment in patients with longstanding recurrent laryngeal nerve palsy or bilateral vocal fold atrophy. It is a time-tested procedure that yields excellent voice and swallowing function improvement by restoring glottal competence. The procedure is usually reserved for patients that have not had recovery of vocal fold mobility after 9 months to 1 year of initial nerve injury or patients with significant vocal atrophy that desire a long-term solution for symptoms of glottal insufficiency. Patients who have documented iatrogenic injury or tumor involvement of the recurrent laryngeal or vagal nerve are candidates for early medialization thyroplasty. The most common materials used for medialization are carved silastic implants or Gore-Tex strips.

Laryngeal framework surgery is preferably performed under conscious sedation with local anesthesia in the operating room. The skin of the neck, the deep soft tissues and the strap muscles around the thyroid cartilage, the hyoid bone, and the cricoid cartilage are anesthetized with a mixture of 5 mL Marcaine with 5 mL 1% lidocaine and 1:100,000 epinephrine. Topical nasal decongestion with cocaine or any other vasoconstrictive agent with anesthetic should be performed, facilitating the use of indirect flexible laryngoscopy during the procedure. Indirect laryngoscopy is used to confirm the side of vocal fold immobility, visualize the position of the implant, and help determine whether arytenoid repositioning would improve closure of a glottal gap. A 3-cm horizontal neck skin incision is performed in a midpoint between the hyoid bone and the cricoid cartilage. The procedure begins with a standard approach to neck surgery by elevating subplatysmal flaps. Superior and inferior dissections proceed to the level of the hyoid bone and the cricoid cartilage. The strap muscles are divided at the midline and the thyroid cartilage is exposed by blunt dissection of the infrahyoid musculature most superficial to the cartilage. The thyrohyoid muscle is divided for improved exposure of the thyroid cartilage on the side of the paralysis. An inferiorly or superiorly based perichondral flap is elevated. The inferior anterior corner of the window is measured 2 to 3 mm above the inferior border of the thyroid cartilage. In men this anterior inferior extent of the window should be positioned 7 mm from the midline of the cartilage and in women it should be positioned 5 mm from the midline of the cartilage. The cartilage is drilled or excised to create a window until the inner cortex of the thyroid cartilage is removed and the perichondrium is sharply incised, revealing the paraglottic space. The carved silastic or Gore-Tex implant is inserted and modified as needed until an adequate voice result or adequate glottal closure is achieved (**Fig. 2**).

Additional medial displacement of the vocal fold can be achieved with arytenoid repositioning. However, this requires access to the posterior portion of the thyroid cartilage, division of the inferior constrictor muscles, and dissection of the pyriform sinus to reveal the muscular process of the posterior cricoarytenoid muscle. A 4-0 double-needle Prolene is sutured with a figure-of-8 stitch to the vocal process.

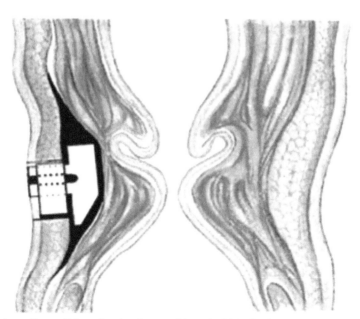

Fig. 2. Schematic rendition of an implant positioned within the fenestra and secured with a shim. (*From* Fakhry C, Flint PW, Cummings CW. Medialization thyroplasty. In: Flint PW, Haughey BH, Lund VJ, et al, editors. Cummings otolaryngology—head and neck surgery. 5th edition. New York: Elsevier; 2010. p. 904–11; with permission.)

Then, dissection of all of the paraglottic space from inner table of thyroid cartilage is performed. The sutures are passed anteriorly through the window and secured around the anterior inferior border of the thyroid cartilage at the midline. The purpose of this is to displace the vocal process medially and inferiorly, bringing the vocal fold position medially. This procedure in combination with a vocal fold implant causes improved closure in the setting of glottal insufficiency. Steven Zeitels has also described a medialization procedure combined with arytenopexy and cricothyroid subluxation that also elongates the vocal fold in a medial position. The results of this procedure are comparable to medialization thyroplasty and arytenoid adduction.

Laryngeal framework surgery for the treatment of UVFI is a long-term solution in patients who have dysphagia related to glottal insufficiency. In comparison to injection laryngoplasty, patients usually undergo a single procedure for improvement of glottal closure. Another advantage of the procedure is the use of conscious sedation instead of general anesthesia, making it a reasonable option in patients with significant comorbidities.

PHARYNGOPLASTY

Patients with high vagal paralysis that have an ipsilateral dilated pyriform sinus with pooling of secretions are ideal candidates for this procedure. Swallowing maneuvers to overcome a dilated pyriform sinus involve turning the head toward the affected side while performing a chin tuck during the swallow, thus obliterating the affected pyriform sinus. The goal of the surgery is to re-create this maneuver permanently so that the bolus of food tends toward the dominant pyriform sinus. Once access to the posterior larynx is gained as described previously, the dilated pyriform sinus is pulled gently. A gastrointestinal anastomosis stapler is placed over the sac and multiple passes are performed to obliterate the pyriform sinus. The goal of the surgery is to reduce the amount of space on the impaired side of the hypopharynx.

CRICOPHARYNGEAL MYOTOMY

The UES is made up of the cricopharynx muscle that is in a state of constant contraction. Discoordination and decreased laryngeal sensory input during the swallow occur in patients with high vagal lesions, which results in delayed relaxation of the UES. In patients with an insensate larynx and UVFI, failure of the bolus to enter the esophagus properly may place them at a higher risk of aspiration.

Endoscopic CP myotomy is performed using a Weerda or bivalved diverticuloscope. The scope is inserted in the postcricoid area and opened to displace the larynx anteriorly. The muscle bar is usually seen on the posterior wall of the esophagus. CO_2 laser is preferred because of its sharp precision and its hemostatic capabilities. The mucosa is incised vertically and the muscle is exposed; all the fibers of the cricopharyngeal muscle are excised until the prevertebral fatty tissue is seen. The main disadvantage of a cricopharyngeal myotomy is the risk of mediastinitis that is potentially life-threatening.

SUMMARY

Glottal insufficiency occurs as a result of UVFI, vocal fold atrophy, and PIPI. Surgical options for the treatment of these include injection laryngoplasty and medialization thyroplasty with or without arytenoid repositioning. High-vagal paralysis patients may also benefit from pharyngoplasty or CP mytotomy.

REFERENCES

1. Arviso LC, Klein A, Johns MM. The management of post-intubation phonatory insufficiency. J Voice 2012;26(4):530–3.
2. Flint PW, Purcell LL, Cummings CW. Pathophysiology and indications for medialization thyroplasty in patients with dysphagia and aspiration. Otolaryngol Head Neck Surg 1997;116(3):349–54.
3. Perie S, Coiffer L, Laccourreye L, et al. Swallowing disorders in paralysis of the lower cranial nerves: a functional analysis. Ann Otol Rhinol Laryngol 1999; 108(6):606–11.
4. Sulica L. The natural history of idiopathic unilateral vocal fold paralysis: evidence and problems. Laryngoscope 2008;118(7):1303–7.
5. Sulica L, Rosen C, Postma G, et al. Current practice in injection augmentation of the vocal folds: indications, treatment principles, techniques and complications. Laryngoscope 2010;120(2):319–25.
6. Takes RP, van den Hoogen FJ, Marres HA. Endoscopic myotomy of the cricopharyngeal muscle with CO_2 laser surgery. Head Neck 2005;27(8):703–9.
7. Woodson G. Cricopharyngeal myotomy and arytenoids adduction in the management of combined laryngeal and pharyngeal paralysis. Otolaryngol Head Neck Surg 1997;116(3):339–43.
8. Franco R. Adduction arytenopexy, hypopharyngoplasty, medialization laryngoplasty and cricothyroid subluxation for the treatment of paralytic dysphonia and dysphagia. Operative Tech Otolaryn 2012;23:164–72.

Special Populations and Considerations

Special Groups: Head and Neck Cancer

Loni C. Arrese, MS[a],*, Cathy L. Lazarus, PhD[b]

KEYWORDS

• Head and neck cancer • Dysphagia • Rehabilitation • Human papillomavirus

KEY POINTS

- Persistent human papillomavirus (HPV) infection of the oral cavity may lead to genetic damage and altered immune function, promoting progression to cancer; specifically squamous cell carcinoma of the tonsils and base of tongue.
- Radiation and chemotherapy can have adverse effects on overall function and quality of life.
- Surgery can have devastating effects on swallow functioning, but results are somewhat predictable and dependent on the location of resection and clinical T stage.

INTRODUCTION

The incidence of head and neck cancer (HNC) has increased significantly over the past decade. According to the American Cancer Society, in 2012 an estimated 92,860 new cancer cases involved the oral cavity and pharynx, tongue, mouth, pharynx, other oral cavity, and larynx (**Fig. 1**).[1]

The steady increase in incidence rates of oropharyngeal cancer over the past several decades has been attributed to the growing number of human papillomavirus (HPV)–related cancers. More than 90% of HPV-positive oropharyngeal cancers are associated with 2 oncogenic high-risk HPV types: HPV 16 and HPV 18.[2] Subtype HPV 16 has been associated with 85% to 90% of all HPV-positive oropharyngeal cancers.[2–4] Persistent HPV infection of the oral cavity may lead to genetic damage and altered immune function, promoting progression to cancer; specifically squamous cell carcinoma of the tonsil and base of tongue.[5,6]

Disclosures: None.
Conflict of Interest: None.
[a] Department of Otolaryngology, JamesCare Head & Neck Clinic, JamesCare Voice and Swallowing Disorders Clinic, The Ohio State University Comprehensive Cancer Center, Arthur G. James Cancer Hospital, Richard J. Solove Research Institute, The Ohio State University, 300 West 10th Avenue, Columbus, OH 43210, USA; [b] Department of Otorhinolaryngology Head & Neck Surgery, Thyroid Head and Neck Research Center, Thyroid Head and Neck Cancer (THANC) Foundation, Beth Israel Medical Center, Albert Einstein College of Medicine, Yeshiva University, 10 Union Square East, Suite 5B, New York, NY 10003, USA
* Corresponding author.
E-mail address: Loni.arrese@osumc.edu

Otolaryngol Clin N Am 46 (2013) 1123–1136
http://dx.doi.org/10.1016/j.otc.2013.08.009
0030-6665/13/$ – see front matter © 2013 Elsevier Inc. All rights reserved.

Abbreviations: Head and Neck Cancer	
BOT	Base of tongue
CRT	Chemotherapy
HNC	Head and neck cancer
HPV	Human papillomavirus
IMRT	Intensity-modulated radiotherapy
MDADI	MD Anderson dysphagia inventory
TL	Total laryngectomy
XRT	Radiation therapy

HPV status has been strongly associated with therapeutic response and overall survival in patients with oropharyngeal cancer.[7] In general, survival rates for HPV-related oropharyngeal cancer are higher than those for HPV-unrelated oropharyngeal cancers, with 2-year survival rates ranging from 80% to 95% versus 50% to 65%, respectively.[4,7] However, treatment for HPV-related and HPV-unrelated oropharyngeal cancers are currently commensurate. To date, little research has been conducted to determine if functional outcomes, including swallowing physiology, are similar among these heterogeneous groups.

Surgery, chemoradiotherapy or a combination of treatment can alter both the anatomy and tissue characteristics of those structures and muscles involved in swallowing. Radiotherapy can affect muscles, nerves, and the vascular system. Injury to the neuromuscular junctures and radiation-induced neuropathy can result in impairment in nerve conduction, muscle fiber atrophy, necrosis, and impairment in muscle contraction with an increase in connective tissue.[8,9] Vascular changes following irradiation have been found which result in tissue fibrosis[10] as well as loss of muscle fibers, decreased fiber size and necrosis.[10] The late effects of tissue fibrosis[11,12] can have a negative impact on swallow functioning,[13,14] with impairment in tongue and tongue base strength and range of motion, pharyngeal constrictor motion,

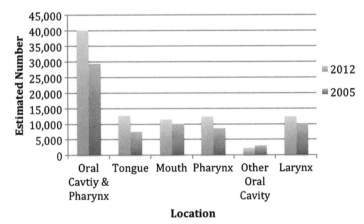

Fig. 1. Estimated new number of head & neck cancer cases by location in 2012 versus 2005 according to the American Cancer Society. (*Data from* American Cancer Society. Cancer Facts & Figures 2012. Atlanta (GA): American Cancer Society; 2012. Available at: http://www.cancer.org/acs/groups/content/@epidemiologysurveilance/documents/document/acspc-031941.pdf.)

Table 1
Common characteristics of dysphagia after radiation therapy ± chemotherapy

Oral	Impairment
Trismus	Inability to open mouth to accept oral intake Impaired chewing
Dry mouth	Reduced range of motion of oral structures Impaired oral transit Difficulty breaking down food without saliva enzymes Increased risk of caries
Lingual weakness	Impaired bolus formation Impaired anteroposterior transport and bolus clearance leading to oral residue Lateral sulci residue

Pharyngeal	Impairment
Decreased base of tongue retraction	Impaired bolus propulsion Pharyngeal residue Increased number of swallows

Reduced laryngeal
   elevation/excursion
	Impaired epiglottic inversion
	Impaired airway protection
	Penetration/aspiration
	Reduced opening of the cricopharyngeal segment
	   resulting in pharyngeal residue

Impaired contraction of
   the pharyngeal constrictors
	Impaired bolus transport and clearance through the
	   pharynx
	Reduced opening of the cricopharyngeal segment
	   resulting in pharyngeal residue

Stenosis of the
   cricopharyngeal segment
	Reduced or absent bolus clearance resulting in
	   pharyngeal residue

reduced laryngeal motion for airway protection and upper esophageal sphincter opening and reduced bolus clearance through the pharynx.[13,14,15] A reduction in both speed, strength and degree of structural movement within the oral cavity and pharynx can impact on bolus flow and clearance. Altered head and neck anatomy following

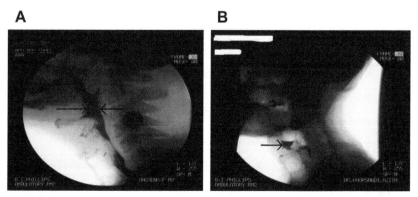

Fig. 2. Postchemotherapy deficits. (*A*) *Arrows* shows the reduced base of tongue retraction. (*B*) *Arrow* shows the reduced laryngeal elevation and airway closure.

Table 2
Studies assessing prophylactic swallowing exercises for patient undergoing definitive radiation therapy for head and neck cancer

Author	Outcome Measures	Therapy Exercises	Onset of Exercises	Results
Van der Molen et al,[26] 2011[a]	Pretreatment and 10 wk posttreatment: VFSS BMI FOIS score Weight changes Pain scale Study-specific questionnaire	Jaw exercises Gargle Masako Super-supraglottic swallow vs TheraBite stretch TheraBite swallow	2 wk before chemoradiation	Significant decrease in mouth opening, weight loss, and oral intake for both groups No significant difference between the pretreatment and posttreatment PAS scores
Carnaby-Mann et al,[27] 2012[a]	Pretreatment, after treatment, and 6 mo posttreatment: Muscle size and composition (determined by T2-weighted MRI) Functional swallowing ability Dietary intake Chemosensory function Salivation Nutritional status Occurrence of dysphagia-related complications	Supervised feeding and safe swallowing precautions/ education vs Buccal extension maneuver Dietary modification vs Falsetto Tongue press Hard swallow Jaw resistance/strengthening using the Therabite Jaw Motion Rehabilitation System Dietary modification	At the start of chemoradiation	Significant differences were seen in superior muscle maintenance and functional swallowing ability
Kulbersh et al,[28] 2006	9 mo posttreatment (range, 6–12 mo): MDADI	Falsetto Masako Mendelsohn Shaker Lingual resistance (all participants)	2 wk before radiation ± chemotherapy	Improved QOL measures: physical, emotional, global No improved QOL in the functional domain

Study	Intervention	Timing	Outcomes	Results
Carroll et al,[29] 2008	Effortful swallow Masako Mendelsohn Shaker Lingual resistance (treatment group) vs Unspecified swallowing exercises (control)	2 wk before chemoradiation vs Postchemoradiation	3 mo posttreatment: VFSS 12 mo posttreatment: PEG status	Significant differences in epiglottic inversion and tongue position during swallow No difference in PEG removal
Kotz et al,[30] 2012	No treatment vs Effortful swallow 2 tongue base retraction exercises Super-supraglottic swallow technique Mendelsohn maneuver	At the start of chemoradiation	Baseline, immediately after treatment, and at 3, 6, 9, and 12 mo posttreatment: FOIS score PSS-HN score	FOIS and PSS-HN: no significant difference immediately after CRT or at 9 or 12 mo after CRT Significant differences at 3 and 6 mo after CRT

Abbreviations: BMI, body mass index; FOIS, Functional Oral Intake Scale; MDADI, MD Anderson Dysphagia Inventory; MRI, magnetic resonance imaging; PAS, Penetration Aspiration Scale; PEG, percutaneous endoscopic gastrostomy tube; PSS-HN, Performance Status Scale for Head and Neck Cancer Patients; QOL, quality of life; VFSS, videofluoroscopic swallow study.

[a] Randomized controlled trials.

Data from Refs.[26-30]

surgery can result in swallowing deficits within the oral and pharyngeal phases of swallowing, depending on the specific structures resected. However, across treatment type, patients often exhibit impairment in bolus propulsion and clearance through the oral cavity and pharynx, as well as impairment in airway protection due to reduced glottic and supraglottic closure. Any of these deficits can result in bolus mis-direction and aspiration before, during or after the swallow.

RADIATION THERAPY

Improvements in radiation therapy, including intensity-modulated radiotherapy (IMRT), and the addition of chemotherapy agents have dramatically shifted the care for HNC. The use of radiation therapy (XRT) ± chemotherapy, either as an adjunct to surgery or as a definitive treatment, has allowed for the development of organ-sparing treatments without a decrease in overall survival. However, these treatment modalities can have adverse effects on overall function and quality of life, causing side effects such as radiation dermatitis, pain, mucositis, soft tissue edema, weight loss, xerostomia, loss of taste, hoarseness, fibrosis, trismus, and dysphagia.[16] Dysphagia is often the most problematic short-term and long-term effect seen in this population. Long-term dysphagia often results in critical consequences, including aspiration and dietary inadequacies, leading to malnutrition and its associated adverse effects.[16]

The reported incidence rates of dysphagia after XRT and chemotherapy are highly variable. Nguyen and colleagues[17] reported an average incidence of dysphagia of 50% after chemotherapy for advanced-stage HNC. Others have reported as many as two-thirds of all patients with HNC are left with permanent swallowing problems.[18] These problems directly impact an individual's nutritional status, hydration, and pulmonary health in addition to having a major impact on quality of life.[19,20]

Characteristics of dysphagia secondary to XRT or chemotherapy depend primarily on tumor size and the presence or absence of metastatic neck disease. These features greatly impact the radiation field and dose required for definitive treatment. Common physiologic deficits and their impact on bolus transport are outlined in **Table 1**. Impaired base of tongue retraction and reduced hyolaryngeal elevation have been identified as 2 of the most salient features of dysphagia after XRT (**Fig. 2**).[21] Lingual strength in patients with oral and oropharyngeal cancer treated with primary chemotherapy has been found to be lower than in that seen in healthy controls.[22,23] Lingual strength has also been found to correlate with aspiration.[24]

Radiation treatment for HNC has shifted primarily to IMRT over the past decade. This shift has allowed for the delivery of nonuniform radiation intensities to various structures, thus protecting structures important for swallowing when possible. A recent study has compared physiologic measures of swallow functioning after IMRT versus conventional radiotherapy.[25] Results indicate that individuals treated with IMRT maintain better swallow function with regard to timing, efficiency, and airway protection compared with individuals treated with conventional radiotherapy.[25]

Undoubtedly, given the incidence of dysphagia in the population and the negative impact on swallow function and safety, the potential role of intervention during treatment is increasingly recognized as a means of maintaining oropharyngeal function. Although early treatment is recommended, it has not been operationally defined at this time. Few studies have looked at prophylactic swallowing intervention by way of muscle strengthening. However, only 2 of these studies were randomized controlled trials, with only 1 including a control group.[26,27] All studies differed in outcome measures. These studies are outlined in **Table 2**.

SURGICAL INTERVENTION

Surgery can have devastating effects on swallow functioning, but results are somewhat predictable and depend on the location of resection and clinical T stage.[31] Surgery has been shown to have a major impact on speech, swallowing, and quality of life.[32–36] One important difference between surgical and radiation treatment is that swallowing function after surgery typically improves over time, whereas it tends to worsen after irradiation.[37,38] Functional deficits caused by surgical intervention are limited to specific anatomic and/or neurophysiologic changes induced by the resection.[39] See **Tables 3–5** for an overview of surgical procedures associated with treatment of HNC, the potential swallowing impairments, and corresponding compensatory and therapeutic interventions.

Glossectomy

Lingual strength and mobility have been correlated with dietary intake and aspiration.[22,24] Thus, glossectomy procedures can greatly impact swallowing function. However, the pharyngeal phase of swallow is not typically impacted when resection is limited to the anterior tongue and oral cavity.[32] Reconstruction of the lingual deficit after glossectomy may contribute to the consequential dysphagia in the initial postoperative phase. However, several articles have reported a return to baseline status by

Table 3
Dysphagia after surgery for common oral cancers, with compensatory strategies and therapeutic maneuvers and exercise

Location	Potential Impairment	Compensatory Strategy	Therapeutic Maneuver and Exercise
Tongue resection	Difficulty with bolus control (pooling/pocketing on surgical side) Impaired bolus preparation Impaired anteroposterior transport (loss of anterior tongue driving force); impaired propulsion into the pharynx Premature spillage into the pharynx Drooling	Food placement on stronger side; head tilt to stronger side or back (rely on gravity); slurp and swallow	Lingual range of motion; lingual strengthening; supraglottic swallow if premature spill occurs
Floor of mouth	Tethering of the anterior tongue Loss of glossoalveolar sulcus Loss of dentition Reduced mouth opening	Food placement on stronger side; head tilt to stronger side	Lingual range of motion; lingual strengthening; lingual control; jaw range of motion
Buccal	Reduced mouth opening Impaired chewing	Food placement of stronger side	Mouth extension and lateralization
Mandible	Loss of dentition Impaired bite force Reduced driving force of the tongue Reduced mouth opening Reduced laryngeal elevation	Food placement of stronger side; puree or soft consistency foods	Lingual range of motion; lingual strengthening; lingual control; jaw range of motion; Mendelsohn maneuver

Table 4
Dysphagia after surgery for common oropharyngeal cancers with compensatory strategies and therapeutic maneuvers and exercise

Location	Potential Impairment	Compensatory Maneuver	Therapeutic Maneuver and Exercise
Soft palate	Velopharyngeal insufficiency → nasal regurgitation Loss of oropharyngeal pressure → reduced bolus propulsion	Obturator; head tilt back	Non-applicable
Tonsil	May result in premature spillage immediately postoperatively	Chin tuck	Non-applicable
Base of tongue (BOT)	Loss of sensation, may include insensate flap reconstruction Impaired bolus propulsion and impaired/incomplete BOT to posterior pharyngeal wall contact Reduced laryngeal elevation Retention in the vallecular space	Head tilt back; head turn to weaker side if unilateral; chin tuck; chin tuck combined with head turn to weaker side; multiple swallows; liquid wash	Oral tongue strengthening; tongue-hold (ie, Masako maneuver); Mendelsohn maneuver; effortful swallow

Table 5
Dysphagia after surgery for common hypopharyngeal, pharyngeal, and laryngeal cancers with compensatory strategies and therapeutic maneuvers and exercise

Location	Potential Impairment	Compensatory Maneuver	Therapeutic Maneuver and Exercise
Posterior pharyngeal wall	Impaired pharyngeal contraction Insensate flap reconstruction Reduced laryngeal elevation	Head turn to weaker side; multiple swallows; liquid wash	Effortful swallow; Mendelsohn maneuver; laryngeal glides (ie, falsetto exercise)
Pyriform sinuses	Loss of natural recess, resulting in spill over into the larynx Weakness or scarring of the lateral pharyngeal wall Reduced/impaired cricopharyngeal opening	Head turn to the weaker side	Super-supraglottic swallow; effortful swallow; Mendelsohn maneuver; Shaker maneuver
Supraglottis	Loss of anatomic airway protection (ie, epiglottis) Delayed pharyngeal swallow from loss of sensation Reduced laryngeal elevation	Chin tuck	Super-supraglottic swallow; laryngeal adduction exercises; Mendelsohn maneuver
Glottis	Impaired glottic closure	Head rotation to the weaker side; chin tuck	Super-supraglottic swallow; laryngeal adduction exercises

1 year.[40,41] Lingual reconstruction can consist of primary closure, skin grafts, local and regional tissue flaps, or microvascular ± osteocutaneous free flaps (**Figs. 3**A, B and **4**). Tissue flaps are used to conserve bulk in the oral cavity and/or oropharynx necessary for intelligible speech production, bolus transfer, propulsion, and contact between the base of tongue or neo–base of tongue and the posterior pharyngeal wall. A palatal drop prosthesis may also be used to improve oral contacts for anteroposterior bolus movement and speech production (see **Fig. 3**C).

Severe swallowing deficits, including significant aspiration, are often seen when total glossectomy is required. These adverse effects are directly related to impaired driving force on the bolus, loss of oral sensation, and impaired laryngeal elevation from removal of the suprahyoid musculature (ie, mylohyoid, geniohyoid).[39] Laryngeal suspension at the time of total glossectomy may accommodate for the reduced laryngeal motion and aid with overall airway protection.

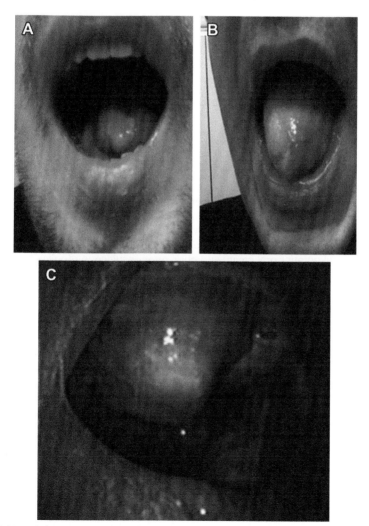

Fig. 3. (*A*) Hemiglossectomy with radial forearm free flap. (*B*) Partial glossectomy with radial forearm free flap. (*C*) Palatal drop prosthesis.

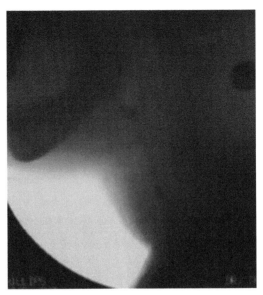

Fig. 4. Esophageal stenosis.

Mandibulectomy

A mandibulectomy often results in profound changes to the tongue and floor of mouth.[39] The extent of the postoperative functional deficit is directly related to the extent of surgical resection. Disruption to the normal mandibular structure may result in impaired occlusion, which can have an impact on mastication and overall jaw stability required for efficient swallowing, oral containment, and laryngeal elevation. However, mandibular reconstruction with a microvascular osteocutaneous flap can improve outcome in terms of chewing, swallowing, and cosmesis.[42] Neurophysiologic changes caused by an insult to V3 (inferior alveolar nerve) can cause loss of sensation to the ipsilateral anterior oral cavity and chin, often resulting in drooling.[39]

Total Laryngectomy

Despite common thought, the incidence of dysphagia after total laryngectomy (TL) has been reported as high as 72%.[43,44] The cause of dysphagia is a direct result of impaired pharyngeal contraction and propulsive forces combined with increased resistance to bolus flow through the pharyngoesophageal segment.[44] One retrospective study showed that 33% of the patients who had both a TL and XRT had evidence of esophageal stenosis on fluoroscopy, with all requiring esophageal dilation for symptom relief.[45] Additionally, if radiation is used, the risk of developing dysphagia has been suggested to be higher for those who receive XRT followed by salvage TL compared with those who receive postoperative XRT after total laryngectomy.[45] Significant differences in self-reported voice and swallowing outcomes were found among individuals who underwent TL alone compared with those who received adjuvant XRT. Those who received TL alone had significantly better self-reported outcomes on the Voice Symptom Scale and MD Anderson Dysphagia Inventory.[46]

Partial Laryngectomy

A partial laryngectomy procedure may be performed when surgical resection of the tumor is possible while maintaining a functional larynx. Partial procedures include

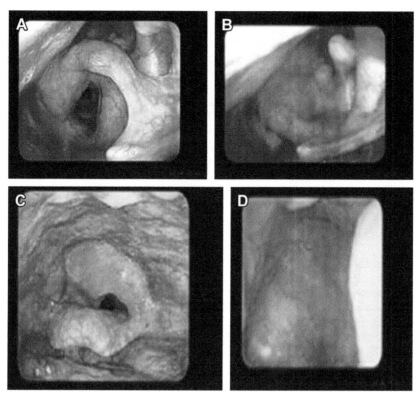

Fig. 5. (A) Vertical partial laryngectomy. (B) Airway closure with head turn (*Right*). (C) Supracricoid laryngectomy. (D) Airway closure with breath hold and head glide back.

supraglottic laryngectomy (horizontal partial laryngectomy), a vertical hemilaryngectomy, and a supracricoid laryngectomy. These procedures can significantly alter airway, necessitating rehabilitation in the postoperative phase. Patients undergoing supraglottic laryngectomy typically need instruction in the super-supraglottic swallow maneuver to establish tongue base to arytenoid contact for airway entrance closure. Patients who undergo hemilaryngectomy often need only a compensatory strategy (ie, chin tuck or head rotation to the surgical side) or a combined posture and breath-hold maneuver (**Fig.** 5B, see **Table 5**).

SUMMARY

Dysphagia can be a devastating consequence of HNC treatment, and can be present regardless of treatment modality (surgery and/or radiation ± chemotherapy). Treatment of these cancers has shifted to organ-sparing techniques over the past few decades. Further research incorporating functional outcomes is warranted to determine the most effective treatments to achieve quantity and quality of life.

REFERENCES

1. American Cancer Society. Cancer Facts & Figures 2012. Atlanta (GA): American Cancer Society; 2012. Available at: http://www.cancer.org/acs/groups/content/@

epidemiologysurveilance/documents/document/acspc-031941.pdf.   Accessed May 29, 2013.
2. Cleveland JL, Junger ML, Saraiya M, et al. The connection between human papillomavirus and oropharyngeal squamous cell carcinomas in the United States Implications for dentistry. J Am Dent Assoc 2011;142(8):915–24.
3. Kreimer AR, Clifford GM, Boyle P, et al. Human papillomavirus types in head and neck squamous cell carcinomas worldwide: a systematic review. Cancer Epidemiol Biomarkers Prev 2005;14(2):467–75.
4. Chaturvedi AK, Engels EA, Anderson WF, et al. Incidence trends for human papillomavirus-related and -unrelated oral squamous cell carcinomas in the United States. J Clin Oncol 2008;26(4):612–9.
5. Herrero R, Castellsague X, Pawlita M, et al. Human papillomavirus and oral cancer: the International Agency for Research on Cancer multicenter study. J Natl Cancer Inst 2003;95(23):1772–83.
6. Marur S, D'Souza G, Westra WH, et al. HPV-associated head and neck cancer: a virus-related cancer epidemic. Lancet Oncol 2010;11(8):781–9.
7. Fakhry C, Westra WH, Li S, et al. Improved survival of patients with human papillomavirus–positive head and neck squamous cell carcinoma in a prospective clinical trial. J Natl Cancer Inst 2008;100(4):261–9.
8. Gorodetsky R, Amir G, Yarom R. Effect of ionizing radiation on neuromuscular junctions in mouse tongues. Int J Radiat Biol 1992;61(4):539–44.
9. Love S, Gomez S. Effects of experimental radiation-induced hypomyelinating neuropathy on motor end-plates and neuromuscular transmission. J Neurol Sci 1984;65(1):93–109.
10. Remy J, et al. Long-term overproduction of collagen in radiation-induced fibrosis. Radiat Res 1991;125(1):14–9.
11. Bentzen SM, Thames HD, Overgaard M. Latent-time estimation for late cutaneous and subcutaneous radiation reactions in a single-follow-up clinical study. Radiother Oncol 1989;15(3):267–74.
12. Stinson SF, et al. Acute and long-term effects on limb function of combined modality limb sparing therapy for extremity soft tissue sarcoma. Int J Radiat Oncol Biol Phys 1991;21(6):1493–9.
13. Lazarus CL, et al. Swallowing and tongue function following treatment for oral and oropharyngeal cancer. J Speech Lang Hear Res 2000;43(4):1011–23.
14. Watkin KL, et al. Ultrasonic quantification of geniohyoid cross-sectional area and tissue composition: a preliminary study of age and radiation effects. Head Neck 2001;23(6):467–74.
15. Pauloski BR, Logemann JA. Impact of tongue base and posterior pharyngeal wall biomechanics on pharyngeal clearance in irradiated postsurgical oral and oropharyngeal cancer patients. Head Neck 2000;22(2):120–31.
16. Murphy BA, Gilbert J. Dysphagia in head and neck cancer patients treated with radiation: assessment, sequelae, and rehabilitation. Semin Radiat Oncol 2009;19(1):35–42.
17. Nguyen NP, Sallah S, Karlsson U, et al. Combined chemotherapy and radiation therapy for head and neck malignancies. Cancer 2002;94(4):1131–41.
18. Staar S, Rudat V, Stuetzer H, et al. Intensified hyperfractionated accelerated radiotherapy limits the additional benefit of simultaneous chemotherapy—results of a multicentric randomized German trial in advanced head-and-neck cancer. Int J Radiat Oncol Biol Phys 2001;50(5):1161–71.
19. Grobbelaar EJ, Owen S, Torrance AD, et al. Nutritional challenges in head and neck cancer. Clin Otolaryngol Allied Sci 2004;29(4):307–13.

20. Eisbruch A, Lyden T, Bradford CR, et al. Objective assessment of swallowing dysfunction and aspiration after radiation concurrent with chemotherapy for head-and-neck cancer. Int J Radiat Oncol Biol Phys 2002;53(1):23–8.
21. Logemann JA, Pauloski BR, Rademaker AW, et al. Swallowing disorders in the first year after radiation and chemoradiation. Head Neck 2008;30(2): 148–58.
22. Lazarus CL, Logemann JA, Pauloski BR, et al. Swallowing and tongue function following treatment for oral and oropharyngeal cancer. J Speech Lang Hear Res 2000;43(4):1011–23.
23. Lazarus C, Logemann JA, Pauloski BR, et al. Effects of radiotherapy with or without chemotherapy on tongue strength and swallowing in patients with oral cancer. Head Neck 2007;29(7):632–7.
24. Butler SG, Stuart A, Leng X, et al. The relationship of aspiration status with tongue and handgrip strength in healthy older adults. J Gerontol A Biol Sci Med Sci 2011; 66(4):452–8.
25. Pauloski B, Rademaker A, Logemann J, et al. Comparison of swallowing function after two forms of chemoradiation for head and neck cancer. Presented at the Annual Dysphagia Research Society Meeting. Seattle, March 8, 2013.
26. Van der Molen L, van Rossum MA, Burkhead LM, et al. A randomized preventive rehabilitation trial in advanced head and neck cancer patients treated with chemoradiotherapy: feasibility, compliance, and short-term effects. Dysphagia 2011; 26(2):155–70.
27. Carnaby-Mann G, Crary MA, Schmalfuss I, et al. "Pharyngocise": randomized controlled trial of preventative exercises to maintain muscle structure and swallowing function during head-and-neck chemoradiotherapy. Int J Radiat Oncol Biol Phys 2012;83(1):210–9.
28. Kulbersh BD, Rosenthal EL, McGrew BM, et al. Pretreatment, preoperative swallowing exercises may improve dysphagia quality of life. Laryngoscope 2006; 116(6):883–6.
29. Carroll WR, Locher JL, Canon CL, et al. Pretreatment swallowing exercises improve swallow function after chemoradiation. Laryngoscope 2008;118(1):39–43.
30. Kotz T, Federman AD, Kao J, et al. Prophylactic swallowing exercises in patients with head and neck cancer undergoing chemoradiation: a randomized trial. Arch Otolaryngol Head Neck Surg 2012;138(4):376–82.
31. Colangelo LA, Logemann JA, Pauloski BR, et al. T stage and functional outcome in oral and oropharyngeal cancer patients. Head Neck 1996;18(3):259–68.
32. Pauloski BR, Logemann JA, Rademaker AW, et al. Speech and swallowing function after anterior tongue and floor of mouth resection with distal flap reconstruction. J Speech Hear Res 1993;36(2):267–76.
33. Furia CL, Kowalski LP, Latorre MR. Speech intelligibility after glossectomy and speech rehabilitation. Arch Otolaryngol Neck Surg 2001;127(7):877–83.
34. Biazevic MG, Antunes JL, Togni J, et al. Survival and quality of life of patients with oral and oropharyngeal cancer at 1-year follow-up of tumor resection. J Appl Oral Sci 2010;18(3):279–84.
35. Dwivedi RC, Chisholm EJ, Khan AS, et al. An exploratory study of the influence of clinico-demographic variables on swallowing and swallowing-related quality of life in a cohort of oral and oropharyngeal cancer patients treated with primary surgery. Eur Arch Otorhinolaryngol 2012;269(4):1233–9.
36. Yang Z, Chen W, Huang H, et al. Quality of life of patients with tongue cancer 1 year after surgery. J Oral Maxillofac Surg 2010;68(9):2164–8.

37. Pauloski BR, Logemann JA, Rademaker AW, et al. Speech and swallowing function after oral and oropharyngeal resections: one-year follow-up. Head Neck 1994;16(4):313–22.
38. Pauloski BR, Rademaker AW, Logemann JA, et al. Speech and swallowing in irradiated and nonirradiated postsurgical oral cancer patients. Otolaryngol Head Neck Surg 1998;118(5):616–24.
39. Kronenberger MB, Meyers AD. Dysphagia following head and neck cancer surgery. Dysphagia 1994;9(4):236–44.
40. O'Connell DA, Rieger J. Swallowing function in patients with base of tongue cancers treated with primary surgery and reconstructed with a modified radial forearm free flap. Arch Otolaryngol Head Neck Surg 2008;134(8):857–64.
41. Brown L, Rieger JM. A longitudinal study of functional outcomes after surgical resection and microvascular reconstruction for oral cancer: tongue mobility and swallowing function. J Oral Maxillofac Surg 2010;68(11):2690–700.
42. Buchbinder D, Urken ML, Vickery C, et al. Functional mandibular reconstruction of patients with oral cancer. Oral Surg Oral Med Oral Pathol 1989;68(4 Pt 2): 499–503 [discussion: 503–4].
43. Armstrong E, Isman K, Dooley P, et al. An investigation into the quality of life of individuals after laryngectomy. Head Neck 2001;23(1):16–24.
44. Maclean J, Szczesniak M, Cotton S, et al. Impact of a laryngectomy and surgical closure technique on swallow biomechanics and dysphagia severity. Otolaryngol Head Neck Surg 2011;144(1):21–8.
45. Vu KN, Day TA, Gillespie MB, et al. Proximal esophageal stenosis in head and neck cancer patients after total laryngectomy and radiation. ORL J Otorhinolaryngol Relat Spec 2008;70(4):229–35.
46. Robertson SM, Yeo JC, Dunnet C, et al. Voice, swallowing, and quality of life after total laryngectomy: results of the west of Scotland laryngectomy audit. Head Neck 2012;34(1):59–65.

Dysphagia in Stroke, Neurodegenerative Disease, and Advanced Dementia

Kenneth W. Altman, MD, PhD[a],*, Amanda Richards, MBBS, FRACS[b],
Leanne Goldberg, MS, CCC-SLP[b], Steven Frucht, MD[c],
Daniel J. McCabe, DMA, CCC-SLP[b]

KEYWORDS

- Stroke • Neurodegenerative disease • Dementia • Dysphagia • Myasthenia gravis
- Muscular dystrophy • Multiple sclerosis

KEY POINTS

- Stroke, neurodegenerative disease, and dementia are disorders that have a high incidence of dysphagia.
- There are similarities and differences, but common themes associated with an aging population prevail.
- Aspiration risk varies with the severity of disease and is a challenge to rehabilitate based on presbypharynges, cognitive status, and level of nutrition.
- It is important to screen for dysphagia in these high-risk groups and to assess aspiration risk early in order to maintain nutrition with pertinent food consistencies.
- In the case of global laryngeal dysfunction, surgical options are available.

INTRODUCTION

Central and peripheral neurologic diseases have a profound impact on deglutition, whether it is traumatic, inflammatory, infectious, autoimmune, or caused by secondary effects of the aging process. Although the causes of stroke, neuromuscular degenerative diseases, and advanced dementia are different, they have several commonalities regarding the presentation of dysphagia:

1. They typically occur in an aging population
2. There is potential for cognitive impairment (through direct effects of the disease, comorbidities, or indirect effects of medication)

---

[a] Department of Otolaryngology Head & Neck Surgery, Eugen Grabscheid MD Voice Center, The Icahn School of Medicine at Mount Sinai, One Gustave L. Levy Place, Box 1189, New York, NY 10029, USA; [b] Department of Otolaryngology Head & Neck Surgery, The Icahn School of Medicine at Mount Sinai, One Gustave L. Levy Place, Box 1189, New York, NY 10029, USA; [c] Department of Neurology, The Icahn School of Medicine at Mount Sinai, One Gustave L. Levy Place, New York, NY 10029, USA
* Corresponding author.
E-mail address: kenneth.altman@mountsinai.org

Otolaryngol Clin N Am 46 (2013) 1137–1149
http://dx.doi.org/10.1016/j.otc.2013.08.005
0030-6665/13/$ – see front matter © 2013 Elsevier Inc. All rights reserved.

Abbreviations: Neurodegenerative Dysphagia

AD	Alzheimer disease
ADL	Activity of daily living
ALS	Amyotrophic lateral sclerosis (also known as motor neuron disease)
DMD	Duchenne muscular dystrophy
FEES	Functional endoscopic evaluation of swallowing
GI	Gastrointestinal
MBS	Modified barium swallow
MG	Myasthenia gravis
MS	Multiple sclerosis
NG	Nasogastric
NPO	Nil per os
PD	Parkinson's disease
PEG	Percutaneous endoscopic gastrostomy

---

3. Neuromuscular atrophy is often present and progressive
4. Discoordination is also present from deconditioning and central neurologic disease
5. Patients eventually become less active and have a sedentary lifestyle
6. They are associated with predominantly oropharyngeal dysphagia and aspiration risk

The initial presentation for an acute-onset event such as stroke is different than the chronic disease presentation, which often involves increasing aspiration risk with time. As the diseases progress with age, there is also an increasing nutritional requirement to stave off muscular atrophy. This requirement leads to increased need for oral intake, further taxing the vulnerable deglutition and increasing aspiration risk. This article reviews commonly encountered central and peripheral neurologic diseases presenting with dysphagia, discusses the likelihood of encountering dysphagia, and introduces a management approach that focuses on preserving nutritional requirements and quality of life.

DYSPHAGIA IN STROKE

Dysphagia is a frequently under-recognized complication of acute stroke, despite its prevalence of up to 78%.[1] It adversely affects outcomes as determined by length of hospitalization, and also increases the risk of mortality.[2–5] It is most prevalent in the acute phase, with about half of patients recovering spontaneously (or dying) in the first week.[2] The severity of dysphagia relates to the degree of pharyngeal representation in the unaffected cerebral hemisphere, with the most severe problems in those with an involved dominant hemisphere.[6] The rate of dysphagia in hemispheric strokes is lower than in those affecting the brainstem.[1] Recovery is thought to be related to neuroplasticity in the nonaffected hemisphere.[7]

Prolonged hospital stay in patients who are dysphagic after stroke is most evident in those with hemorrhagic disease, with a 55% increase in the duration of stay.[3] The discharge destination of patients after stroke is also dramatically altered when there is comorbid dysphagia, with more than double the rate of patients requiring long-term care.[2]

Pneumonia represents a major cause of morbidity and is associated with 24% to 30% of deaths in patients after acute stroke.[5,8] Those with dysphagia have a 3-fold increase in pneumonia (RR, 3.17), and aspiration shown on videofluoroscopy markedly increases the risk of pneumonia (RR, 11.56).[1] As a consequence, stroke mortality in dysphagic patients approaches 40%.[5] The effects of dysphagia on patients who have had strokes through their hospitalization are listed in **Table 1**.

The potential for rehabilitation of deglutition following stroke depends on many factors, primarily the geographic distribution and extent of the stroke. If a patient shows progress with cognition, mobility, and dysphagia in the first week following a stroke, then there should be further potential for significant rehabilitation. In general, the less time it takes a patient to show such progress, the better the prognosis for full recovery. Therapy is aimed at oral sensation, oromotor manipulation, and compensatory maneuvers to protect from aspiration. It is also vital to recognize and monitor aspiration risk with certain food consistencies, and to maintain adequate nutrition during the rehabilitation period.

NEURODEGENERATIVE DISEASE

Neurodegenerative diseases are among the most important and most common causes of dysphagia in patients seen by neurologists. Muscular dystrophy is a prototypical example of a peripheral degenerative disease affecting muscle that causes dysphagia in the advanced stages of illness. MG is an autoimmune neuromuscular disease, degenerative in the sense that there is increasing damage to the neuromuscular junction over time. Dysphagia may be prominent in some patients with myasthenia, and all myasthenic patients are at risk for dysphagia because of side effects from their medications and intercurrent respiratory illness, which may exacerbate their symptoms. MS is a central demyelinating disorder with a high incidence of dysphagia, particularly when white matter lesions affect the brainstem. Amyotrophic lateral sclerosis (ALS), otherwise known as Lou Gehrig disease, uniformly produces dysphagia, and management of speech and swallowing are important early discussions in the ALS clinic. In addition, patients with PD frequently develop swallowing difficulty later in their course, often without recognition by the patients or their families. **Table 2** summarizes these important neurodegenerative diseases with relevance to dysphagia, listing the incidence in the general population, associated prevalence of dysphagia, and the aspect of deglutition affected.

Muscular Dystrophy

DMD is an X-linked disease affecting 1 in 3600 to 1 in 6000 live male births.[9] Mutations of the dystrophin gene (Xp21.2) result in progressive muscle degeneration[9–11] and replacement with interstitial fat and fibrosis.[11] Diagnosis at presentation is typically around age 5 years and precipitated by divergent physical ability compared with

Table 1		
Acute stroke and the impact of dysphagia		
	No Dysphagia (%)	Dysphagia (%)
Prevalence assessed clinically/instrumentally	22–70	30–78
Average hospital length of stay ≤7 d	85.34	55.39
Average hospital length of stay >7 d	14.66	44.61
Discharge destination: home	59.79	20.72
Discharge destination: long-term care	15.7	33.93
Incidence of pneumonia	2–16	16–33
Mortality	6	37

Data from Refs.[1,2,5]

Table 2
Neurodegenerative diseases and their effect on deglutition

Disease	Incidence in General Population	Prevalence of Dysphagia (%)	Aspect of Deglutition Effected	Risk of Aspiration
Muscular dystrophy	17–28:100,000	18	Oral>pharyngeal	Low early stages, high late stages
MG	1.7–10.4:1,000,000	40	Pharyngeal>oral	High (35%)
MS	2–7:100,000	24–65	Oral/Pharyngeal Cortical	High
ALS	2:100,000	83	Oral>pharyngeal cortical	High
Parkinson's disease	13:100,000	82	Esophageal>oral/ pharyngeal cortical	High

Data from Refs.[9–11,13–16,18–22,24,25,27,28]

peers. Children commonly have progressive muscle weakness resulting in loss of ambulation. In late stages, cardiopulmonary sequelae result in life-threatening complications and, in the absence of intervention, the mean age of death is 19 years.[9]

Dysphagia in DMD is most symptomatic in the late nonambulatory phase of disease. Aloysius and colleagues[10] evaluated the role of videofluoroscopy in children with DMD and feeding difficulties. Oral phase difficulties predominated and resulted from masticatory muscle weakness, malocclusion, and macroglossia. The swallow trigger was mildly delayed and weak pharyngeal propulsion resulted in pharyngeal residue. Patients were also desensitized to residue. Choking episodes occurred with more advanced disease, although no patients showed aspiration on videofluoroscopy. van den Engel-Hoek and colleagues[11] examined dystrophic changes in the oral muscles of swallow in patients with DMD. They found that increased echogenicity in digastric muscles, geniohyoid, and superior longitudinal muscles was associated with reduction in strength and a need for multiple swallows to clear the oral cavity. Weakened anterosuperior excursion of the hyoid results in a reduction of laryngeal protection and delayed opening of the upper esophageal sphincter. Early recognition of these findings facilitates a greater role for supportive care during these advanced stages.

Myasthenia Gravis

MG is an autoimmune postsynaptic neuromuscular junction disorder.[12] It predominantly affects women in the third and fourth decades, although male patients show a bimodal peak in the third and sixth decades.[12] Anti–acetylcholine receptor antibodies reduce the available number of acetylcholine receptors and result in subthreshold endplate potentials.[12,13] The clinical features involve painless weakness of striated muscle. Although ocular manifestations are the most common, bulbar weakness may be the presenting symptom in up to 6% to 15%.[13,14] Patients may also present with dysphonia characterized by vocal weakness and fatigue, and may even have vocal fold paresis with consequent increased aspiration to liquids. Natural history of the disease is progression to maximum severity within 2 years.[13]

Colton-Hudson and colleagues[15] found that the oral preparatory phase was affected with poor bolus formation, extended chewing, and reduced buccal tension. Oral phase abnormalities included slow transit, piecemeal deglutition, increased residue, and poor seal. The most common findings were in the pharyngeal phase, and included delays in initiation and a reduction in tongue base and epiglottic mobility. Weak constrictor muscles result in pharyngeal residue. Laryngeal penetration was common (35%) and often silent. EMG studies[14] reveal prolongation of suprahyoid laryngeal elevators in MG, which may compensate in those with subclinical swallow impairment. In this disorder, cricopharyngeal muscle function is usually normal. Proper diagnosis is critical to management of the disease, and aggressive medical therapy should result in dramatic improvement of dysphagia.

Multiple Sclerosis

MS is a central, demyelinating, immune-mediated disease with a female predominance. Incidence is 2 in 100,000 to 7 in 100,000 and peaks at around 30 years.[16] MS is triggered by environmental factors in genetically at-risk patients, and a focal lymphocytic infiltrate results in myelin and axonal damage. Median time to death is approximately 30 years from disease onset.[17]

The incidence of dysphagia varies depending on the severity of the disability from 24% to 65%,[18–20] and is most severe in those with brainstem involvement.[18,19] Aspiration pneumonia is consequently the leading cause of death in MS.[19] Abnormalities include reduced lingual control and tongue base retraction, delayed swallow trigger, reduced laryngeal closure and pharyngeal contraction, and diminished sensation.[19,20] The oral phase is more often affected in those with severe dysphagia.[18] Oromotor impairment also results in the characteristic dysphonia with scanning speech. Upper esophageal sphincter dysfunction is common and most pronounced with disease progression,[19,20] with reduced compliance rather than deficient traction as the postulated mechanism.[20] As a result, coughing and choking episodes were reported in most patients with dysphagia.[20] In addition to these aspects of dysphagia, patients with MS have impaired motor control of their limbs and hands resulting in compromised ability to feed themselves.

Amyotrophic Lateral Sclerosis

ALS (also known as motor neuron disease) is an idiopathic neurodegenerative disorder. Its incidence is approximately 2 in 100,000 and it affects men more than women.[21,22] Peak onset of sporadic disease (approximately 90%–95% of cases) occurs at 58 to 63 years, with familial disease approximately 1 decade earlier.[22] Familial disease has mendelian inheritance.[21,22] Pathophysiology involves degeneration and loss of motor neurons with astrocytic gliosis.[23]

The hallmark clinical feature is the presence of upper and lower motor neuron features involving the brainstem and spinal cord. Fifty percent of patients die within 30 months of symptom onset, but the prognosis is better in those with isolated bulbar disease.[22] Presentation with limb-onset disease predominates (70%), but bulbar onset occurs in approximately 25%. The tongue is disproportionately affected compared with other musculature and therefore oral preparatory and oral phase are most affected. Upper motor neuron dysfunction results in a brisk gag and jaw jerk, whilst lower motor neuron involvement causes tongue fasciculation, wasting and weakness, palatal weakness, and poor cough.[22]

Ertekin and colleagues[24] investigated the pathophysiologic mechanisms of dysphagia in ALS. They concluded that the swallow trigger reflex was delayed, disordered, and eventually absent, but that reflexive swallow was preserved until the end-stage disease. The cricopharyngeus muscle became hyper-reflexive and hypertonic, with a resultant loss of coordination during voluntary swallow initiation and laryngeal protection. Aspiration risk is high, and there are premier roles for supportive care and family support.

Parkinson's Disease

PD is a common progressive bradykinetic disorder with an incidence of approximately 13 in 100,000[25] and a 1.5% lifetime risk of development.[26] Median age of onset is 60 years and mean duration of disease is 15 years, with aspiration pneumonia the most common cause of death.[26] The disease is characterized by bradykinesia, and one of muscular rigidity, a 4-Hz- to 6-Hz resting tremor, or postural instability. The underlying pathophysiology is severe loss of dopaminergic neurons in the pars compacta nigral cells of the basal ganglia.[26] However, atypical PD and Parkinson plus syndromes such as progressive supranuclear palsy are increasingly recognized. The prototypical parkinsonian voice is weak, soft, and hypokinetic.

EMG and esophageal scintigraphy studies[27] reveal that there is a high rate of objective dysphagia, even in asymptomatic patients, and objective pooled prevalence rates of dysphagia are 82%.[28] Potulska and colleagues[27] noted prolongation of lower esophageal bolus transport in all patients. The oral preparatory and oral phases became affected later in the disease, reflecting the progression of tremor, bradykinesia, and rigidity. The dorsal motor nucleus of vagus and esophageal myenteric plexus degenerate, and this results in both pharyngeal and esophageal phase dysphagia.

Although there are increasing options for the treatment of PD medically and surgically with brainstem electrical stimulation, there are hallmark on-off effects of medication that limit seamless management of dysphagia. For example, timing of traditional medication results in a peak of agility followed by a decline in function until the next dose is used, so swallowing is safer during the period of agility rather than when the medication is wearing off. Fatigue is also a common problem with patients with PD, and similarly affects aspiration risk during the part of the day when present.

ADVANCED DEMENTIA

In 2001 there were 24.3 million people in the world with dementia, whereas in 2040 the number is estimated to increase to more than 81 million. The prevalence of dementia is estimated to double every 5 years after 65 years of age, and at age 85 years the prevalence is approximately 50%.[29] Dementia is a leading cause of death in the United States, with mortality affected by aspiration, hydration, and nutritional status. Data in the year 2000 show approximately 4.5 million people in North America with a diagnosis of dementia, and more than half progressed to the moderate to severe stages of their disease.[29]

Dementia is a terminal diagnosis. Alzheimer disease and other related illnesses causing dementia are progressive, incurable, and lead to a complete loss of cognitive function and subsequent death. A characteristic feature of the final phase of dementia, which can last from 6 months to 2 years, is loss of interest in eating, dysphagia, or both. An estimated 60% of nursing home residents have dementia, with approximately half (480,000) in the last stages of their disease.[30] The prognosis and progressive clinical course affects these important decisions.

Mean survival after dementia diagnosis varies between 1 and 16 years, whereas one-third of these individuals live to advanced stages.[30] Activity of daily living (ADLs) are typically lost in a hierarchical fashion, and the severe phase of dementia is characterized by loss of capacity to provide self-care in basic ADLs such as eating, bathing, and walking independently. Advanced stages of dementia are listed in **Table 3**.[31] In these stages there are also many behavioral symptoms that compromise quality of life for both patients and caregivers and are sources of great stress, with institutionalization being the ultimate consequence.

Table 3		
Advanced stages of dementia		
Stage	**Manifestations**	**Mean Duration (y)**
6a	Ability to perform ADLs becomes compromised (eg, putting clothing on correctly)	2.5
6b	Loss of ability to bathe independently	2.5
6c	Loss of ability to manage the mechanics of toileting correctly	2.5
6d	Urinary incontinence	2.5
6e	Fecal incontinence Speech overtly breaks down in the ability to articulate. Stuttering neologisms, and/or an increased paucity of speech are noted. Still able to respond to nonverbal stimuli and communicate pleasure and pain via behavior	2.5
7a	Evident rigidity on examination of the passive range of motion of major joints, such as the elbow, in most patients with AD Require continuous assistance with basic ADLs for survival Speech is limited to 6 or fewer intelligible words	1
7b	Approximately 40% of patients with AD manifest contractures of the elbow, wrists, and fingers to the extent that they cannot move a major joint more than halfway Speech limited to a single intelligible word	1.5
7c	Loss of ability to ambulate independently Speech is lost	1
7d	Loss of ability to sit up independently	1
7e	Loss of ability to smile; only grimacing facial movements are observed	1.5
7f	Loss of ability to hold up the head independently	—

Many patients and their families have limited understanding of the terminal nature of a dementia diagnosis. Because of the complexity that characterizes advanced dementia, many moral, ethical, religious, and medical decisions arise; these include appreciating the risks, benefits, and alternatives to adjunctive enteral feeding percutaneous endoscopic gastrostomy (PEG), nil per os (NPO) status, and the role of comfort care or compassionate oral intake. A recent systematic review concluded that there is no objective evidence showing that PEG prolongs life in this population,[32] but the investigators concluded that it provides a reliable route for medications and may help maintain nutritional and hydration status.

SENTINEL INDICATORS OF DECLINE WITH DYSPHAGIA AND ASPIRATION RISK

Depending on the level of monitoring, advancing disease in combination with the aging process frequently leads to an aspiration event that requires hospitalization, and reassessment of swallowing function at that time shows the aspiration. The treatment team is then faced with the dilemma of supplying the patient's nutritional needs in the presence of the aspiration risk, and often recommends NPO status, along with placement of a PEG. However, PEG tube placement has not been shown to eliminate aspiration, because oral secretions and backflow from the tube feedings can still be aspirated.[33–35] Important aspects not often recognized by the treatment team include the role of fatigue when eating; that is, when patients have limited muscular, coordination, and cognitive abilities, they may safely tolerate some oral intake but not be able to provide for all of their nutritional and hydration needs.

It is therefore beneficial to recognize early indicators of decline that pose greater risk to the patients before a definitive aspiration event, thereby prolonging some oral intake. In this approach, there is a role for supplemental PEG feeding to maintain baseline nutritional and hydration status but also allowing compassionate oral intake. Quantifying the level of aspiration risk also allows patients and their families to decide whether to pursue PEG. Although this approach may not prolong life, the quality of life is expected to be enhanced by enjoying the consistency and taste of foods, as well as the ritual human interaction at mealtime. Recognizing the indicators of decline (listed in **Table 4**) provides opportunities to maximize patient status with preferred food consistencies, and allows the initiation of compensatory maneuvers during this transition period.

SCREENING AND MANAGEMENT PROTOCOL FOR HIGH-RISK PATIENTS

The development of screening protocols for dysphagia is a key step in early identification of the patient at high risk for aspiration and the consequences of dysphagia, such as malnutrition and dehydration. High-risk patients should be considered following stroke, with neurodegenerative disease, late stages of dementia, advanced age, and certain other medical and surgical conditions.[3] Such protocols not only reduce the complication rates of stroke but they are also designed to reduce the economic burden of disease.[2,3] Protocols should not substitute for specialty medical care but should offer guidance that standardizes their approach and creates opportunity for measuring results. **Fig. 1** shows a clinical algorithm for dysphagia evaluation and management. Although this was initially designed for hospitalized patients, its use can be applied to those in an ambulatory practice setting.

Patients with dysphagia may be identified through demographic and disease-related risk factors, and further defined with a nursing screen. Following identification, an interdisciplinary partnership is ideal with (1) the speech and swallowing pathologist to perform bedside/radiographic evaluation and treatment of oral/pharyngeal contributions to dysphagia, and (2) the otolaryngologist to visualize laryngeal anatomy and function, and partner with endoscopic evaluation of swallowing. The use of bedside swallow evaluation, functional endoscopic evaluation of swallowing (FEES), fluoroscopic modified barium swallow (MBS), or formal barium esophagogram depend on the individual clinical situation and availability of resources. The nutritionist,

Table 4
Sentinel indicators of decline in deglutition with increased aspiration risk

Demographic	History	Physical Examination	Swallowing Evaluation
Advanced age	Falls	Impaired cognition	Decreased oral bolus manipulation
Medical comorbidities	Wheelchair bound	Drooling	Delayed initiation of tongue thrust
Poor nutritional status	Recent hospitalization	Wet voice	Decreased laryngeal sensation
Depression/anxiety	Recent surgery	Weak voice	Pooled secretions in the pyriforms
Nursing home resident	Respiratory symptoms	Cough	Decreased or absent swallow reflex
	Fatigue and weakness	Dysarthria	Gross aspiration or microaspiration

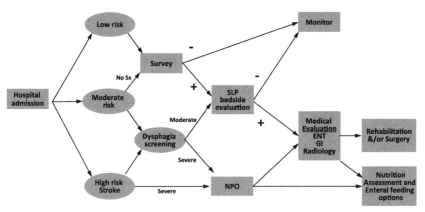

Fig. 1. Protocol for dysphagia screening. (*Adapted from* Altman KW. Dysphagia evaluation and care in the hospital setting: the need for protocolization. Otolaryngol Head Neck Surg 2011;145(6):895–8; with permission.)

neurologist, gastrointestinal radiologist, social worker, and others also play important roles and should be integrated into such a pathway.

After determining a variety of factors contributing to dysphagia, the otolaryngologist, gastroenterologist, and general/thoracic surgeon may each be involved with screening the esophagus, performing a more thorough evaluation of the gastrointestinal tract, providing a variety of surgical procedures, and accessing interim and longer-term enteral feeding ports. Although the algorithm presented here may take many forms, it is important to define an institutional approach in order to measure outcomes and improve access to standardized care.

THERAPEUTIC INTERVENTIONS AND NEUROPLASTICITY

Treatment options for those with neurodegenerative dysphagia include:

1. Compensations (diet/liquid consistency alterations, compensatory maneuvers, supplemental/alternative routes for intake)
2. Exercises to regain muscle coordination/strength
3. Treatments that may more directly stimulate neuroplastic changes in the swallow mechanism

Compensations and exercises are discussed more fully elsewhere in this issue by Murry and colleagues. Although compensatory measures have some efficacy in improving the safe per oral intake of foods and liquid,[36] they are traditionally used to help regain health in persons with dysfunctional swallowing. Because of altered/absent sensory abilities after cerebrovascular accident, any compensatory maneuver should be tested for effect with FEES or MBS before including it in the treatment plan.

Exercises and treatments that may directly stimulate neuroplastic changes in the swallow mechanism have been studied more closely over the past decade, and show promise for regaining lost abilities.[37] Head and neck exercises have traditionally been used to strengthen discrete muscles of the swallow mechanism in isolation. However, there is growing evidence to suggest that targeting the entire mechanism during swallowing better preserves the timing and interaction of sensory and motoric aspects of this complex activity.[38,39] Patients with reversible muscle weakness are better candidates for rehabilitation with both muscle strengthening and neuroplasticity, than those patients with neurodegenerative disorders in whom sustained muscle recruitment is diminished. MG, MS, ALS, and late-stage dementia changes may prove to be contraindications for success with strengthening exercises.

Interesting work has been done on methods for passive stimulation of central and peripheral pathways to enhance neuroplasticity in patients with dysphagia. There continues to be contradictory evidence for the efficacy of surface stimulation of the neck and submental regions such as E-Stim, perhaps because of the nondiscrete activation of many muscles all at once. However, surface EMG has been shown to significantly improve swallowing outcomes when used as supplemental biofeedback.[40,41] Recent studies into the use of transcranial neural stimulation have also proved to have positive effects on swallowing.[42–44] Dosing and location issues (affected vs nonaffected hemispheres) remain to be refined.[45,46] Another frontier that will benefit from study may be the resensitization of laryngeal/tracheal afferents that might allow those with acquired laryngeal desensitization to better protect their airways and prevent aspiration. The development of stronger functional magnetic resonance imaging and algorithms will greatly help in developing new treatments for restoring central functioning of the swallow process.

TREATMENT OPTIONS FOR GLOBAL LARYNGEAL DYSFUNCTION

In patients with acute stroke and those with advanced-stage neurodegenerative disease, the resulting global laryngeal dysfunction can result in major morbidity and mortality. Although a significant proportion of patients who have had strokes recover from their dysphagia within a week, approximately 50% of dysphagic patients are left with swallowing deficits.[2]

Following early risk stratification, those patients with significant penetration or aspiration should be made NPO and provided with enteral feeding methods, which allows adequate nutrition while oral intake is then cautiously advanced, if appropriate.[4] Although NG or PEG feeding have not been shown to reduce aspiration pneumonia, their role in adequate nutrition and hydration is clear.[47] Early NG feeding reduces mortality,[47] although early PEG insertion has been associated with an increased mortality.[48] PEG should therefore be considered when dysphagia persists, but can initially be delayed in the acute stages of illness.

Tracheotomy can improve secretion management and pulmonary toilet,[2] and patients with advanced neurodegenerative disease may already require a tracheostomy for respiratory support. However, the tracheotomy tube can only limit aspiration, and secretions and thin liquids can still bypass the cuff.[2] Despite the traditional view that tracheotomy causes laryngeal dysfunction, the underlying neurologic dysfunction is more likely to be the overriding factor.[49] In select patients who fail to respond to more conservative measures, tracheoesophageal diversion and laryngotracheal separation can be considered. Because of the radical nature of these procedures, they are largely reserved for the pediatric population in desperate circumstances.[50] Total laryngectomy has the benefit of eliminating aspiration because there is no conduit connecting the mouth to the trachea. However, it is rarely performed because many patients with global laryngeal dysfunction also have significant cognitive impairment and oromotor and oropharyngeal components to their dysphagia.

SUMMARY

Stroke, neurodegenerative disease, and advanced dementia are all characterized by the prominent role of dysphagia. The nature of the baseline diseases both causes the dysphagia and makes the patients more prone to the consequences. Early recognition through a systematic approach helps avoid aspiration, maintains nutrition, and seeks to preserve quality of life.

REFERENCES

1. Martino R, Foley N, Bhogal S, et al. Dysphagia after stroke: incidence, diagnosis, and pulmonary complications. Stroke 2005;36(12):2756–63.
2. Altman KW, Schaefer SD, Yu GP, et al. The voice and laryngeal dysfunction in stroke: a report from the Neurolaryngology Subcommittee of the AAO-HNS. Otolaryngol Head Neck Surg 2007;136(6):873–81.
3. Altman KW, Yu GP, Schaefer SD. Consequences of dysphagia in the hospitalized patient. Arch Otolaryngol Head Neck Surg 2010;136(8):784–9.
4. Altman KW. Dysphagia evaluation and care in the hospital setting: the need for protocolization. Otolaryngol Head Neck Surg 2011;145(6):895–8.
5. Smithard DG, O'Neill PA, Park C, et al. Complications and outcome after acute stroke does dysphagia matter? Stroke 1996;27(7):1200–4.
6. Hamdy S, Aziz Q, Rothwell JC, et al. Explaining oropharyngeal dysphagia after unilateral hemispheric stroke. Lancet 1997;350(9079):686–92.
7. Hamdy S, Aziz Q, Rothwell JC, et al. Recovery of swallowing after dysphagic stroke relates to functional reorganization in the intact motor cortex. Gastroenterology 1998;115(5):1104–12.
8. Katzan IL, Cebul RD, Husak SH, et al. The effect of pneumonia on mortality among patients hospitalized for acute stroke. Neurology 2003;60(4):620–5.
9. Bushby K, Finkel R, Birnkrant DJ, et al. Diagnosis and management of Duchenne muscular dystrophy, part 1: diagnosis, and pharmacological and psychosocial management. Lancet Neurol 2010;9(1):77–93.
10. Aloysius A, Born P, Kinali M, et al. Swallowing difficulties in Duchenne muscular dystrophy: indications for feeding assessment and outcome of videofluoroscopic swallow studies. Europ J Paediatr Neurol 2008;12(3):239–45.
11. van den Engel-Hoek L, Erasmus CE, Hendriks JC, et al. Oral muscles are progressively affected in Duchenne muscular dystrophy: implications for dysphagia treatment. J Neurol 2013. http://dx.doi.org/10.1007/s00415-012-6793-y.
12. Meyer A, Levy Y. Geoepidemiology of myasthenia gravis. Autoimmun Rev 2010; 9(5):A383–6.
13. Meriggioli MN, Sanders DB. Autoimmune myasthenia gravis: emerging clinical and biological heterogeneity. Lancet Neurol 2009;8(5):475–90.
14. Ertekin C, Yüceyar N, Aydogdu I. Clinical and electrophysiological evaluation of dysphagia in myasthenia gravis. J Neurol Neurosurg Psychiatry 1998;65(6): 848–56.
15. Colton-Hudson A, Koopman WJ, Moosa T, et al. A prospective assessment of the characteristics of dysphagia in myasthenia gravis. Dysphagia 2002;17(2): 147–51.
16. Koch-Henriksen N, Soelberg Sørensen P. The changing demographic pattern of multiple sclerosis epidemiology. Lancet Neurol 2010;9:520–32.
17. Compston A, Coles A. Multiple sclerosis. Lancet 2008;372(9648):1502–17.
18. Calcagno P, Ruoppolo G, Grasso MG, et al. Dysphagia in multiple sclerosis – prevalence and prognostic factors. Acta Neurol Scand 2002;105:40–3.
19. Prosiegel M, Schelling A, Wagner-Sonntag E. Dysphagia and multiple sclerosis. Int MS J 2004;11(1):22–31.
20. De Pauw A, Dejaeger E, D'hooghe B, et al. Dysphagia in multiple sclerosis. Clin Neurol Neurosurg 2002;104(4):345–51.

21. Mitchell JD, Borasio GD. Amyotrophic lateral sclerosis. Lancet 2007;369(9578): 2031–41.
22. Kiernan MC, Vucic S, Cheah BC, et al. Amyotrophic lateral sclerosis. Lancet 2011;377(9769):942–55.
23. Rowland LP, Shneider NA. Amyotrophic lateral sclerosis. N Engl J Med 2001; 344(22):1688–700.
24. Ertekin C, Aydogdu I, Yüceyar N, et al. Pathophysiological mechanisms of oropharyngeal dysphagia in amyotrophic lateral sclerosis. Brain 2000; 123(Pt 1):125–40.
25. Van Den Eeden SK, Tanner CM, Bernstein AL, et al. Incidence of Parkinson's disease: variation by age, gender, and race/ethnicity. Am J Epidemiol 2003; 157(11):1015–22.
26. Lees AJ, Hardy J, Revesz T. Parkinson's disease. Lancet 2009;373(9680): 2055–66.
27. Potulska A, Friedman A, Królicki L, et al. Swallowing disorders in Parkinson's disease. Parkinsonism Relat Disord 2003;9(6):349–53.
28. Kalf JG, de Swart BJ, Bloem BR, et al. Prevalence of oropharyngeal dysphagia in Parkinson's disease. Parkinsonism Relat Disord 2012;18(4):311–5.
29. Prince M. Epidemiology of dementia. Psychiatry 2007;6:488–90.
30. Gillick M. When the nursing home resident with advanced dementia stops eating: what is the medical director to do? J Am Med Dir Assoc 2001;2(5): 259–63.
31. Reisberg B. The encyclopedia of visual medicine series. An atlas of Alzheimer's disease. Pearl River (NY): Parthenon; 1999.
32. Goldberg L, Altman KW. The role of gastrostomy tube placement in advanced dementia with dysphagia: a critical review [abstract]. Dysphagia Research Society 20th Annual Meeting. Toronto, March 8–10, 2012.
33. Cardin F. Special considerations for endoscopists on PEG indications in older patients. ISRN Gastroenterol 2012;2012:607149.
34. Leibovitz A, Plotnikov G, Habot B, et al. Pathogenic colonization of oral flora in frail elderly patients fed by nasogastric tube of percutaneous enterogastric tube. J Gerontol 2003;58(1):52–5.
35. Langmore SE, Skarupski KA, Park PS, et al. Predictors of aspiration pneumonia in nursing home residents. Dysphagia 2002;17(4):298–307.
36. Ashford J, McCabe D, Wheeler-Hegland K, et al. Evidence-based systematic review: oropharyngeal dysphagia behavioral treatments. Part III–impact of dysphagia treatments on populations with neurological disorders. J Rehabil Res Dev 2009;46(2):195–204.
37. Robbins J, Butler SG, Daniels SK, et al. Swallowing and dysphagia rehabilitation: translating principles of neural plasticity into clinically oriented evidence. J Speech Lang Hear Res 2008;51(1):S276–300.
38. Crary MA, Carnaby GD, LaGorio LA, et al. Functional and physiological outcomes from an exercise-based dysphagia therapy: a pilot investigation of the McNeill Dysphagia Therapy Program. Arch Phys Med Rehabil 2012;93(7):1173–8.
39. Crary MA. A direct intervention program for chronic neurogenic dysphagia secondary to brainstem stroke. Dysphagia 1995;10:6–18.
40. Bryant M. Biofeedback in the treatment of a selected dysphagic patient. Dysphagia 1991;6:140–4.
41. Crary MA, Carnaby Mann GD, Groher ME, et al. Functional benefits of dysphagia therapy using adjunctive sEMG biofeedback. Dysphagia 2004;19: 160–4.

42. Park JW, Oh JC, Lee JW, et al. The effect of 5Hz high-frequency rTMS over contralesional pharyngeal motor cortex in post-stroke oropharyngeal dysphagia: a randomized controlled study. Neurogastroenterol Motil 2013;25(4):324-e250.
43. Oh BM, Kim DY, Paik NJ. Recovery of swallowing function is accompanied by the expansion of the cortical map. Int J Neurosci 2007;117(9):1215–27.
44. Barritt AW, Smithard DG. Role of cerebral cortex plasticity in the recovery of swallowing function following dysphagic stroke. Dysphagia 2009;24(1):83–90.
45. Michou E, Mistry S, Jefferson S, et al. Targeting unlesioned pharyngeal motor cortex improves swallowing in healthy individuals and after dysphagic stroke. Gastroenterology 2012;142(1):29–38.
46. Hiscock A, Miller S, Rothwell J, et al. Informing dose-finding studies of repetitive transcranial magnetic stimulation to enhance motor function: a qualitative systematic review. Neurorehabil Neural Repair 2008;22(3):228–49.
47. Singh S, Hamdy S. Dysphagia in stroke patients. Postgrad Med J 2006;82(968): 383–91.
48. Dennis MS, Lewis SC, Warlow C, FOOD Trial Collaboration. Effect of timing and method of enteral tube feeding for dysphagic stroke patients (FOOD): a multicentre randomised controlled trial. Lancet 2005;365(9461):764–72.
49. Donzelli J, Brady S, Wesling M, et al. Effects of the removal of the tracheotomy tube on swallowing during the fiberoptic endoscopic exam of the swallow (FEES). Dysphagia 2005;20(4):283–9.
50. Cook SP. Candidate's thesis: laryngotracheal separation in neurologically impaired children: long-term results. Laryngoscope 2009;119(2):390–5.

Index

Note: Page numbers of article titles are in **boldface** type.

A

Achalasia, 1048–1049
Aerodigestive tract, areas/spaces of, 936–940
    evolution of, in course of human evolution, 931–933
    of mammals, 924–926
    of newborn humans, 929
Airway, protection of, complex brainstem circuits for, computational modeling of, 959–960
      importance of, 947–948
Amyotrophic lateral sclerosis, dysphagia in, 1139
Aspiration, prevention during swallowing, 956

B

Barium swallow, modified, advantages and disadvantages of, 1019
      and functional endoscopic evaluation of swallowing, **1009–1021**
        compared, 1015–1020
      clinical indicators for, 1016–1017
      clinical outcomes of, 1017–1018
      compensatory strategies/swallowing interventions during, 1018–1019
      equipment for, 1012–1013
      in pediatric patients, 1020
      radiation exposure and, 1013
      results of, factors affecting, 1019–1020
      technique and protocol for, 1010–1012
Bones and cartilages, in swallowing, 936
Botulinum toxin injection, in cricopharyngeus muscle dysfunction, 1091–1093
Brainstem circuits, complex, for computational modeling of airway protection, 959–960

C

Cervical osteophytes, 1042–1043
Chagas disease, 1048
Chemotherapy, and/or radiation, characteristics of dysphagia after, 1123
Chronic obstructive pulmonary disease, 956
Cough and breathing, neurophysiology of, 957–958
Cricopharyngeal bar, 1043–1144
Cricopharyngeus muscle, anatomy of, 1100
Cricopharyngeus muscle dysfunction, evaluation of, 1086–1094
    management of, **1085–1097**
      botulinum toxin injection in, 1091–1093
      esophageal dilation in, 1091
      myotomy in, 1093–1094
      nonsurgical, 1090–1091

Otolaryngol Clin N Am 46 (2013) 1151–1157
http://dx.doi.org/10.1016/S0030-6665(13)00200-4
0030-6665/13/$ – see front matter © 2013 Elsevier Inc. All rights reserved.

oto.theclinics.com

Moving?

Make sure your subscription moves with you!

To notify us of your new address, find your **Clinics Account Number** (located on your mailing label above your name), and contact customer service at:

Email: journalscustomerservice-usa@elsevier.com

800-654-2452 (subscribers in the U.S. & Canada)
314-447-8871 (subscribers outside of the U.S. & Canada)

Fax number: 314-447-8029

Elsevier Health Sciences Division
Subscription Customer Service
3251 Riverport Lane
Maryland Heights, MO 63043

*To ensure uninterrupted delivery of your subscription, please notify us at least 4 weeks in advance of move.

Printed and bound by CPI Group (UK) Ltd, Croydon, CR0 4YY

03/10/2024

01040493-0007